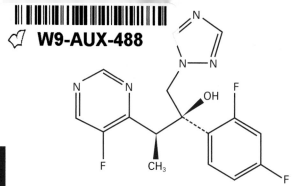

2015

Nelson's Pediatric Antimicrobial Therapy

21st Edition

John S. Bradley, MD
Editor in Chief

John D. Nelson, MD
Emeritus

Joseph B. Cantey, MD
David W. Kimberlin, MD
John A.D. Leake, MD, MPH
Paul E. Palumbo, MD
Jason Sauberan, PharmD
William J. Steinbach, MD
Contributing Editors

American Academy of Pediatrics

DEDICATED TO THE HEALTH OF ALL CHILDREN™

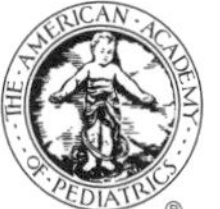

American Academy of Pediatrics Departments of Publishing and Marketing and Sales Staff

Mark Grimes, Director, Department of Publishing
Alain Park, Senior Product Development Editor
Carrie Peters, Editorial Assistant
Sandi King, MS, Director, Division of Editorial and Production Services
Shannan Martin, Publishing and Production Services Specialist
Linda Diamond, Manager, Art Direction and Production
Jason Crase, Manager, Editorial Services
Houston Adams, Digital Content and Production Specialist
Mary Lou White, Director, Department of Marketing and Sales
Linda Smessaert, MSIMC, Brand Manager, Clinical and Professional Publications

Published by the American Academy of Pediatrics
141 Northwest Point Blvd, Elk Grove Village, IL 60007-1019
847/434-4000
Fax: 847/434-8000
www.aap.org

ISSN: 2164-9278 (print)
ISSN: 2164-9286 (electronic)
ISBN: 978-1-58110-918-4
eBook: 978-1-58110-917-7
MA0746

The recommendations in this publication do not indicate an exclusive course of treatment or serve as a standard of medical care. Variations, taking into account individual circumstances, may be appropriate.

This book has been developed by the American Academy of Pediatrics. The authors, editors, and contributors are expert authorities in the field of pediatrics. No commercial involvement of any kind has been solicited or accepted in the development of the content of this publication.

Every effort has been made to ensure that the drug selection and dosages set forth in this text are in accordance with the current recommendations and practice at the time of the publication. It is the responsibility of the health care professional to check the package insert of each drug for any change in indications or dosage and for added warnings and precautions.

Brand names are furnished for identifying purposes only. No endorsement of the manufacturers or products listed is implied.

Please see our Web site for content-related notices and updates: www.aap.org/nelsonsabx.

First edition published in 1975.
9-360

1 2 3 4 5 6 7 8 9 10

Editor in Chief

John S. Bradley, MD
Professor of Pediatrics
Chief, Division of Infectious Diseases, Department of Pediatrics
University of California, San Diego, School of Medicine
Director, Division of Infectious Diseases, Rady Children's Hospital San Diego
San Diego, CA

Emeritus

John D. Nelson, MD
Professor Emeritus of Pediatrics
The University of Texas
Southwestern Medical Center at Dallas
Southwestern Medical School
Dallas, TX

Contributing Editors

Joseph B. Cantey, MD
Assistant Professor of Pediatrics
Divisions of Neonatology and Infectious Diseases, Department of Pediatrics
UT Southwestern
Dallas, TX

David W. Kimberlin, MD
Professor of Pediatrics
Codirector, Division of Pediatric Infectious Diseases
Sergio Stagno Endowed Chair in Pediatric Infectious Diseases
University of Alabama at Birmingham
Birmingham, AL

John A.D. Leake, MD, MPH
Professor of Pediatrics
Division of Infectious Diseases, Department of Pediatrics
University of California, San Diego, School of Medicine
Division of Infectious Diseases, Rady Children's Hospital San Diego
San Diego, CA

Paul E. Palumbo, MD
Professor of Pediatrics and Medicine
Geisel School of Medicine at Dartmouth
Director, International Pediatric HIV Program
Dartmouth-Hitchcock Medical Center
Lebanon, NH

Jason Sauberan, PharmD
Assistant Clinical Professor
University of California, San Diego, Skaggs School of Pharmacy and Pharmaceutical Sciences
Rady Children's Hospital San Diego
San Diego, CA

William J. Steinbach, MD
Associate Professor of Pediatrics, Division of Pediatric Infectious Diseases
Associate Professor of Molecular Genetics and Microbiology
Director, International Pediatric Fungal Network
Duke University School of Medicine
Durham, NC

Contents

Introduction

Welcome to the 21st edition: *Nelson's Pediatric Antimicrobial Therapy 2015!* Our collaboration with the American Academy of Pediatrics (AAP) has become stronger and more integrated as we work closely with our AAP editor, Alain Park. The book is at a crossroads, trying to decide whether to stay small and concise or to expand and give our contributing editors free rein to make recommendations as well as tell us all why the recommendations are being made. In addition, the AAP has interviewed a number of health care professionals who own this book to provide some valuable advice on which sections should be expanded and which should be deleted, helping us write a more focused set of chapters. Along those lines, we have created some new tables that provide a quick at-a-glance overview of bacterial and fungal pathogen susceptibilities to commonly used antimicrobials.

The iPhone/iPad app has been very successful. The Android version of the app (which we have used) was not updated for the 2014 edition of the book, but if we get enough requests for this version of the app in the future, we may develop one for subsequent editions. However, we were very pleased to learn in our survey that many still prefer the book format.

The collective advice and experience of the editors is still backed up by grading our recommendations: our assessment of how strongly we feel about a recommendation and the strength of the evidence to support our recommendation (noted below).

Strength of Recommendation	Description
A	Strongly recommended
B	Recommended as a good choice
C	One option for therapy that is adequate, perhaps among many other adequate therapies
Level of Evidence	**Description**
I	Based on well-designed, prospective, randomized, and controlled studies in an appropriate population of children
II	Based on data derived from prospectively collected, small comparative trials, or noncomparative prospective trials, or reasonable retrospective data from clinical trials in children, or data from other populations (eg, adults)
III	Based on case reports, case series, consensus statements, or expert opinion for situations in which sound data do not exist

For this edition, Joseph B. (JB) Cantey is taking over work on Chapter 5, Antimicrobial Therapy for Newborns, from Pablo Sanchez, whose role on creating the chapter on newborns goes back decades. We wish Pablo the best of luck in his new position in Columbus, OH. JB follows in Pablo's footsteps with expertise as a double-trained infectious diseases/neonatologist. Jason Sauberan continues to carefully update the Antimicrobial Dosages for Neonates with the tremendous amount of new information becoming available. The neonatal pharmacology field gets ever more complicated with new drugs and our increasing understanding of organ system maturation and drug distribution. We are very happy to have John van den Anker, a neonatologist/pharmacologist from Children's National Medical Center, working with us again this year on the neonatal dosage table; he is personally responsible for much of the new information we have on neonatal developmental pharmacology.

We are extremely fortunate to have as editors some of the best clinicians in pediatric infectious diseases out there. They take the time to partner with the AAP and provide amazing advice and insight in their particular areas of interest, knowledge, and experience. David Kimberlin, John Leake, Jason Sauberan, and Bill Steinbach are each exceptionally talented and *collaborative!*

As we state each year, many of the recommendations by the editors for specific situations have not been systematically evaluated in controlled, prospective, comparative clinical trials. Many of the recommendations may be supported by published data, but for many possible reasons, the data have never been presented to or reviewed by the US Food and Drug Administration (FDA) and therefore are not in the package label. We in pediatrics find ourselves in this situation frequently. Many of us are working closely with the FDA to try to narrow the gap in our knowledge of antimicrobial agents between adults and children.

We are deeply grateful for the hard work and tireless efforts of Alain Park, our AAP senior product development editor, who challenges us to come up with new ways to share our information with pediatric health care professionals. How about an AAP Nelson's Editors' Infectious Diseases Update continuing medical education program? We have wonderful supporters in the AAP Departments of Marketing and Publications—Jeff Mahony, Mark Grimes, Linda Smessaert, and Maureen DeRosa—who make certain that all our recommendations make it to everyone as effectively and effortlessly as possible.

John S. Bradley, MD, FAAP

John D. Nelson, MD

1. Choosing Among Antibiotics Within a Class: Beta-lactams, Macrolides, Aminoglycosides, and Fluoroquinolones

New drugs should be compared with others in the same class regarding (1) antimicrobial spectrum; (2) degree of antibiotic exposure (a function of the pharmacokinetics of the nonprotein-bound drug at the site of infection and the pharmacodynamic properties of the drug); (3) demonstrated efficacy in adequate and well-controlled clinical trials; (4) tolerance, toxicity, and side effects; and (5) cost. If there is no substantial benefit for efficacy or safety, one should opt for using an older, more familiar, and less expensive drug with the narrowest spectrum of activity required to treat the infection.

Beta-lactams

Oral Cephalosporins (cephalexin, cefadroxil, cefaclor, cefprozil, cefuroxime, cefixime, cefdinir, cefpodoxime, cefditoren [tablet only], and ceftibuten). As a class, the oral cephalosporins have the advantages over oral penicillins of somewhat greater safety and greater palatability of the suspension formulations (penicillins have a bitter taste). The serum half-lives of cefpodoxime, ceftibuten, and cefixime are greater than 2 hours. This pharmacokinetic feature accounts for the fact that they may be given in 1 or 2 doses per day for certain indications, particularly otitis media, where the middle-ear fluid half-life is likely to be much longer than the serum half-life. Cefaclor, cefprozil, cefuroxime, cefdinir, cefixime, cefpodoxime, and ceftibuten have the advantage over cephalexin and cefadroxil (the "first-generation cephalosporins") of enhanced coverage for *Haemophilus influenzae* (including beta-lactamase–producing strains) and some enteric gram-negative bacilli; however, ceftibuten and cefixime in particular have the disadvantage of less activity against *Streptococcus pneumoniae* than the others, particularly against penicillin (beta-lactam) non-susceptible strains. None of the currently available oral cephalosporins have activity against *Pseudomonas* or methicillin-resistant *Staphylococcus aureus* (MRSA). The palatability of generic versions of these products may not have the same pleasant characteristics as the original products.

Parenteral Cephalosporins. First-generation cephalosporins, such as cefazolin, are used mainly for treatment of gram-positive infections (excluding MRSA) and for surgical prophylaxis; the gram-negative spectrum is limited. Cefazolin is well tolerated on intramuscular or intravenous injection.

A second-generation cephalosporin (cefuroxime) and the cephamycins (cefoxitin and cefotetan) provide increased activity against many gram-negative organisms, particularly *Haemophilus* and *Escherichia coli*. Cefoxitin has, in addition, activity against approximately 80% of strains of *Bacteroides fragilis* and can be considered for use in place of metronidazole, clindamycin, or carbapenems when that organism is implicated in non–life-threatening disease.

Third-generation cephalosporins (cefotaxime, ceftriaxone, and ceftazidime) all have enhanced potency against many enteric gram-negative bacilli. They are inactive against enterococci and *Listeria* and only ceftazidime has significant activity against *Pseudomonas*. Cefotaxime and ceftriaxone have been used very successfully to treat meningitis caused by pneumococcus (mostly penicillin-susceptible strains), *H influenzae* type b (Hib), meningococcus, and small numbers of young infants with susceptible strains of *E coli* meningitis. These drugs have the greatest usefulness for treating gram-negative bacillary infections due to their safety, compared with other classes of antibiotics. Because ceftriaxone is excreted to a large extent via the liver, it can be used with little dosage adjustment in patients with renal failure. Further, it has a serum half-life of 4 to 7 hours and can be given once a day for all infections caused by susceptible organisms, including meningitis.

Cefepime, a fourth-generation cephalosporin approved for use in children, exhibits the antipseudomonal activity of ceftazidime, the gram-positive activity of second-generation cephalosporins, and better activity against gram-negative enteric bacilli such as *Enterobacter* and *Serratia* than is documented with cefotaxime and ceftriaxone.

Ceftaroline is a fifth-generation cephalosporin, the first of the cephalosporins with activity against MRSA. Ceftaroline was approved by the US Food and Drug Administration (FDA) in December 2010 for adults with complicated skin infections (including MRSA) and community-acquired pneumonia (with insufficient numbers of adult patients with MRSA pneumonia to be able to comment on efficacy). The pharmacokinetics of ceftaroline have been evaluated in all groups, including neonates; clinical studies for community-acquired pneumonia and complicated skin infection are currently underway for children.

Penicillinase-Resistant Penicillins (dicloxacillin [capsules only]; nafcillin and oxacillin [parenteral only]). "Penicillinase" refers specifically to the beta-lactamase produced by *S aureus* in this case and not those produced by gram-negative bacteria. These antibiotics are active against penicillin-resistant *S aureus* but not against MRSA. Nafcillin differs pharmacologically from the others in being excreted primarily by the liver rather than by the kidneys, which may explain the relative lack of nephrotoxicity compared with methicillin, which is no longer available in the United States. Nafcillin pharmacokinetics are erratic in persons with liver disease.

Antipseudomonal Beta-lactams (ticarcillin/clavulanate, piperacillin, piperacillin/tazobactam, aztreonam, ceftazidime, cefepime, meropenem, imipenem, and doripenem). Timentin (ticarcillin/clavulanate) and Zosyn (piperacillin/tazobactam) represent combinations of 2 beta-lactam drugs. One beta-lactam drug in the combination, known as a "beta-lactamase inhibitor" (clavulanic acid or tazobactam in these combinations), binds irreversibly to and neutralizes specific beta-lactamase enzymes produced by the organism, allowing the second beta-lactam drug (ticarcillin or piperacillin) to act as the active antibiotic to bind effectively to the intracellular target site, resulting in death of the organism. Thus, the combination only adds to the spectrum of the original antibiotic when the mechanism of resistance is a beta-lactamase enzyme and only when the beta-lactamase inhibitor is capable of binding to and inhibiting that particular organism's beta-lactamase. The combinations extend the spectrum of activity to include many beta-lactamase–positive bacteria, including some strains of enteric gram-negative bacilli (*E coli, Klebsiella,* and *Enterobacter*), *S aureus,* and *B fragilis.* Timentin and Zosyn have no significant activity against *Pseudomonas* beyond that of ticarcillin or piperacillin because their beta-lactamase inhibitors do not effectively inhibit all of the many relevant beta-lactamases of *Pseudomonas.*

Pseudomonas has an intrinsic capacity to develop resistance following exposure to any beta-lactam, based on the activity of several inducible chromosomal beta-lactamases, upregulated efflux pumps, and changes in the cell wall. Because development of resistance during therapy is not uncommon (particularly beta-lactamase resistance against ticarcillin, piperacillin, or ceftazidime), an aminoglycoside such as tobramycin is often used in combination. Cefepime, meropenem, and imipenem are relatively stable to the beta-lactamases induced while on therapy and can be used as single-agent therapy for most *Pseudomonas* infections, but resistance may still develop to these agents based on other mechanisms of resistance. For *Pseudomonas* infections in compromised hosts or in life-threatening infections, these drugs, too, should be used in combination with an aminoglycoside or a second active agent.

Aminopenicillins (amoxicillin and amoxicillin/clavulanate [oral formulations only, in the United States], ampicillin [oral and parenteral], and ampicillin/sulbactam [parenteral only]). Amoxicillin is very well absorbed, good tasting, and associated with very few side effects. Augmentin is a combination of amoxicillin and clavulanate (see previous text regarding beta-lactam/beta-lactamase inhibitor combinations) that is available in several fixed proportions that permit amoxicillin to remain active against many beta-lactamase–producing bacteria, including *H influenzae* and *S aureus* (but not MRSA). Amoxicillin/clavulanate has undergone many changes in formulation since its introduction. The ratio of amoxicillin to clavulanate was originally 4:1, based on susceptibility data of pneumococcus and *Haemophilus* during the 1970s. With the emergence of penicillin-resistant pneumococcus, recommendations for increasing the dosage of amoxicillin, particularly for upper respiratory tract infections, were made. However, if one increases the dosage of clavulanate even slightly, the incidence of diarrhea increases dramatically. If one keeps the dosage of clavulanate constant while increasing the dosage of amoxicillin, one can treat the relatively resistant pneumococci while not increasing gastrointestinal side effects. The original 4:1 ratio is present in suspensions containing 125-mg and 250-mg amoxicillin/5 mL and the 125-mg and 250-mg chewable tablets. A higher 7:1 ratio is present in the suspensions containing 200-mg and 400-mg amoxicillin/5 mL and in the 200-mg and 400-mg chewable tablets. A still higher ratio of 14:1 is present in the suspension formulation Augmentin ES-600 that contains 600-mg amoxicillin/5 mL; this preparation is designed to deliver 90 mg/kg/day of amoxicillin, divided twice daily, for the treatment of ear (and sinus) infections. The high serum and middle ear fluid concentrations achieved with 45 mg/kg/dose, combined with the long middle ear fluid half-life of amoxicillin, allow for a therapeutic antibiotic exposure to pathogens in the middle ear with a twice-daily regimen. However, the prolonged half-life in the middle ear fluid is not necessarily found in other infection sites (eg, skin, lung tissue, joint tissue), for which dosing of amoxicillin and Augmentin should continue to be 3 times daily for most susceptible pathogens.

For older children who can swallow tablets, the amoxicillin to clavulanate ratios are as follows: 500-mg tablet (4:1); 875-mg tablet (7:1); 1,000-mg tablet (16:1).

Sulbactam, another beta-lactamase inhibitor like clavulanate, is combined with ampicillin in the parenteral formulation Unasyn. The cautions regarding spectrum of activity for Timentin and Zosyn with respect to the limitations of the beta-lactamase inhibitor in increasing the spectrum of activity (see Antipseudomonal Beta-lactams) also apply to Unasyn.

Carbapenems. Meropenem, imipenem, doripenem, and ertapenem are carbapenems with a broader spectrum of activity than any other class of beta-lactam currently available. Meropenem, imipenem, and ertapenem are approved by the FDA for use in children, while doripenem is under investigation in children. At present, we recommend them for treatment of infections caused by bacteria resistant to standard therapy or for mixed infections involving aerobes and anaerobes. Imipenem has greater central nervous system irritability compared with other carbapenems, leading to an increased risk of seizures in children with meningitis. Meropenem was not associated with an increased rate of seizures, compared with cefotaxime in children with meningitis. Imipenem and meropenem are active against virtually all coliform bacilli, including cefotaxime-resistant (extended spectrum beta-lactamase [ESBL]–producing or ampC-producing) strains, against *Pseudomonas aeruginosa* (including most ceftazidime-resistant strains), and against anaerobes, including *B fragilis.* While ertapenem lacks the excellent activity against *P aeruginosa* of the other carbapenems, it has the advantage of a prolonged serum half-life, which allows for once-daily dosing in adults and children aged 13 years and older and twice-daily dosing in younger children. Newly emergent strains of *Klebsiella pneumoniae* contain *K pneumoniae* carbapenemases that degrade and inactivate all the carbapenems. While the current strains involve adults predominantly in the Northeast United States, they have begun to spread to other areas of the country, reinforcing the need to keep track of your local antibiotic susceptibility patterns.

Macrolides

Erythromycin is the prototype of macrolide antibiotics. Almost 30 macrolides have been produced, but only 3 are FDA approved for children in the United States: erythromycin, azithromycin (also called an azalide), and clarithromycin, while a fourth, telithromycin (also called a ketolide), is approved for adults and only available in tablet form. As a class, these drugs achieve greater concentrations in tissues than in serum, particularly with azithromycin and clarithromycin. As a result, measuring serum concentrations is usually not clinically useful. Gastrointestinal intolerance to erythromycin is caused by the breakdown products of the macrolide ring structure. This is much less of a problem with azithromycin and clarithromycin. Azithromycin, clarithromycin, and telithromycin extend the activity of erythromycin to include *Haemophilus;* azithromycin and clarithromycin also have substantial activity against certain mycobacteria. Azithromycin is also active in vitro and effective against many enteric gram-negative pathogens including *Salmonella* and *Shigella.*

Aminoglycosides

Although 5 aminoglycoside antibiotics are available in the United States, only 3 are widely used for systemic therapy of aerobic gram-negative infections and for synergy in the treatment of certain gram-positive infections: gentamicin, tobramycin, and amikacin. Streptomycin and kanamycin have more limited utility due to increased toxicity. Resistance in gram-negative bacilli to aminoglycosides is caused by bacterial enzyme adenylation, acetylation, or phosphorylation. The specific activities of each enzyme in each pathogen are highly variable. As a result, antibiotic susceptibility tests must be done for each aminoglycoside drug separately. There are small differences in comparative toxicities of these aminoglycosides to the kidneys and eighth cranial nerve hearing/vestibular function, although it is uncertain whether these small differences are clinically significant. For all children receiving a full treatment course, it is advisable to monitor peak and trough serum concentrations early in the course of therapy, as the degree of drug exposure correlates with toxicity and elevated trough concentrations predict impending drug accumulation. With amikacin, desired peak concentrations are 20 to 35 µg/mL and trough drug concentrations are less than 10 µg/mL; for gentamicin and tobramycin, depending on the frequency of dosing, peak concentrations should be 5 to 10 µg/mL and trough concentrations less than 2 µg/mL. Children with cystic fibrosis require greater dosages to achieve therapeutic serum concentrations. Inhaled tobramycin has been very successful in children with cystic fibrosis as an adjunctive therapy of gram-negative bacillary infections. The role of inhaled aminoglycosides in other gram-negative pneumonias (eg, ventilator-associated pneumonia) has not yet been defined.

Once-Daily Dosing of Aminoglycosides. Once-daily dosing of 5 to 7.5 mg/kg gentamicin or tobramycin has been studied in adults and in some neonates and children; peak serum concentrations are greater than those achieved with dosing 3 times daily. Aminoglycosides demonstrate concentration-dependent killing of pathogens, suggesting a potential benefit to higher serum concentrations achieved with once-daily dosing. Regimens giving the daily dosage as a single infusion, rather than as traditionally split doses every 8 hours, are effective and safe for normal adult hosts and immune-compromised hosts with fever and neutropenia and may be less toxic. Experience with once-daily dosing in children is increasing, with similar results as noted for adults. Once-daily dosing should be considered as effective as multiple, smaller doses per day and may be safer for children.

Fluoroquinolones

More than 30 years ago, toxicity to cartilage in weight-bearing joints in experimental juvenile animals was documented to be dose and duration of therapy dependent. Pediatric studies were, therefore, not initially undertaken with ciprofloxacin or other fluoroquinolones (FQs). However, with increasing antibiotic resistance in pediatric pathogens and an accumulating database in pediatrics suggesting that joint toxicity may be uncommon, the FDA allowed prospective studies to proceed in 1998. As of July 2014, no cases of documented FQ-attributable joint toxicity have occurred in children with FQs that are approved for use in the United States. However, no published data are available from prospective, blinded studies to accurately assess this risk. Unblinded studies with levofloxacin for respiratory tract infections and unpublished randomized studies comparing ciprofloxacin versus other agents for complicated urinary tract infection suggest the possibility of uncommon, reversible, FQ-attributable arthralgia, but these data should be interpreted with caution. Prospective, randomized, double-blind studies of moxifloxacin, in which cartilage injury is being assessed, are currently underway. The use of FQs in situations of antibiotic resistance where no other active agent is available is reasonable, weighing the benefits of treatment against the low risk of toxicity of this class of antibiotics. The use of an oral FQ in situations in which the only alternative is parenteral therapy is also justified (Bradley JS, et al. *Pediatrics.* 2011;128[4]:e1034–e1045).

Ciprofloxacin usually has very good gram-negative activity (with great regional variation in susceptibility) against enteric bacilli (*E coli, Klebsiella, Enterobacter, Salmonella,* and *Shigella*) and against *P aeruginosa.* However, it lacks substantial gram-positive coverage and should not be used to treat streptococcal, staphylococcal, or pneumococcal infections. Newer-generation FQs are more active against these pathogens; levofloxacin has documented efficacy and short-term safety in pediatric clinical trials for respiratory tract infections (acute otitis media and community-acquired pneumonia). None of the newer-generation FQs are more active against gram-negative pathogens than ciprofloxacin. Quinolone antibiotics are bitter tasting. Ciprofloxacin and levofloxacin are currently available in a suspension form; ciprofloxacin is FDA approved in pediatrics for complicated urinary tract infections and inhalation anthrax, while levofloxacin is approved for inhalation anthrax only, as the sponsor chose not to apply for approval for pediatric respiratory tract infections. For reasons of safety and to prevent the emergence of widespread resistance, FQs should still not be used for primary therapy of pediatric infections and should be limited to situations in which safe and effective oral therapy with other classes of antibiotics does not exist.

2. Choosing Among Antifungal Agents: Polyenes, Azoles, and Echinocandins

Polyenes

Amphotericin B (AmB) is a polyene antifungal antibiotic that has been available since 1958 for the treatment of invasive fungal infections. Its name originates from the drug's amphoteric property of reacting as an acid as well as a base. Nystatin is another polyene antifungal, but, due to systemic toxicity, it is only used in topical preparations. It was named after the research laboratory where it was discovered, the New York State Health Department Laboratory. AmB remains the most broad-spectrum antifungal available for clinical use. This lipophilic drug binds to ergosterol, the major sterol in the fungal cell membrane, and creates transmembrane pores that compromise the integrity of the cell membrane and create a rapid fungicidal effect through osmotic lysis. Toxicity is likely due to the cross-reactivity with the human cholesterol bi-lipid membrane, which resembles ergosterol. The toxicity of the conventional formulation, AmB deoxycholate (AmB-D), is substantial from the standpoints of systemic reactions (fever, rigors) and acute and chronic renal toxicity. Premedication with acetaminophen, diphenhydramine, and meperidine is often required to prevent systemic reactions during infusion. Renal dysfunction manifests primarily as decreased glomerular filtration with a rising serum creatinine concentration, but substantial tubular nephropathy is associated with potassium and magnesium wasting, requiring supplemental potassium for many neonates and children, regardless of clinical symptoms associated with infusion. Fluid loading with saline pre– and post–AmB-D infusion seems to mitigate renal toxicity.

Three lipid preparations approved in the mid-1990s decrease toxicity with no apparent decrease in clinical efficacy. Decisions on which lipid AmB preparation to use should, therefore, largely focus on side effects and costs. Two clinically useful lipid formulations exist: one in which ribbon-like lipid complexes of AmB are created (amphotericin B lipid complex [ABLC]), Abelcet, and one in which AmB is incorporated into true liposomes (liposomal amphotericin B [L-AmB]), AmBisome. The standard dosage used of these preparations is 5 mg/kg/day, in contrast to the 1 mg/kg/day of AmB-D. In most studies, the side effects of L-AmB were somewhat less than those of ABLC, but both have significantly fewer side effects than AmB-D. The advantage of the lipid preparations is the ability to safely deliver a greater overall dose of the parent AmB drug. The cost of conventional AmB-D is substantially less than either lipid formulation. A colloidal dispersion of AmB in cholesteryl sulfate, Amphotec, is also available, with decreased nephrotoxicity, but infusion-related side effects are closer to AmB-D than to the lipid formulations. The decreased nephrotoxicity of the 3 lipid preparations is thought to be due to the preferential binding of its AmB to high-density lipoproteins, compared to AmB-D binding to low-density lipoproteins. Despite in vitro concentration-dependent killing, a clinical trial comparing L-AmB at doses of 3 mg/kg/day versus 10 mg/kg/day found no efficacy benefit for the higher dose and only greater toxicity.[1] Therefore, it is generally not recommended to use any AmB preparations at higher dosages (>5 mg/kg/day), as it will likely only incur greater toxicity with no real therapeutic advantage. AmB has a long terminal half-life and, coupled with the concentration-dependent killing, the agent is best used as single daily doses. If the overall AmB exposure needs to be decreased due to toxicity, it is best to increase the dosing interval (eg, 3 times weekly) but retain the full mg/kg dose for optimal pharmacokinetics.

AmB-D has been used for nonsystemic purposes, such as in bladder washes, intraventricular instillation, intrapleural instillation, and other modalities, but there are no firm data supporting those clinical indications, and it is likely that the local toxicities outweigh the theoretical benefits. Due to the lipid chemistry, the L-AmB does not interact well with renal tubules, so there is a theoretical concern with using a lipid formulation, as opposed to AmB-D, when treating isolated urinary fungal disease. Importantly, there are several pathogens that are inherently or functionally resistant to AmB, including *Candida lusitaniae, Trichosporon* spp, *Aspergillus terreus, Fusarium* spp, and *Pseudalescheria boydii* (*Scedosporium apiospermum*) or *Scedosporium prolificans.*

Azoles

This class of systemic agents was first approved in 1981 and is divided into imidazoles (ketoconazole), triazoles (fluconazole, itraconazole), and second-generation triazoles (voriconazole, posaconazole, and isavuconazole) based on the number of nitrogens in the azole ring. All of the azoles work by inhibition of ergosterol synthesis (fungal cytochrome P450 [CYP] sterol 14-demethylation) that is required for fungal cell membrane integrity. While the polyenes are rapidly fungicidal, the azoles are fungistatic against yeasts and fungicidal against molds. However, it is important to note that ketoconazole and fluconazole have no mold activity. The only systemic imidazole is ketoconazole, which is primarily active against *Candida* spp and is available in an oral formulation.

Fluconazole is active against a broader range of fungi than ketoconazole and includes clinically relevant activity against *Cryptococcus, Coccidioides,* and *Histoplasma.* Like most other azoles, fluconazole requires a double loading dose on the first day, which has been nicely studied in neonates[2] and is likely also required, but not definitively proven yet, in children. Fluconazole achieves relatively high concentrations in urine and cerebrospinal fluid (CSF) compared with AmB due to its low lipophilicity, with urinary concentrations often so high that treatment against even "resistant" pathogens that are isolated only in the urine is possible. Fluconazole remains one of the most active, and so far the safest, systemic antifungal agents for the treatment of most *Candida* infections. *Candida albicans* remains generally sensitive to fluconazole, although some resistance is present in many non-*albicans Candida* spp as well as in *C albicans* in children repeatedly exposed to fluconazole. *Candida krusei* is considered inherently resistant to fluconazole, and *Candida glabrata* demonstrates dose-dependent resistance to fluconazole. Fluconazole is available in parenteral and oral (with >90% bioavailability) formulations and toxicity is unusual and primarily hepatic.

Itraconazole is active against an even broader range of fungi and, unlike fluconazole, includes molds such as *Aspergillus.* It is currently available as a capsule or oral solution (the intravenous [IV] form was discontinued); the oral solution provides higher, more consistent serum concentrations than capsules and should be used preferentially.

Absorption using itraconazole oral solution is improved on an empty stomach (unlike the capsule form, which is best administered under fed conditions), and monitoring itraconazole serum concentrations, like most azole antifungals, is a key principal in management. In adult patients, itraconazole is recommended to be loaded at 200 mg twice daily for 2 days, followed by 200 mg daily starting on the third day. Itraconazole is indicated in adults for therapy of mild/moderate disease with blastomycosis, histoplasmosis, and others. Although it possesses antifungal activity, itraconazole is not indicated as primary therapy against invasive aspergillosis, as voriconazole is a far better option. Itraconazole is not active against *Zygomycetes* (eg, mucormycosis). Limited pharmacokinetic data are available in children; itraconazole has not been approved by the US Food and Drug Administration (FDA) for pediatric indications. Toxicity in adults is primarily hepatic.

Voriconazole was approved in 2002 and is only FDA approved for children 12 years and older, although there are now substantial pharmacokinetic data and experience for children aged 2 to 12 years.[3] Voriconazole is a fluconazole derivative, so think of it as having the greater tissue and CSF penetration of fluconazole but the added antifungal spectrum to include molds. While the bioavailability of voriconazole in adults is approximately 96%, it is only approximately 50% in children, requiring clinicians to carefully monitor voriconazole trough concentrations, especially in patients taking the oral formulation. Voriconazole serum concentrations are tricky to interpret, confounded by great interpatient variability, but monitoring concentrations is essential to using this drug, like all azole antifungals, and especially important in circumstances of suspected treatment failure or possible toxicity. Most experts suggest voriconazole trough concentrations of 1 to 2 µg/mL or greater, which would generally exceed the pathogen's minimum inhibitory concentration, but generally toxicity will not be seen until concentrations of approximately 6 µg/mL or greater. One important point is the acquisition of an accurate trough concentration, one obtained just before the next dose is due and not obtained through a catheter infusing the drug. These simple trough parameters will make interpretation possible. The fundamental voriconazole pharmacokinetics are different in adults versus children; in adults, voriconazole is metabolized in a nonlinear fashion, whereas in children, the drug is metabolized in a linear fashion. This explains the increased pediatric starting dosing for voriconazole at 9 mg/kg/dose versus loading with 6 mg/kg/dose in adult patients. Children, most especially younger children, require higher dosages of voriconazole and also have a larger therapeutic window for dosing. However, many studies have shown an inconsistent relationship between dosing and levels, highlighting the need for close monitoring after the initial dosing scheme and then dose adjustment as needed. Given the poor clinical and microbiological response of *Aspergillus* infections to AmB, voriconazole is now the treatment of choice for invasive aspergillosis and many other mold infections (eg, pseudallescheriasis, fusariosis). Importantly, infections with Zygomycetes (eg, mucormycosis) are resistant to voriconazole. Voriconazole retains activity against most *Candida* spp, including some that are fluconazole resistant, but it is unlikely to replace fluconazole for treatment of fluconazole-susceptible *Candida* infections. Importantly, there are increasing reports of *C glabrata* resistance to voriconazole. Voriconazole produces some unique transient visual field abnormalities in about 10% of adults and children. There are an increasing number of reports, seen in as high as 20% of patients, of a photosensitive sunburn-like erythema that is not aided by sunscreen (only sun avoidance). In some rare long-term (mean of 3 years of therapy) cases this voriconazole phototoxicity has developed into cutaneous squamous cell carcinoma. Discontinuing voriconazole is recommended in patients experiencing chronic phototoxicity. The rash is the most common indication for switching from voriconazole to posaconazole if a triazole antifungal is required. Hepatotoxicity is uncommon, occurring only in 2% to 5% of patients. Voriconazole is CYP metabolized (CYP2C19), and allelic polymorphisms in the population have shown that some Asian patients can achieve higher toxic serum concentrations than other patients. Voriconazole also interacts with many similarly P450 metabolized drugs to produce some profound changes in serum concentrations of many concurrently administered drugs.

Posaconazole, an itraconazole derivative, was FDA approved in 2006 as an oral suspension for children 13 years and older. An extended-release tablet formulation was approved in November 2013, also for 13 years and older, and an IV formulation was approved in March 2014 for patients 18 years and older. Effective absorption of the oral suspension strongly requires taking the medication with food, ideally a high-fat meal; taking posaconazole on an empty stomach will result in approximately one-fourth of the absorption as in the fed state. The tablet formulation has better absorption due to its delayed release in the small intestine, but absorption will still be slightly increased with food. If the patient is unable to take food, the tablet is recommended. Due to the low pH (<5) of IV posaconazole, a central venous catheter is required for administration. The IV formulation contains only slightly lower amounts of the cyclodextrin vehicle than does voriconazole, so similar theoretical renal accumulation concerns exist. The exact pediatric dosing for posaconazole has not been completely determined and requires consultation with a pediatric antifungal expert. The pediatric oral suspension dose recommended by some experts for treating invasive disease is 24 mg/kg/day divided twice daily. In adult patients, IV posaconazole is loaded at 300 mg twice daily on the first day, then 300 mg once daily starting on the second day. Similarly, in adult patients the extended-release tablet is dosed as 300 mg twice daily on the first day, then 300 mg once daily starting on the second day. In adult patients, the maximum amount of posaconazole oral suspension given is 800 mg per day due to its excretion, and that has been given as 400 mg twice daily or 200 mg 4 times a day in severely ill patients due to findings of a marginal increase in exposure with more frequent dosing. Greater than 800 mg per day is not indicated in any patient. Like voriconazole and itraconazole, trough levels should be monitored, and most experts feel that posaconazole levels for treatment should be at least greater than 700 ng/mL (0.7 µg/mL). The in vitro activity of posaconazole against *Candida* spp is better than that of fluconazole and similar to voriconazole. Overall activity against *Aspergillus* is also equivalent to voriconazole, but notably it is the first triazole with substantial activity against some Zygomycetes, including *Rhizopus* spp and *Mucor* spp, as well as activity against *Coccidioides, Histoplasma,* and *Blastomyces* and the pathogens of phaeohyphomycosis. Posaconazole treatment of invasive aspergillosis in patients with chronic granulomatous disease appears to be superior to voriconazole in this specific patient population for an unknown reason. Posaconazole is eliminated by hepatic glucuronidation but does demonstrate inhibition of the CYP3A4 enzyme system, leading to many drug interactions with other P450 metabolized drugs. It is currently approved for prophylaxis of *Candida* and *Aspergillus* infections in high-risk adults and for treatment of *Candida* oropharyngeal disease or esophagitis in adults. Posaconazole, like itraconazole, has generally poor CSF penetration.

Isavuconazole is a new triazole that is expected to be FDA approved for clinical use soon with oral and IV formulations. Isavuconazole has a similar antifungal spectrum as voriconazole and some activity against the *Zygomycetes* (yet not as potent against *Zygomycetes* as posaconazole). A phase 3 clinical trial in adult patients demonstrated non-inferiority versus voriconazole against invasive aspergillosis and other mold infections. No pediatric dosing data exist for isavuconazole yet.

Echinocandins

This class of systemic antifungal agents was first approved in 2001. The echinocandins inhibit cell wall formation (in contrast to acting on the cell membrane by the polyenes and azoles) by noncompetitively inhibiting beta-1,3-glucan synthase, an enzyme present in fungi but absent in mammalian cells. These agents are generally very safe, as there is no beta-1,3-glucan in humans. The echinocandins are not metabolized through the CYP system, so fewer drug interactions are problematic, compared with the azoles. There is no need to dose-adjust in renal failure, but one needs a lower dosage in the setting of very severe hepatic dysfunction. As a class, these antifungals generally have poor CSF penetration, although animal studies have shown adequate brain parenchyma levels, and do not penetrate the urine well. While the 3 clinically available echinocandins each individually have some unique and important dosing and pharmacokinetic parameters, especially in children, efficacy is generally equivalent. Opposite the azole class, the echinocandins are fungicidal against yeasts but fungistatic against molds. The fungicidal activity against yeasts has elevated the echinocandins to the preferred therapy against *Candida* in a neutropenic or critically ill patient. Echinocandins are thought to be best utilized against invasive aspergillosis as salvage therapy if a triazole fails or in a patient with suspected triazole resistance. Improved efficacy with combination therapy with the echinocandins and the triazoles against *Aspergillus* infections is unclear, with disparate results in multiple smaller studies and a definitive clinical trial demonstrating no clear benefit over voriconazole monotherapy. Some experts have used combination therapy in invasive aspergillosis with a triazole plus echinocandin only during the initial phase of waiting for triazole drug levels to be appropriate. There are reports of echinocandin resistance in *Candida* spp, as high as 12% in *C glabrata* in some studies, and the echinocandins as a class are often somewhat less active against *Candida parapsilosis* isolates (approximately 10%–15% respond poorly, but most are still susceptible).

Caspofungin received FDA approval for children aged 3 months to 17 years in 2008 for empiric therapy of presumed fungal infections in febrile, neutropenic children; treatment of candidemia as well as *Candida* esophagitis, peritonitis, and empyema; and for salvage therapy of invasive aspergillosis. Due to its earlier approval, there are generally more reports with caspofungin than the other echinocandins. Caspofungin dosing in children is calculated according to body surface area, with a loading dose on the first day of 70 mg/m^2, followed by daily maintenance dosing of 50 mg/m^2, and not to exceed 70 mg regardless of the calculated dose. Significantly higher doses of caspofungin have been studied in adult patients without any clear added benefit in efficacy, but if the 50 mg/m^2 dose is tolerated and does not provide adequate clinical response, the daily dose can be increased to 70 mg/m^2.

Micafungin was approved in adults in 2005 for treatment of candidemia, *Candida* esophagitis and peritonitis, and prophylaxis of *Candida* infections in stem cell transplant recipients, and in 2013 for pediatric patients aged 4 months and older. Micafungin has the most pediatric and neonatal data available of all 3 echinocandins, including more extensive pharmacokinetic studies surrounding dosing and several efficacy studies.[4–6] Micafungin dosing in children is age dependent, as clearance increases dramatically in the younger age groups (especially neonates), necessitating higher doses for younger children. Doses in children are generally thought to be 2 to 4 mg/kg/day, with higher doses likely needed for younger patients, and premature neonates dosed at 10 mg/kg/day. Adult micafungin dosing (100 or 150 mg once daily) is to be used in patients who weigh more than 40 kg. Unlike the other echinocandins, a loading dose is not required for micafungin.

Anidulafungin was approved for adults for candidemia and *Candida* esophagitis in 2006 and is not officially approved for pediatric patients. Like the other echinocandins, anidulafungin is not P450 metabolized and has not demonstrated significant drug interactions. Limited clinical efficacy data are available in children, with only some pediatric pharmacokinetic data suggesting weight-based dosing.[7] The adult dose for invasive candidiasis is a loading dose of 200 mg on the first day, followed by 100 mg daily.

3. How Antibiotic Dosages Are Determined Using Susceptibility Data, Pharmacodynamics, and Treatment Outcomes

Factors Involved in Dosing Recommendations

Our view of how to use antimicrobials is continually changing. As the published literature and our experience with each drug increase, our recommendations evolve as we compare the efficacy, safety, and cost of each drug in the context of current and previous data from adults and children. Every new antibiotic must demonstrate some degree of efficacy and safety in adults before we attempt to treat children. Occasionally, unanticipated toxicities and unanticipated clinical failures modify our initial recommendations.

Important considerations in any new recommendations we make include (1) the susceptibilities of pathogens to antibiotics, which are constantly changing, are different from region to region, and are hospital- and unit-specific; (2) the antibiotic concentrations achieved at the site of infection over a 24-hour dosing interval; (3) the mechanism of how antibiotics kill bacteria; (4) how often the dose we select produces a clinical and microbiological cure; (5) how often we encounter toxicity; and (6) how likely the antibiotic exposure will lead to antibiotic resistance in the treated child and in the population in general.

Susceptibility

Susceptibility data for each bacterial pathogen against a wide range of antibiotics are available from the microbiology laboratory of virtually every hospital. This antibiogram can help guide you in antibiotic selection for empiric therapy. Many hospitals can separate the inpatient culture results from outpatient results, and many can give you the data by ward of the hospital (eg, pediatric ward vs neonatal intensive care unit vs adult intensive care unit). Susceptibility data are also available by region and by country from reference laboratories or public health laboratories. The recommendations made in *Nelson's Pediatric Antimicrobial Therapy* reflect overall susceptibility patterns present in the United States. Wide variations may exist for certain pathogens in different regions of the United States and the world.

Drug Concentrations at the Site of Infection

With every antibiotic, we can measure the concentration of antibiotic present in the serum. We can also directly measure the concentrations in specific tissue sites, such as spinal fluid or middle ear fluid. Because free, nonprotein-bound antibiotic is required to inhibit and kill pathogens, it is also important to calculate the amount of free drug available at the site of infection. While traditional methods of measuring antibiotics focused on the peak concentrations in serum and how rapidly the drugs were excreted, complex models of drug distribution and elimination now exist not only for the serum but for other tissue compartments as well. Antibiotic exposure to pathogens at the site of infection can be described in many ways: (1) the percentage of time in a 24-hour dosing interval that the antibiotic concentrations are above the minimum inhibitory concentration (MIC; the antibiotic concentration required for inhibition of growth of an organism) at the site of infection (%T>MIC); (2) the mathematically calculated area below the serum concentration-versus-time curve (area under the curve [AUC]); and (3) the maximal concentration of drug achieved at the tissue site (Cmax). For each of these 3 values, a ratio of that value to the MIC of the pathogen in question can be calculated and provides more useful information on specific drug activity against a specific pathogen than simply looking at the MIC. It allows us to compare the exposure of different antibiotics (that achieve quite different concentrations in tissues) to a pathogen (where the MIC for each drug may be different) and to assess the activity of a single antibiotic that may be used for empiric therapy to the many different pathogens that may be causing an infection at that tissue site.

Pharmacodynamics

Pharmacodynamic data provide the clinician with information on how the bacterial pathogens are killed (see Suggested Reading). Beta-lactam antibiotics tend to eradicate bacteria following prolonged exposure of the antibiotic to the pathogen at the site of infection, usually expressed as noted previously, as the percent of time over a dosing interval that the antibiotic is present at the site of infection in concentrations greater than the MIC (%T>MIC). For example, amoxicillin needs to be present at the site of pneumococcal infection at a concentration above the MIC for only 40% of a 24-hour dosing interval. Remarkably, neither higher concentrations of amoxicillin nor a more prolonged exposure will substantially increase the cure rate. On the other hand, gentamicin's activity against *Escherichia coli* is based primarily on the absolute concentration of free antibiotic at the site of infection, in the context of the MIC of the pathogen (Cmax:MIC). The more antibiotic you can deliver to the site of infection, the more rapidly you can sterilize the tissue; we are only limited by the toxicities of gentamicin. For fluoroquinolones like ciprofloxacin, the antibiotic exposure best linked to clinical and microbiologic success is the AUC:MIC.

Assessment of Clinical and Microbiological Outcomes

In clinical trials of anti-infective agents, most adults and children will hopefully be cured, but a few will fail therapy. For those few, we may note inadequate drug exposure (eg, more rapid drug elimination in a particular patient) or infection caused by a pathogen with a particularly high MIC. By analyzing the successes and the failures based on the appropriate exposure parameters outlined previously (%T>MIC, AUC:MIC, or Cmax:MIC), we can often observe a particular value of exposure, above which we observe a higher rate of cure and below which the cure rate drops quickly. Knowing this target value (the "antibiotic exposure break point") allows us to calculate the dosage that will create treatment success in most children. It is this dosage that we subsequently offer to you (if we have it) as one likely to cure your patient.

Suggested Reading

Bradley JS, et al. *Pediatr Infect Dis J.* 2010;29(11):1043–1046 PMID: 20975453

4. Community-Associated Methicillin-Resistant *Staphylococcus aureus*

Community-associated methicillin-resistant *Staphylococcus aureus* (CA-MRSA) is a community pathogen for children (that can also spread from child to child in hospitals) that first appeared in the United States in the mid-1990s and currently represents 30% to 80% of all community isolates in various regions of the United States (check your hospital microbiology laboratory for your local rate); it is increasingly present in many areas of the world, with some strain variation documented. This CA-MRSA, like the hospital-associated MRSA strain that has been prevalent for the past 40 years, is resistant to methicillin and to all other beta-lactam antibiotics, except for the newly US Food and Drug Administration (FDA)-approved fifth-generation cephalosporin antibiotic, ceftaroline, for which there are only limited published pediatric data on pharmacokinetics, safety, and efficacy (as of publication date). There are an undetermined number of pathogenicity factors that make CA-MRSA more aggressive than methicillin-susceptible *S aureus* (MSSA), which used to be a standard pediatric pathogen for decades. Community-associated MRSA seems to cause greater tissue necrosis, an increased host inflammatory response, an increased rate of complications, and an increased rate of recurrent infections compared with MSSA. Response to therapy with non–beta-lactam antibiotics (eg, vancomycin, clindamycin) seems to be slower, and it is unknown whether longer courses of these alternative agents that seem to be needed for clinical cure are due to a hardier, better-adapted, more resistant CA-MRSA or whether these alternative agents are just not as effective against MRSA as beta-lactam agents are against MSSA. Recent guidelines have been published by the Infectious Diseases Society of America.[1]

Therapy for CA-MRSA

Vancomycin (intravenous [IV]) has been the mainstay of parenteral therapy of MRSA infections for the past 4 decades and continues to have activity against more than 98% of strains isolated from children. A few cases of intermediate resistance and "heteroresistance" (transient moderately increased resistance based on thickened staphylococcal cell walls) have been reported, most commonly in adults who are receiving long-term therapy or who have received multiple exposures to vancomycin. Unfortunately, the response to therapy using standard vancomycin dosing of 40 mg/kg/day in the treatment of the new CA-MRSA strains has not been as predictably successful as in the past with MSSA. Increasingly, data in adults suggest that serum trough concentrations of vancomycin in treating serious CA-MRSA infections should be kept in the range of 15 to 20 µg/mL, which frequently causes toxicity in adults. For children, serum trough concentrations of 15 to 20 µg/mL can usually be achieved using the old pediatric "meningitis dosage" of vancomycin of 60 mg/kg/day. Although no prospectively collected data are available, it appears that this dosage in children is reasonably effective and not associated with the degree of nephrotoxicity observed in adults. For vancomycin, the area under the curve–minimum inhibitory concentration (MIC) ratio that best predicts a successful outcome is about 400 or greater, which is achievable for CA-MRSA strains with in vitro MIC values of 1 µg/mL or less but difficult to achieve for strains with 2 µg/mL or greater.[2] Strains with MIC values of 4 µg/mL or greater should generally be considered resistant to vancomycin.

At these higher "meningitis" treatment dosages, one needs to follow renal function for the development of toxicity.

Clindamycin (oral [PO] or IV) is active against approximately 70% to 90% of strains, with great geographic variability (again, check with your hospital laboratory). The dosage for moderate to severe infections is 30 to 40 mg/kg/day, in 3 divided doses, using the same mg/kg dose PO or IV. Clindamycin is not as bactericidal as vancomycin but achieves higher concentrations in abscesses. Some CA-MRSA strains are susceptible to clindamycin on initial testing but have inducible clindamycin resistance (methylase-mediated) that is usually assessed by the "D-test." Within each population of these CA-MRSA organisms, a rare organism will have a mutation that allows for constant (rather than induced) resistance. Although still somewhat controversial, clindamycin should be effective therapy for infections that have a relatively low organism load (cellulitis, small abscesses) and are unlikely to contain a significant population of these mutants. Infections with a high organism load (empyema) may have a greater risk of failure against strains positive on the D-test (as a large population is more likelihood to have a significant number of truly resistant organisms), and clindamycin should not be used as the preferred agent. Some laboratories no longer report the D-test results but simply call the organism "resistant."

Clindamycin is used to treat most CA-MRSA infections that are not life-threatening, and, if the child responds, therapy can be switched from IV to PO (although the oral solution is not very well tolerated). *Clostridium difficile* enterocolitis is a concern as a clindamycin-associated complication; however, despite a great increase in the use of clindamycin in children during the past decade, there are no recent published data on a clinically significant increase in the rate of this complication in children.

Trimethoprim/sulfamethoxazole (TMP/SMX) (PO, IV), Bactrim/Septra, is active against CA-MRSA in vitro. New, prospective comparative data on treatment of skin or skin structure infections in adults and children (presented at IDWeek, October 2013) document efficacy equivalent to clindamycin. Given our current lack of prospective, comparative information in MRSA bacteremia, pneumonia, and osteomyelitis, TMP/SMX should not be used routinely to treat these more serious infections.

Linezolid, Zyvox (PO, IV), active against virtually 100% of CA-MRSA strains, is another reasonable alternative but is considered bacteriostatic and has relatively frequent hematologic toxicity in adults (neutropenia, thrombocytopenia) and some infrequent neurologic toxicity (peripheral neuropathy, optic neuritis), particularly when used for courses of 2 weeks or longer (a complete blood cell count should be checked every week or 2 in children receiving prolonged linezolid therapy). It is still under patent, so the cost is substantially more than clindamycin or vancomycin.

Daptomycin (IV), FDA approved for adults for skin infections and bacteremia/endocarditis, is a new class of antibiotic, a lipopeptide, and is highly bactericidal. Daptomycin should be considered for treatment of skin infection and bacteremia in failures with other, better studied antibiotics. Daptomycin should not be used to treat pneumonia, as it is inactivated by pulmonary surfactant. Pediatric studies for skin infections, bacteremia, and osteomyelitis are under way. Some new animal toxicity data suggest additional caution for the use of daptomycin in infants younger than 1 year. Pediatric clinical trial investigations in these younger infants are not proceeding at this time.

Tigecycline and fluoroquinolones, both of which may show in vitro activity, are not generally recommended for children if other agents are available and are tolerated due to potential toxicity issues for children with tetracyclines and fluoroquinolones and rapid emergence of resistance with fluoroquinolones.

Ceftaroline, a fifth-generation cephalosporin antibiotic, is the first beta-lactam antibiotic to be active against MRSA. The gram-negative coverage is similar to cefotaxime, with no activity against *Pseudomonas.* As of publication date, pediatric pharmacokinetic data have been collected for all age groups, and studies for skin and skin structure infections and community-acquired pneumonia are completed in children and are being analyzed. The efficacy and toxicity profile in adults is what one would expect from most cephalosporins.

Combination therapy for serious infections, with vancomycin and rifampin (for deep abscesses) or vancomycin and gentamicin (for bacteremia), is often used, but no data exist on improved efficacy over single antibiotic therapy. Some experts use vancomycin and clindamycin in combination, particularly for children with a toxic-shock clinical presentation.

Life-Threatening and Serious Infections

If any CA-MRSA is present in your community, empiric therapy for presumed staphylococcal infections that are life-threatening or infections for which any risk of failure is unacceptable (eg, meningitis) should follow the recommendations for CA-MRSA and include high-dose vancomycin, clindamycin, or linezolid, as well as nafcillin or oxacillin (beta-lactam antibiotics are considered better than vancomycin or clindamycin for MSSA).

Moderate Infections

If you live in a location with greater than 10% methicillin resistance, consider using the CA-MRSA recommendations for hospitalized children with presumed staphylococcal infections of any severity, and start empiric therapy with clindamycin (usually active against >90% of CA-MRSA), vancomycin, or linezolid IV.

In skin and skin structure abscesses, drainage of the abscess may be completely curative in some children, and antibiotics may not be necessary following incision and drainage.

Mild Infections

For nonserious, presumed staphylococcal infections in regions with significant CA-MRSA, empiric topical therapy with mupirocin (Bactroban) or retapamulin (Altabax) ointment, or oral therapy with trimethoprim/sulfamethoxazole or clindamycin, are preferred. For older children, doxycycline and minocycline are also options based on data in adults.

Recurrent Infections

For children with problematic, recurrent infections, no well-studied, prospectively collected data provide a solution. Bleach baths (one-half cup of bleach in one-quarter–filled bathtub[3]) seem to be able to transiently decrease the numbers of colonizing organisms. Bathing with chlorhexidine (Hibiclens, a preoperative antibacterial skin disinfectant) daily or a few times each week should provide topical anti-MRSA activity for several hours following a bath. Nasal mupirocin ointment (Bactroban) designed to eradicate colonization may also be used. All of these measures have advantages and disadvantages and need to be used together with environment measures (eg, washing towels frequently, using hand sanitizers, not sharing items of clothing). Helpful advice can be found on the Centers for Disease Control and Prevention Web site at www.cdc.gov/mrsa.

5. Antimicrobial Therapy for Newborns

NOTES

- Prospectively collected data in newborns continue to become available, thanks in large part to federal legislation (including the US Food and Drug Administration [FDA] Safety and Innovation Act of 2012 that mandates neonatal studies). In situations of inadequate data, suggested doses are based on efficacy, safety, and pharmacologic data from older children or adults. These may not account for the effect of developmental changes (effect of ontogeny) on drug metabolism that occur during early infancy and among premature and full-term newborns.[1] These values may vary widely, particularly for the unstable premature newborn. Oral convalescent therapy for neonatal infections has not been well studied but may be used cautiously in non–life-threatening infections in adherent families with ready access to medical care.[2]
- The recommended antibiotic dosages and intervals of administration are given in the tables at the end of this chapter.
- **Adverse drug reaction:** Neonates should not receive intravenous (IV) ceftriaxone while receiving IV calcium-containing products including parenteral nutrition by the same or different infusion lines, as fatal reactions with ceftriaxone-calcium precipitates in lungs and kidneys in neonates have occurred. There are no data on interactions between IV ceftriaxone and oral calcium-containing products or between intramuscular ceftriaxone and IV or oral calcium-containing products. Current information is available on the FDA Web site.[3] Cefotaxime is preferred over ceftriaxone for neonates.[4]
- **Abbreviations:** 3TC, lamivudine; ABLC, lipid complex amphotericin; ABR, auditory brainstem response; AmB, amphotericin B; AmB-D, AmB deoxycholate; ALT, alanine transaminase; amox/clav, amoxicillin/clavulanate; AOM, acute otitis media; AST, aspartate transaminase; bid, twice daily; CBC, complete blood cell count; CLD, chronic lung disease; CMV, cytomegalovirus; CNS, central nervous system; CSF, cerebrospinal fluid; div, divided; ECHO, echocardiogram; ECMO, extracorporeal membrane oxygenation; ESBL, extended spectrum beta-lactamase; FDA, US Food and Drug Administration; GA, gestational age; GBS, group B streptococcus; G-CSF, granulocyte colony stimulating factor; HIV, human immunodeficiency virus; HSV, herpes simplex virus; ID, infectious diseases; IM, intramuscular; IV, intravenous; IVIG, intravenous immune globulin; L-AmB, liposomal AmB; MRSA, methicillin-resistant *Staphylococcus aureus;* MSSA, methicillin-susceptible *S aureus;* NEC, necrotizing enterocolitis; NICU, neonatal intensive care unit; NVP, nevirapine; PCR, polymerase chain reaction; pip/tazo, piperacillin/tazobactam; PO, orally; RSV, respiratory syncytial virus; spp, species; ticar/clav, ticarcillin/clavulanate; tid, 3 times daily; TIG, tetanus immune globulin; TMP/SMX, trimethoprim/sulfamethoxazole; UTI, urinary tract infection; VCUG, voiding cystourethrogram; VDRL, Venereal Disease Research Laboratories; ZDV, zidovudine.

A. RECOMMENDED THERAPY FOR SELECTED NEWBORN CONDITIONS

Condition	Therapy (evidence grade) *See Table 5B-D for neonatal dosages.*	Comments
Conjunctivitis		
– Chlamydial[5–8]	Azithromycin 10 mg/kg/day PO for 1 day, then 5 mg/kg/day PO for 4 days (AII), or erythromycin ethylsuccinate PO for 10–14 days (AII)	Macrolides PO preferred to topical eye drops to prevent development of pneumonia; association of erythromycin and pyloric stenosis in young neonates.[9] Alternative: 3-day course of higher-dose azithromycin at 10 mg/kg/dose once daily, although safety not well defined in neonates (CIII). Oral sulfonamides may be used after the immediate neonatal period for infants who do not tolerate erythromycin.
– Gonococcal[10–14]	Ceftriaxone 25–50 mg/kg (max 125 mg) IV, IM once (AI) (Longer treatment may be used for severe cases.)	Saline irrigation of eyes. Alternative: cefotaxime may be used in neonates with hyperbilirubinemia. Evaluate for chlamydial infection. All neonates born to mothers with untreated gonococcal infection (regardless of symptoms) require therapy. Cefixime and ciprofloxacin no longer recommended for empiric maternal therapy.
– *Staphylococcus aureus*[15–17]	Topical therapy sufficient for mild *S aureus* cases (AII), but oral or IV therapy may be considered for moderate to severe conjunctivitis. MSSA: oxacillin/nafcillin IV or cefazolin (for non-CNS infections) IM, IV for 7 days. MRSA: vancomycin IV or clindamycin IV, PO.	Neomycin or erythromycin (BIII) ophthalmic drops or ointment No prospective data for MRSA conjunctivitis (BIII) Cephalexin PO for mild-moderate disease caused by MSSA Increased *S aureus* resistance with ciprofloxacin/levofloxacin ophthalmic formulations (AII)
– *Pseudomonas aeruginosa*[18–20]	Ceftazidime IM, IV AND tobramycin IM, IV for 7–10 days (alternatives: meropenem, cefepime, pip/tazo) (BIII)	Aminoglycoside or polymyxin B–containing ophthalmic drops or ointment as adjunctive therapy

– Other gram-negative	Aminoglycoside or polymyxin B–containing ophthalmic drops or ointment if mild (AII) Systemic therapy if moderate to severe or unresponsive to topical therapy (AIII)	Duration of therapy dependent on clinical course and may be as short as 5 days if clinically resolved.
Cytomegalovirus		
– Congenital[21–24]	For symptomatic neonates with congenital infection syndrome and multisystem disease: oral valganciclovir at 16 mg/kg/dose PO bid for 6 mo[24] (AI); IV ganciclovir 6 mg/kg/dose IV q12h can be used for some or all of the first 6 wk of therapy if oral therapy not advised (AII).	Benefit for hearing loss and neurodevelopmental outcomes (AI). Treatment recommended for neonates with symptomatic congenital CMV disease, with or without CNS involvement. Neutropenia in 20% (oral valganciclovir) to 68% (IV ganciclovir) of neonates on long-term therapy (responds to G-CSF or temporary discontinuation of therapy). Treatment for congenital CMV should start within the first month of life. CMV-IVIG not recommended.
– Perinatally or postnatally acquired[23]	Ganciclovir 12 mg/kg/day IV div q12h for 14–21 days (AIII)	Antiviral treatment has not been studied in this population but can be considered in patients with acute, severe, visceral (end-organ) disease such as pneumonia, hepatitis, encephalitis, necrotizing enterocolitis, or persistent thrombocytopenia. If such patients are treated with parenteral ganciclovir, a reasonable approach is to treat for 2 wk and then reassess responsiveness to therapy. If clinical data suggest benefit of treatment, an additional 1 wk of parenteral ganciclovir can be considered if symptoms and signs have not fully resolved. Observe for possible relapse after completion of therapy (AIII).

A. RECOMMENDED THERAPY FOR SELECTED NEWBORN CONDITIONS (cont)

Condition	Therapy (evidence grade) *See Table 5B-D for neonatal dosages.*	Comments
Fungal infections (See Chapter 8.)		
– Candidiasis[25–33]	L-AmB/ABLC (5 mg/kg/day) or AmB-D (1 mg/kg/day). If urinary tract involvement is excluded, then can use L-AmB/ABLC due to theoretical concerns of lipid formulations not penetrating kidneys adequately for treatment. For susceptible strains, fluconazole is usually effective. For treatment of neonates, load with 25 mg/day for day 1, then continue with 12 mg/kg/day (BI).[34] For treatment of neonates and young infants (<120 days) on ECMO, fluconazole load with 35 mg/kg on day 1, followed by 12 mg/kg/day (BII). If used for prophylaxis, fluconazole 6 mg/kg/day twice a week in high-risk neonates (birth weight <1,000 g) in centers where incidence of disease is high (generally thought to be >10%). If used for prophylaxis in neonates and young infants (<120 days) on ECMO, fluconazole 25 mg/kg once weekly (BII).	Prompt removal of all catheters essential (AII). Evaluate for other sites of infection: CSF analysis, cardiac echo, abdominal ultrasound to include bladder; retinal eye examination. Persistent disease requires evaluation of catheter removal or search for disseminated sites. Antifungal susceptibility testing is suggested with persistent disease. (*Candida krusei* inherently resistant to fluconazole; *Candida parapsilosis* may be less susceptible to echinocandins; *Candida glabrata* demonstrates increasing resistance to fluconazole and echinocandins). No proven benefit for combination antifungal therapy in candidiasis. Change from AmB or fluconazole to micafungin/caspofungin if cultures persistently positive (BIII). Although fluconazole has been shown to reduce colonization, it has not reduced the rate of invasive candidiasis or death.[28] Role of flucytosine (5-FC) orally in neonates with *Candida* meningitis is not well defined and not routinely recommended due to toxicity concerns. Length of therapy dependent on disease (BIII), usually 3 wk. Limited data in humans exist on echinocandin CSF/brain penetration. Animal studies suggest adequate penetration, but clinical utility in the CSF/brain is unclear. Higher echinocandin doses needed in the smallest infants. Antifungal bladder washes not indicated.
– Aspergillosis (usually cutaneous infection with systemic dissemination)[35–37]	Voriconazole (18 mg/kg/day div q12h load, then continue with 16 mg/kg/day; very important to maintain trough serum concentrations ≥2 mg/L). Duration depends on severity of disease and success of local debridement (BIII).	Aggressive antifungal therapy, early debridement of skin lesions (AIII) Goal serum trough levels are between 2 and 6 µg/ml. Trough levels should be obtained before sixth dose and then intermittently to ensure adequate levels.

Gastrointestinal infections		
– NEC or peritonitis secondary to bowel rupture[38–43]	Ampicillin IV AND gentamicin IM, IV for ≥10 days (AII). Alternatives: pip/tazo AND gentamicin (AII); ceftazidime/cefotaxime AND gentamicin ± metronidazole (BIII); OR meropenem (BI). ADD fluconazole if known to have gastrointestinal colonization with *Candida* (BIII).	Surgical drainage (AII). Definitive antibiotic therapy based on culture results (aerobic, anaerobic, and fungal); meropenem or cefepime if ceftazidime-resistant gram-negative bacilli isolated. Vancomycin rather than ampicillin if MRSA prevalent. Bacteroides colonization may occur as early as the first week of life (AIII).[43] Duration of therapy dependent on clinical response and risk of persisting intra-abdominal abscess (AIII). Probiotics may prevent NEC in neonates born <1,500 g, but agent, dose, and safety not fully known.[40]
– *Salmonella*[44]	Ampicillin IM, IV (if susceptible) OR cefotaxime IM, IV for 7–10 days (AII)	Observe for focal complications (eg, meningitis, arthritis) (AIII)
Herpes simplex infection		
– CNS and disseminated disease[45–47]	Acyclovir IV for 21 days (AII) (if eye disease present, ADD topical 1% trifluridine, 0.1% idoxuridine, or 0.15% ganciclovir ophthalmic gel) (AII)	For CNS disease, perform CSF HSV PCR near end of 21 days of therapy and continue acyclovir until PCR negative. Serum AST/ALT may help identify early disseminated infection. Foscarnet for acyclovir-resistant disease. Acyclovir PO (300 mg/m^2/dose tid) suppression for 6 mo recommended following parenteral therapy (AI).[48] Monitor for neutropenia during suppressive therapy. Different dosages than those listed in Table B have been modeled, but there are no safety or efficacy data in humans to support them.[49]
– Skin, eye, or mouth disease[45–47]	Acyclovir IV for 14 days (AII) (if eye disease present, ADD topical 1% trifluridine, 0.1% idoxuridine, or 0.15% ganciclovir ophthalmic gel) (AII). Obtain CSF PCR for HSV to assess for CNS infection.	Acyclovir PO (300 mg/m^2/dose tid) suppression for 6 mo recommended following parenteral therapy (AI).[48] Monitor for neutropenia during suppressive therapy.

A. RECOMMENDED THERAPY FOR SELECTED NEWBORN CONDITIONS (cont)

Condition	Therapy (evidence grade) *See Table 5B-D for neonatal dosages.*	Comments
Human immunodeficiency virus infection[50,51]	There has been recent interest in using "treatment" antiretroviral regimens for high-risk, exposed neonates in an attempt to achieve a remission or possibly even a cure. This was initially stimulated by the experience of a baby from Mississippi: high-risk neonate treated within the first 2 days of life with subsequent infection documentation; off therapy at 18 mo of age without evidence of circulating virus until 4 y of age, at which point HIV became detectable. While a clinical trial is ongoing to study issues further, full treatment dosing of high-risk neonates is not currently recommended due to lack of safety and dosing data and lack of defined efficacy.	
	Peripartum presumptive preventive therapy for HIV-exposed newborns: ZDV for the first 6 wk of age (AI). GA ≥35 wk: ZDV 8 mg/kg/day PO div bid OR 6 mg/kg/day IV div q6h for 6 wk. GA <35 wk but >30 wk: ZDV 4 mg/kg/day PO (OR 3 mg/kg/day IV) div q12h. Increase at 2 wk of age to 6 mg/kg/day PO (OR 4.6 mg/kg/day IV) div q12h. GA ≤30 wk: ZDV 3 mg/kg/day IV (OR 4 mg/kg/day PO) div q12h. Increase at 4 wk of age to 6 mg/kg/day PO (OR 4.6 mg/kg/day IV) div q12h. For newborns whose mothers received NO antenatal intervention, add 3 doses of NVP (first dose at 0–48 h; second dose 48 h later; third dose 96 h after second dose) to the 6 wk of ZDV treatment (AI). NVP dose: birth weight 1.5–2 kg: 8 mg/dose PO; birth weight >2 kg: 12 mg/dose PO (AI).[52] The preventive ZDV doses listed above for neonates are also treatment doses for infants with diagnosed HIV infection. Note that antiretroviral treatment doses for neonates are established only for ZDV and 3TC (4 mg/kg/day div q12h). Treatment of HIV-infected neonates should be considered only with expert consultation.	For detailed information: http://aidsinfo.nih.gov/Guidelines (accessed October 9, 2014). National Perinatal HIV Consultation and Referral Service (888/448-8765) provides free clinical consultation. Start therapy at 6–8 h of age if possible (AII). Monitor CBC at birth and 4 wk (AII). Some experts consider the use of ZDV in combination with other antiretroviral drugs in certain situations (eg, mothers with minimal intervention before delivery, has high viral load, or with known resistant virus). Consultation with a pediatric HIV specialist is recommended (BIII). Perform HIV-1 DNA PCR or RNA assays at 14–21 days, 1–2 mo, and 4–6 mo (AI). Initiate prophylaxis for pneumocystis pneumonia at 6 wk of age if HIV infection not yet excluded (AII).

Influenza A and B viruses[53,54]	Preterm, <38 wk postmenstrual age: 1 mg/kg/dose PO bid Preterm, 38–40 wk postmenstrual age: 1.5 mg/kg/dose PO bid Preterm, >40 wk postmenstrual age: 3.0 mg/kg/dose PO bid[54] Term, birth–8 mo: 3.0 mg/kg/dose PO bid[55]	Oseltamivir chemoprophylaxis not recommended for infants <3 mo of age unless the situation is judged critical because of limited safety and efficacy data in this age group.
Omphalitis and funisitis		
– Empiric therapy for omphalitis and necrotizing funisitis direct therapy against coliform bacilli, *S aureus* (consider MRSA), and anaerobes[56–58]	Cefotaxime OR gentamicin, AND clindamycin for ≥10 days (AII)	Need to culture to direct therapy. Alternatives for coliform coverage if resistance likely: cefepime, meropenem. For suspect MRSA: add vancomycin. Alternatives for combined MSSA and anaerobic coverage: pip/tazo or ticar/clav. Appropriate wound management for infected cord and necrotic tissue (AIII).
– Group A or B streptococci[59]	Penicillin G IV for ≥7–14 days (shorter course for superficial funisitis without invasive infection) (AII)	Group A streptococcus usually causes "wet cord" without pus and with minimal erythema; single dose of benzathine penicillin IM adequate. Consultation with pediatric ID specialist is recommended for necrotizing fasciitis (AII).
– *S aureus*[58]	MSSA: oxacillin/nafcillin IV, IM for ≥5–7 days (shorter course for superficial funisitis without invasive infection) (AIII) MRSA: vancomycin (AIII)	Assess for bacteremia and other focus of infection. Alternatives for MRSA: linezolid, clindamycin (if susceptible).
– *Clostridium* spp[60]	Clindamycin OR penicillin G IV for ≥10 days, with additional agents based on culture results (AII)	Crepitance and rapidly spreading cellulitis around umbilicus Mixed infection with other gram-positive and gram-negative bacteria common

A. RECOMMENDED THERAPY FOR SELECTED NEWBORN CONDITIONS (cont)

Condition	Therapy (evidence grade) *See Table 5B-D for neonatal dosages.*	Comments
Osteomyelitis, suppurative arthritis[61–63] Obtain cultures (aerobic; fungal if NICU) of bone or joint fluid before antibiotic therapy. Duration of therapy dependent on causative organism and normalization of erythrocyte sedimentation rate and C-reactive protein; minimum for osteomyelitis 3 wk and arthritis therapy 2–3 wk if no organism identified (AIII). Surgical drainage of pus (AIII); physical therapy may be needed (BIII).		
– Empiric therapy	Nafcillin/oxacillin IV (or vancomycin if MRSA is a concern) AND cefotaxime or gentamicin IV, IM (AIII)	
– Coliform bacteria (eg, *Escherichia coli, Klebsiella* spp, *Enterobacter* spp)	For *E coli* and *Klebsiella:* cefotaxime OR gentamicin OR ampicillin (if susceptible) (AIII). For *Enterobacter, Serratia,* or *Citrobacter:* ADD gentamicin IV, IM to cefotaxime or ceftriaxone, OR use cefepime or meropenem alone (AIII).	Meropenem for ESBL-producing coliforms (AIII). Pip/tazo or cefepime are alternatives for susceptible bacilli (BIII).
– Gonococcal arthritis and tenosynovitis[11–14]	Ceftriaxone IV, IM OR cefotaxime IV for 7–10 days (AII)	Cefotaxime is preferred for neonates with hyperbilirubinemia.
– *S aureus*	MSSA: oxacillin/nafcillin IV (AII) MRSA: vancomycin IV (AIII)	Alternative for MSSA: cefazolin (AIII) Alternatives for MRSA: linezolid, clindamycin (if susceptible) (BIII) Addition of rifampin if persistently positive cultures
– Group B streptococcus	Ampicillin or penicillin G IV (AII)	
– *Haemophilus influenzae*	Ampicillin IV OR cefotaxime IV, IM if ampicillin-resistant	Start with IV therapy and switch to oral therapy when clinically stable. Amox/clav PO OR amoxicillin PO if susceptible (AIII).
Otitis media[64]	No controlled treatment trials in newborns; if no response, obtain middle ear fluid for culture.	In addition to *Pneumococcus* and *Haemophilus,* coliforms and *S aureus* may also cause AOM in neonates (AIII).

– Empiric therapy[65]	Oxacillin/nafcillin AND cefotaxime or gentamicin	Start with IV therapy and switch to oral therapy when clinically stable. Amox/clav (AIII).
– *E coli* (therapy of other coliforms based on susceptibility testing)	Cefotaxime OR gentamicin	Start with IV therapy and switch to oral therapy when clinically stable. For ESBL-producing strains, use meropenem (AII). Amox/clav if susceptible (AIII).
– *S aureus*	MSSA: oxacillin/nafcillin IV (MSSA) MRSA: vancomycin or clindamycin IV (If susceptible)	Start with IV therapy and switch to oral therapy when clinically stable. MSSA: cephalexin PO for 10 days or cloxacillin PO (AIII). MRSA: linezolid PO or clindamycin PO (BIII).
– Group A or B streptococcus	Penicillin G or ampicillin IV, IM	Start with IV therapy and switch to oral therapy when clinically stable. Amoxicillin 30–40 mg/kg/day PO div q8h for 10 days.
Parotitis, suppurative[66]	Oxacillin/nafcillin IV AND gentamicin IV, IM for 10 days; consider vancomycin if MRSA suspected (AIII).	Usually staphylococcal but occasionally coliform. Antimicrobial regimen without incision/drainage is adequate in >75% of cases.
Pulmonary infections		
– Empiric therapy of the neonate with early onset of pulmonary infiltrates (within the first 48–72 h of life)	Ampicillin IV/IM AND gentamicin or cefotaxime IV/IM for 10 days; many neonatologists treat low-risk neonates for ≤7 days (see Comments).	For newborns with no additional risk factors for bacterial infection (eg, maternal chorioamnionitis) who (1) have negative blood cultures, (2) have no need for >8 h of oxygen, and (3) are asymptomatic at 48 h into therapy, 4 days may be sufficient therapy, based on limited data.[67]
– Aspiration pneumonia[68]	Ampicillin IV, IM AND gentamicin IV, IM for 7–10 days (AIII)	Early onset neonatal pneumonia may represent aspiration of amniotic fluid, particularly if fluid is not sterile. Mild aspiration episodes may not require antibiotic therapy.
– *Chlamydia trachomatis*[69]	Azithromycin PO, IV q24h for 5 days OR erythromycin ethylsuccinate PO for 14 days (AII)	Association of erythromycin and pyloric stenosis in young infants
– *Mycoplasma hominis*[70,71]	Clindamycin PO, IV for 10 days (Organisms are resistant to macrolides.)	Pathogenic role in pneumonia not well defined and clinical efficacy unknown; no association with bronchopulmonary dysplasia (BIII)

A. RECOMMENDED THERAPY FOR SELECTED NEWBORN CONDITIONS (cont)

Condition	**Therapy (evidence grade)** *See Table 5B-D for neonatal dosages.*	Comments
Pulmonary infections (cont)		
– Pertussis[72]	Azithromycin 10 mg/kg PO, IV q24h for 5 days OR erythromycin ethylsuccinate PO for 14 days (AII)	Association of erythromycin and pyloric stenosis in young infants; may also occur with azithromycin. Alternatives for >1 mo of age, clarithromycin for 7 days, and for >2 mo of age, TMP/SMX for 14 days.
– *P aeruginosa*[73]	Ceftazidime IV, IM AND tobramycin IV, IM for ≥10–14 days (AIII)	Alternatives: cefepime or meropenem, OR pip/tazo AND tobramycin
– Respiratory syncytial virus[74]	Treatment: see Comments. Prophylaxis: palivizumab (Synagis, a monoclonal antibody) 15 mg/kg IM monthly for these high-risk infants (AI). In first y of life, palivizumab prophylaxis is recommended for infants born before 29 wk, 0 days' gestation. Palivizumab prophylaxis is not recommended for otherwise healthy infants born at ≥29 wk, 0 days' gestation. In first y of life, palivizumab prophylaxis is recommended for preterm infants with CLD of prematurity, defined as birth at <32 wk, 0 days' gestation and a requirement for >21% oxygen for at least 28 days after birth. Clinicians may administer palivizumab prophylaxis in the first year of life to certain infants with hemodynamically significant heart disease.	Aerosol ribavirin (6-g vial to make 20-mg/mL solution in sterile water), aerosolized over 18–20 h daily for 3–5 days (BII), provides little benefit and should only be used for life-threatening infection with RSV. Difficulties in administration, complications with airway reactivity, and concern for potential toxicities to health care workers preclude routine use. Palivizumab does not provide benefit in the treatment of an active RSV infection. Palivizumab may benefit immunocompromised children but is not routinely recommended as benefits not well defined. Palivizumab prophylaxis is not recommended in the second year of life except for children who required at least 28 days of supplemental oxygen after birth and who continue to require medical intervention (supplemental oxygen, chronic corticosteroid, or diuretic therapy). Monthly prophylaxis should be discontinued in any child who experiences a breakthrough RSV hospitalization. Children with pulmonary abnormality or neuromuscular disease that impairs the ability to clear secretions from the upper airways may be considered for prophylaxis in the first y of life.

	Clinicians may administer up to a maximum of 5 monthly doses of palivizumab (15 mg/kg per dose) during the RSV season to infants who qualify for prophylaxis in the first year of life. Qualifying infants born during the RSV season may require fewer doses; eg, infants born in January would receive their last dose in March.	Children <24 mo who will be profoundly immunocompromised during the RSV season may be considered for prophylaxis. Insufficient data are available to recommend palivizumab prophylaxis for children with cystic fibrosis or Down syndrome. The burden of RSV disease and costs associated with transport from remote locations may result in a broader use of palivizumab for RSV prevention in Alaska Native populations and possibly in selected other American Indian populations. Palivizumab prophylaxis is not recommended for prevention of health care–associated RSV disease.
– *S aureus*[17,75–77]	MSSA: oxacillin/nafcillin IV (AIII). MRSA: vancomycin IV OR clindamycin IV if susceptible (AIII). Duration of therapy depends on extent of disease (pneumonia vs pulmonary abscesses vs empyema) and should be individualized with therapy up to 21 days or greater.	Alternative for MSSA: cefazolin IV Addition of rifampin or linezolid if persistently positive cultures (AIII) Thoracostomy drainage of empyema
– Group B streptococcus[78,79]	Penicillin G IV OR ampicillin IV, IM for 10 days (AIII)	For serious infections, ADD gentamicin for synergy until clinically improved. No prospective, randomized data on the efficacy of a 7-day treatment course.
– *Ureaplasma* spp (*urealyticum* or *parvum*)[80]	Azithromycin PO/IV for 5 days or clarithromycin PO for 10 days (BIII)	Pathogenic role of *Ureaplasma* not well defined and no prophylaxis recommended for CLD Many *Ureaplasma* spp resistant to erythromycin Association of erythromycin and pyloric stenosis in young infants

A. RECOMMENDED THERAPY FOR SELECTED NEWBORN CONDITIONS (cont)

Condition	Therapy (evidence grade) *See Table 5B-D for neonatal dosages.*	Comments
Sepsis and meningitis[78,81,82]	**NOTE:** Duration of therapy: 10 days for sepsis without a focus (AIII); minimum of 21 days for gram-negative meningitis (or at least 14 days after CSF is sterile) and 14–21 days for GBS meningitis and other gram-positive bacteria (AIII)	There are no prospective, controlled studies on 5- or 7-day courses for mild or presumed sepsis.
– Initial therapy, organism unknown	Ampicillin IV AND cefotaxime IV (AII), OR ampicillin IV AND gentamicin IV, IM (AII)	Cefotaxime preferred if meningitis suspected or cannot be excluded (AIII). For locations with a high rate (10% or greater) of ESBL-producing *E coli,* and meningitis is suspected, empiric therapy with meropenem (or cefepime) is preferred over cefotaxime. For empiric therapy of sepsis without meningitis, in areas with a high rate of ESBL *E coli,* gentamicin is preferred. Initial empiric therapy of nosocomial infection should be based on each hospital's pathogens and susceptibilities. Always narrow antibiotic coverage once susceptibility data are available.
– *Bacteroides fragilis*	Metronidazole or meropenem IV, IM (AIII)	Alternative: clindamycin, but increasing resistance reported
– *Enterococcus* spp	Ampicillin IV, IM AND gentamicin IV, IM (AIII); for ampicillin-resistant organisms: vancomycin AND gentamicin (AIII)	Gentamicin needed with ampicillin or vancomycin for bactericidal activity; continue until clinical and microbiological response documented (AIII). For vancomycin-resistant enterococci that are also ampicillin resistant: linezolid (AIII).
– *E coli*[81,82]	Cefotaxime IV, IM or gentamicin IV, IM (AII) if no CNS infection	Meropenem (or cefepime) for ESBL-producing organisms (AIII)
– Gonococcal[11–14]	Ceftriaxone IV, IM OR cefotaxime IV, IM (AII)	Duration of therapy not well defined; consider that 5 days cefotaxime is preferred for neonates with hyperbilirubinemia.
– *Listeria monocytogenes*[83]	Ampicillin IV, IM AND gentamicin IV, IM (AIII)	Gentamicin is synergistic in vitro with ampicillin. Continue until clinical and microbiological response documented (AIII).

– *P aeruginosa*	Ceftazidime IV, IM AND tobramycin IV, IM (AIII)	Meropenem, cefepime, and tobramycin are suitable alternatives (AIII). Pip/tazo should not be used for CNS infection.
– *S aureus*[17,75–77,84,85]	MSSA: oxacillin/nafcillin IV, IM, or cefazolin IV, IM (AII) MRSA: vancomycin IV (AIII)	Alternatives for MRSA: clindamycin, linezolid
– *Staphylococcus epidermidis* (or any coagulase-negative staphylococci)	Vancomycin IV (AIII)	If organism susceptible and infection not severe, oxacillin/nafcillin or cefazolin are alternatives for methicillin-susceptible strains. Cefazolin does not enter CNS. Add rifampin if cultures persistently positive. Alternative: linezolid.
– Group A streptococcus	Penicillin G or ampicillin IV (AII)	
– Group B streptococcus[78]	Ampicillin or penicillin G IV AND gentamicin IV, IM (AI)	Continue gentamicin until clinical and microbiological response documented (AIII). Duration of therapy: 10 days for bacteremia/sepsis (AII); minimum of 14 days for meningitis (AII).
Skin and soft tissues		
– Breast abscess[86]	Vancomycin IV (for MRSA) or oxacillin/nafcillin IV, IM (MSSA) AND cefotaxime OR gentamicin if gram-negative rods seen on Gram stain (AIII)	Gram stain of expressed pus guides empiric therapy; vancomycin if MRSA prevalent in community; alternative to vancomycin: clindamycin, linezolid, may need surgical drainage to minimize damage to breast tissue. Treatment duration individualized until clinical findings have completely resolved (AIII).
– Erysipelas (and other group A streptococcal infections)	Penicillin G IV for 5–7 days, followed by oral therapy (if bacteremia not present) to complete a 10-day course (AIII)	Alternative: ampicillin. GBS may produce similar cellulitis or nodular lesions.
– Impetigo neonatorum	MSSA: oxacillin/nafcillin IV, IM OR cephalexin (AIII) MRSA: vancomycin IV for 5 days (AIII)	Systemic antibiotic therapy usually not required for superficial impetigo; local chlorhexidine cleansing may help with or without topical mupirocin (MRSA) or bacitracin (MSSA). Alternatives for MRSA: clindamycin IV, PO, or linezolid IV, PO.

A. RECOMMENDED THERAPY FOR SELECTED NEWBORN CONDITIONS (cont)

Condition	**Therapy (evidence grade)** *See Table 5B-D for neonatal dosages.*	Comments
Skin and soft tissues (cont)		
– *S aureus*[17,75,77,87]	MSSA: oxacillin/nafcillin IV, IM (AII) MRSA: vancomycin IV (AIII)	Surgical drainage may be required. MRSA may cause necrotizing fasciitis. Alternatives for MRSA: clindamycin IV or linezolid IV. Convalescent oral therapy if infection responds quickly to IV therapy.
– Group B streptococcus[78]	Penicillin G IV OR ampicillin IV, IM	Usually no pus formed Treatment course dependent on extent of infection, 7–14 days
Syphilis, congenital (<1 mo of age)[88]	During periods when availability of penicillin is compromised, see www.cdc.gov/std/Treatment/misc/penicillinG.htm.	Evaluation and treatment do not depend on mother's HIV status. Obtain follow-up serology every 2–3 mo until nontreponemal test nonreactive or decreased 4-fold. If CSF positive, repeat spinal tap with CSF VDRL at 6 mo, and if abnormal, re-treat.
– Proven or highly probable disease: (1) abnormal physical examination; (2) serum quantitative nontreponemal serologic titer 4-fold higher than mother's titer; or (3) positive dark field or fluorescent antibody test of body fluid(s)	Aqueous penicillin G 50,000 U/kg/dose q12h (day of life 1–7), q8h (>7 days) IV OR procaine penicillin G 50,000 U/kg IM q24h for 10 days (AII)	Evaluation to determine type and duration of therapy: CSF analysis (VDRL, cell count, protein), CBC and platelet count. Other tests as clinically indicated, including long-bone radiographs, chest radiograph, liver function tests, cranial ultrasound, ophthalmologic examination, and hearing test (ABR). If >1 day of therapy is missed, entire course is restarted.

– Normal physical examination, serum quantitative nontreponemal serologic titer ≤maternal titer, and maternal treatment was (1) none, inadequate, or undocumented; (2) erythromycin, azithromycin, or other non-penicillin regimen; or (3) <4 wk before delivery	Evaluation abnormal or not done completely: aqueous penicillin G 50,000 U/kg/dose q12h (day of life 1–7), q8h (>7 days) IV OR procaine penicillin G 50,000 U/kg IM q24h for 10 days (AII) Evaluation normal: aqueous penicillin G 50,000 U/kg/dose q12h (day of life 1–7), q8h (>7 days) IV OR procaine penicillin G 50,000 U/kg IM q24h for 10 days; OR benzathine penicillin G 50,000 units/kg/dose IM in a single dose (AIII)	Evaluation: CSF analysis, CBC with platelets, long-bone radiographs. If >1 day of therapy is missed, entire course is restarted. Reliable follow-up important if only a single dose of benzathine penicillin given.
– Normal physical examination, serum quantitative nontreponemal serologic titer ≤maternal titer, mother treated adequately during pregnancy and >4 wk before delivery; no evidence of reinfection or relapse in mother	Benzathine penicillin G 50,000 units/kg/dose IM in a single dose (AIII)	No evaluation required. Some experts would not treat but provide close serologic follow-up.

A. RECOMMENDED THERAPY FOR SELECTED NEWBORN CONDITIONS (cont)

Condition	Therapy (evidence grade) *See Table 5B-D for neonatal dosages.*	Comments
– Normal physical examination, serum quantitative nontreponemal serologic titer ≤maternal titer, mother's treatment adequate before pregnancy	No treatment	No evaluation required. Some experts would treat with benzathine penicillin G 50,000 U/kg as a single IM injection, particularly if follow-up is uncertain.
Syphilis, congenital (>1 mo of age)[88]	Aqueous crystalline penicillin G 200,000–300,000 U/kg/day IV div q4–6h for 10 days (AII)	Evaluation to determine type and duration of therapy: CSF analysis (VDRL, cell count, protein), CBC and platelet count. Other tests as clinically indicated, including long-bone radiographs, chest radiograph, liver function tests, neuroimaging, ophthalmologic examination, and hearing evaluation. If no clinical manifestations of disease, CSF examination is normal, and CSF VDRL test result is nonreactive, some specialists would treat with up to 3 weekly doses of benzathine penicillin G 50,000 U/kg IM. Some experts would provide a single dose of benzathine penicillin G 50,000 U/kg IM after 10 days of parenteral treatment, but value of this additional therapy is not well documented.
Tetanus neonatorum[89]	Metronidazole IV/PO (alternative: penicillin G IV) for 10–14 days (AIII) Human TIG 3,000–6,000 U IM for 1 dose (AIII)	Wound cleaning and debridement vital; IVIG (200–400 mg/kg) is an alternative if TIG not available; equine tetanus antitoxin not available in the United States but is alternative to TIG.
Toxoplasmosis, congenital[90,91]	Sulfadiazine 100 mg/kg/day PO div q12h AND pyrimethamine 2 mg/kg PO daily for 2 days (loading dose), then 1 mg/kg PO q24h for 2–6 mo, then 3 times weekly (M-W-F) up to 1 y (AII) Folinic acid (leucovorin) 10 mg 3 times weekly (AII)	Corticosteroids (1 mg/kg/day div q12h) if active chorioretinitis or CSF protein >1 g/dL (AIII). Start sulfa after neonatal jaundice has resolved. Therapy is only effective against active trophozoites, not cysts.

Urinary tract infection[92]	Initial empiric therapy with ampicillin AND gentamicin; OR ampicillin AND cefotaxime pending culture and susceptibility test results for 7–10 days	Investigate for kidney disease and abnormalities of urinary tract: VCUG indicated if renal ultrasound abnormal or after first UTI. Oral therapy acceptable once neonate asymptomatic and culture sterile. No prophylaxis for grades 1–3 reflux.[93] In neonates with reflux, prophylaxis reduces recurrences but does not impact renal scarring.[93]
– Coliform bacteria (eg, *E coli, Klebsiella, Enterobacter, Serratia*)	Cefotaxime IV, IM OR, in absence of renal or perinephric abscess, gentamicin IV, IM for 7–10 days (AII)	Ampicillin used for susceptible organisms
– *Enterococcus*	Ampicillin IV, IM for 7 days for cystitis, may need 10–14 days for pyelonephritis, add gentamicin until cultures are sterile (AIII); for ampicillin resistance, use vancomycin, add gentamicin until cultures are sterile.	Aminoglycoside needed with ampicillin or vancomycin for synergistic bactericidal activity (assuming organisms susceptible to an aminoglycoside)
– *P aeruginosa*	Ceftazidime IV, IM OR, in absence of renal or perinephric abscess, tobramycin IV, IM for 7–10 days (AIII)	Meropenem or cefepime are alternatives.
– *Candida* spp[30–32]	AmB-D IV OR fluconazole (if susceptible) (AII)	Because neonatal *Candida* disease is often systemic with isolated *Candida* UTI less likely to occur, and given that AmB lipid formulations are similarly effective and less toxic than AmB-D, they are preferred. However, the AmB lipid formulations theoretically have less penetration into the renal system compared with AmB-D. Evaluate for other sites in high-risk neonates: CSF analysis; cardiac ECHO; abdominal ultrasound to include kidneys, bladder; eye examination. Other triazoles are alternatives. Echinocandins are not renally eliminated and should not be used to treat isolated neonatal UTI.

B. ANTIMICROBIAL DOSAGES FOR NEONATES—Lead author Jason Sauberan, assisted by the editors and John van der Anker

		Dosages (mg/kg/day) and Intervals of Administration				
		Chronologic Age ≤28 days				
		Body Weight ≤2,000 g		Body Weight >2,000 g		Chronologic Age
Antibiotic	**Route**	**0–7 days old**	**8–28 days old**[a]	**0–7 days old**	**8–28 days old**	**29–60 days**
NOTE: This table contains empiric dosage recommendations for each agent listed. Please see Table A (Recommended Therapy for Selected Newborn Conditions) in this chapter for more precise details of optimal dosages for specific pathogens in specific tissue sites. Given the complexities of maturing organ function and drug elimination during the first few months of life, together with the wide variation in "compartments" for drug diffusion from very premature infants to term infants over the first months of life, these dosing recommendations represent our best estimates, but each infant should be independently evaluated for the appropriate dose. See also Table A for information on anti-influenza and antiretroviral drug dosages.						
Acyclovir	IV[b]	40 div q12h	60 div q8h	60 div q8h	60 div q8h	60 div q8h
	PO[c]	–	900/m²/day div q8h	–	900/m²/day div q8h	900/m²/day div q8h
Amoxicillin/clavulanate	PO	–	–	30 div q12h	30 div q12h	30 div q12h
Amphotericin B						
– deoxycholate	IV	1 q24h	1 q24h	1 q24h	1 q24h	1 q24h
– lipid complex	IV	5 q24h	5 q24h	5 q24h	5 q24h	5 q24h
– liposomal	IV	5 q24h	5 q24h	5 q24h	5 q24h	5 q24h
Ampicillin[d]	IV, IM	100 div q12h	150 div q12h	150 div q8h	150 div q8h	200 div q6h
Anidulafungin[e]	IV	1.5 q24h[e]	1.5 q24h[e]	1.5 q24h[e]	1.5 q24h[e]	1.5 q24h[e]
Azithromycin[f]	PO	10 q24h	10 q24h	10 q24h	10 q24h	10 q24h
	IV	10 q24h	10 q24h	10 q24h	10 q24h	10 q24h
Aztreonam	IV, IM	60 div q12h	90 div q8h	60 div q12h	90 div q8h	120 div q6h
Caspofungin[g]	IV	25/m² q24h	25/m² q24h	25/m² q24h	25/m² q24h	25/m² q24h
Cefazolin	IV, IM	50 div q12h	50 div q12h	50 div q12h	75 div q8h	75 div q8h
Cefepime[h]	IV, IM	100 div q12h	150 div q8h	150 div q8h	150 div q8h	150 div q8h
Cefotaxime	IV, IM	100 div q12h	150 div q8h	100 div q12h	150 div q8h	200 div q6h

Cefoxitin	IV, IM	70 div q12h	100 div q8h	100 div q8h	100 div q8h	120 div q6h
Ceftazidime	IV, IM	100 div q12h	150 div q8h	100 div q12h	150 div q8h	150 div q8h
Ceftriaxone[i]	IV, IM	–	–	50 q24h	50 q24h	50 q24h
Cefuroxime	IV, IM	100 div q12h	150 div q8h	100 div q12h	150 div q8h	150 div q8h
Chloramphenicol[j]	IV, IM	25 q24h	50 div q12h	25 q24h	50 div q12h	50–100 div q6h
Clindamycin	IV, IM, PO	15 div q8h	15 div q8h	21 div q8h	30 div q8h	30 div q8h
Daptomycin (new concerns for neurologic toxicity in the newborn; use cautiously)	IV	12 div q12h	12 div q12h	12 div q12h	12 div q12h	12 div q12h
Erythromycin	PO	20 div q12h	30 div q8h	20 div q12h	30 div q8h	40 div q6h
Fluconazole						
– treatment (start with initial loading dose)[k]	IV, PO	12 q24h[k]	12 q24h[k]	12 q24h[k]	12 q24h[k]	12 q24h[k]
– prophylaxis	IV, PO	6 mg/kg/dose twice weekly	6 mg/kg/dose twice weekly	6 mg/kg/dose twice weekly	6 mg/kg/dose twice weekly	6 mg/kg/dose twice weekly
Flucytosine[l]	PO	75 div q8h	75 div q6h	75 div q6h	75 div q6h	75 div q6h
Ganciclovir	IV	Insufficient data	Insufficient data	12 div q12h	12 div q12h	12 div q12h
Linezolid	IV, PO	20 div q12h	30 div q8h	30 div q8h	30 div q8h	30 div q8h
Meropenem						
– sepsis[m]	IV	40 div q12h	60 div q8h[m]	60 div q8h	90 div q8h[m]	90 div q8h
– meningitis	IV	120 div q8h	120 div q8h	120 div q8h	120 div q8h	120 div q8h
Metronidazole (start with initial loading dose)[n]	IV, PO	15 div q12h	See footnote[n]	22.5 div q8h	30 div q6h	30 div q6h
Micafungin	IV	10 q24h	10 q24h	10 q24h	10 q24h	10 q24h
Nafcillin,[o] oxacillin[o]	IV, IM	50 div q12h	75 div q8h	75 div q8h	100 div q6h	150 div q6h

B. ANTIMICROBIAL DOSAGES FOR NEONATES (cont)—Lead author Jason Sauberan, assisted by the editors and John van der Anker

		Dosages (mg/kg/day) and Intervals of Administration				
		Chronologic Age ≤28 days				
		Body Weight ≤2,000 g		Body Weight >2,000 g		
Antibiotic	Route	0–7 days old	8–28 days old[a]	0–7 days old	8–28 days old	Chronologic Age 29–60 days
Penicillin G benzathine	IM	50,000 U	50,000 U	50,000 U	50,000 U	50,000 U
Penicillin G crystalline (congenital syphilis)	IV	100,000 U div q12h	150,000 U div q8h	100,000 U div q12h	150,000 U div q8h	200,000 U div q6h
Penicillin G crystalline (GBS meningitis)	IV	200,000 U div q12h	300,000 U div q8h	300,000 U div q8h	400,000 U div q6h	400,000 U div q6h
Penicillin G procaine	IM	50,000 U q24h	50,000 U q24h	50,000 U q24h	50,000 U q24h	50,000 U q24h
Piperacillin/tazobactam	IV	300 div q8h	300 div q8h	320 div q6h	320 div q6h	320 div q6h
Rifampin	IV, PO	10 q24h	10 q24h	10 q24h	10 q24h	10 q24h
Ticarcillin/clavulanate	IV	150 div q12h	225 div q8h	150 div q12h	225 div q8h	300 div q6h
Valganciclovir	PO	insufficient data	insufficient data	32 div q12h	32 div q12h	32 div q12h
Voriconazole[p]	IV, PO	16 div q12h	16 div q12h	16 div q12h	16 div q12h	16 div q12h
Zidovudine	IV	3 div q12h[q]	3 div q12h[p]	6 div q12h	6 div q12h	See Table A: HIV
	PO	4 div q12h[q]	4 div q12h[p]	8 div q12h	8 div q12h	See Table A: HIV

[a]Use 0–7 days of age frequency until 14 days of age if birth weight <1,000 g.
[b]Only parenteral acyclovir should be used for the treatment of acute neonatal HSV disease.
[c]Oral suppression therapy for 6 months after initial neonatal HSV treatment. Dosing units are mg/m²/day.
[d]300 mg/kg/day for GBS meningitis; div q8h for all neonates ≤7 days of age and q6h >7 days of age.
[e]Loading dose 3 mg/kg followed 24 hours later by maintenance dose listed.
[f]Azithromycin oral dose for pertussis should be 10 mg/kg once daily for the entire 5-day treatment course, while for other upper respiratory tract infections, 10 mg/kg is given on the first day, followed by 5 mg/kg once daily for 4 days. For CNS disease, 10 mg/kg once daily for entire course.
[g]Dosing units are mg/m². Higher dosage of 50 mg/m² may be needed for *Aspergillus*.
[h]Doses listed are for meningitis or *Pseudomonas* infections. Can give 60 mg/kg/day div q12h for treatment of non-CNS infections caused by enteric bacilli *(eg, E coli, Klebsiella, Enterobacter, Serratia)* as they are more susceptible to cefepime than *Pseudomonas*.
[i]Usually avoided in neonates. Can be considered for transitioning to outpatient treatment of GBS bacteremia in well-appearing neonates at low risk for hyperbilirubinemia.
[j]Desired serum concentration 15–25 mg/mL.
[k]Loading dose 25 mg/kg followed 24 hours later by maintenance dose listed.
[l]Desired serum concentrations peak 50–100 mg/L, trough 25–50 mg/L.
[m]Adjust dosage after 14 days of age instead of after 7 days of age.

[n]Loading dose 15 mg/kg. Maintenance dosage for postmenstrual age <34 wk, 15 mg/kg/day div q12h; for 34–40 wk, 22.5 mg/kg/day div q8h.
[o]Increase to 50 mg/kg/dose for meningitis.
[p]Initial loading dose of 18 div q12h on day 1. Desired serum concentrations, trough 2–6 µg/mL.
[q]Starting dose if gestational age <35+0 wk and postnatal ≤14 days. See Table A HIV for zidovudine dosage after 2 weeks of age and for NVP and 3TC recommendations.

C. AMINOGLYCOSIDES

Empiric Dosage (mg/kg/dose) by Gestational and Postnatal Age

		<32 wk		32–36 wk		≥37 wk (term)	
Medication	**Route**	**0–14 days**	**>14 days**	**0–7 days**	**>7 days[a]**	**0–7 days**	**>7 days[a]**
Amikacin[b]	IV, IM	15 q48h	15 q24h	15 q24h	15 q24h	15 q24h	17.5 q24h
Gentamicin[c]	IV, IM	5 q48h	5 q36h	4 q36h	4 q24h	4 q24h	4 q24h
Tobramycin[c]	IV, IM	5 q48h	5 q36h	4 q36h	4 q24h	4 q24h	4 q24h

[a]At >60 days of age can consider amikacin 15–20 mg/kg q24h and gentamicin/tobramycin 4.5–7.5 mg/kg q24h (see Chapter 11).
[b]Desired serum concentrations: 20–35 mg/L (peak), <7 mg/L (trough).
[c]Desired serum concentrations: 5–10 mg/L (peak), <2 mg/L (trough).

D. VANCOMYCIN[a]

Empiric Dosage[b,c] (mg/kg/dose) by Gestational Age and Serum Creatinine

≤28 wk			>28 wk		
Serum Creatinine	**Dose**	**Frequency**	**Serum Creatinine**	**Dose**	**Frequency**
<0.5	15	q12h	<0.7	15	q12h
0.5–0.7	20	q24h	0.7–0.9	20	q24h
0.8–1	15	q24h	1–1.2	15	q24h
1.1–1.4	10	q24h	1.3–1.6	10	q24h
>1.4	15	q48h	>1.6	15	q48h

[a]Serum creatinine concentrations normally fluctuate and are partly influenced by transplacental maternal creatinine in the first week of age. Cautious use of creatinine-based dosing strategy with frequent reassessment of renal function and vancomycin serum concentrations are recommended in neonates ≤7 days old.
[b]Up through 60 days of age. If >60 days of age, 45–60 mg/kg/day div q8h (see Chapter 11).
[c]Desired serum concentrations vary by pathogen, site of infection, degree of illness; for MRSA aim for a target based on area under the curve–minimum inhibitory concentration of ~400, which will require peak and trough measurement. For coagulase-negative staphylococci and *Enterococcus*, troughs of 5–10 mg/L are likely to be effective.

E. Use of Antimicrobials During Pregnancy or Breastfeeding

The use of antimicrobials during pregnancy should be balanced by the risk of fetal toxicity, including anatomical anomalies. A number of factors determine the degree of transfer of antibiotics across the placenta: lipid solubility, degree of ionization, molecular weight, protein binding, placental maturation, and placental and fetal blood flow. The FDA provides 5 categories to indicate the level of risk to the fetus: (1) Category A: fetal harm seems remote, as controlled studies have not demonstrated a risk to the fetus; (2) Category B: animal reproduction studies have not shown a fetal risk, but no controlled studies in pregnant women have been done, or animal studies have shown an adverse effect that has not been confirmed in human studies (penicillin, amoxicillin, ampicillin, cephalexin/cefazolin, azithromycin, clindamycin, vancomycin, zanamivir); (3) Category C: studies in animals have shown an adverse effect on the fetus, but there are no studies in women; the potential benefit of the drug may justify the possible risk to the fetus (chloramphenicol, ciprofloxacin, gentamicin, levofloxacin, oseltamivir, rifampin); (4) Category D: evidence exists of human fetal risk, but the benefits may outweigh such risk (doxycycline); (5) Category X: the drug is contraindicated because animal or human studies have shown fetal abnormalities or fetal risk (ribavirin).

Fetal serum antibiotic concentrations (or cord blood concentrations) following maternal administration have not been systematically studied.[94] The following commonly used drugs appear to achieve fetal concentrations that are equal to or only slightly less than those in the mother: penicillin G, amoxicillin, ampicillin, sulfonamides, trimethoprim, and tetracyclines, as well as oseltamivir.[95] The aminoglycoside concentrations in fetal serum are 20% to 50% of those in maternal serum. Cephalosporins, carbapenems, nafcillin, oxacillin, clindamycin, and vancomycin[96] penetrate poorly (10%–30%), and fetal concentrations of erythromycin and azithromycin are less than 10% of those in the mother.

The most current, updated information on the safety of antimicrobials and other agents in human milk can be found at the National Library of Medicine LactMed Web site (http://toxnet.nlm.nih.gov/newtoxnet/lactmed.htm, accessed October 9, 2014).[97]

In general, neonatal exposure to antimicrobials in human milk is minimal or insignificant. Aminoglycosides, beta-lactams, ciprofloxacin, clindamycin, macrolides, fluconazole, and agents for tuberculosis are considered safe for the mother to take during breastfeeding.[98] The most common reported neonatal side effect of maternal antimicrobial use during breastfeeding is increased stool output. Clinicians should recommend mothers alert their pediatric health care professional if stool output changes occur. Maternal treatment with sulfa-containing antibiotics should be approached with caution in the breastfed infant who is jaundiced or ill.

6. Antimicrobial Therapy According to Clinical Syndromes

NOTES

- This chapter should be considered a rough guideline for a typical patient. Dosage recommendations are for patients with relatively normal hydration, renal function, and hepatic function. Higher dosages may be necessary if the antibiotic does not penetrate well into the infected tissue (eg, meningitis) or if the child is immunocompromised.
- Duration of treatment should be individualized. Those recommended are based on the literature, common practice, and general experience. Critical evaluations of duration of therapy have been carried out in very few infectious diseases. In general, a longer duration of therapy should be used (1) for tissues in which antibiotic concentrations may be relatively low (eg, undrained abscess, central nervous system [CNS] infection); (2) for tissues in which repair following infection-mediated damage is slow (eg, bone); (3) when the organisms are less susceptible; (4) when a relapse of infection is unacceptable (eg, CNS infections); or (5) when the host is immunocompromised in some way. An assessment after therapy will ensure that your selection of antibiotic, dose, and duration of therapy were appropriate.
- Diseases in this chapter are arranged by body systems. Consult the index for the alphabetized listing of diseases and chapters 7 through 10 for the alphabetized listing of pathogens and for uncommon organisms not included in this chapter.
- A more detailed description of treatment of methicillin-resistant *Staphylococcus aureus* infections is provided in Chapter 4.
- Therapy of *Pseudomonas aeruginosa* systemic infections is evolving from intravenous (IV) ceftazidime plus tobramycin to single drug IV therapy with cefepime due to the relative stability of cefepime to beta-lactamases, compared with ceftazidime. Oral therapy with ciprofloxacin is often replacing IV therapy in otherwise normal children who are compliant and able to take oral therapy.
- **Abbreviations:** AAP, American Academy of Pediatrics; ADH, antidiuretic hormone; AFB, acid-fast bacilli; ALT, alanine transaminase; AmB, amphotericin B; amox/clav, amoxicillin/clavulanate; AOM, acute otitis media; AST, aspartate transaminase; AUC:MIC, area under the curve–minimum inhibitory concentration; bid, twice daily; CA-MRSA, community-associated methicillin-resistant *Staphylococcus aureus;* CDC, Centers for Disease Control and Prevention; CMV, cytomegalovirus; CNS, central nervous system; CRP, C-reactive protein; CSD, cat-scratch disease; CSF, cerebrospinal fluid; CT, computed tomography; DAT, diphtheria antitoxin; div, divided; DOT, directly observed therapy; EBV, Epstein-Barr virus; ELF, epithelial lining fluid (in lung airways); ESBL, extended spectrum beta-lactamase; ESR, erythrocyte sedimentation rate; ETEC, enterotoxin-producing *Escherichia coli;* FDA, US Food and Drug Administration; GI, gastrointestinal; HIV, human immunodeficiency virus; HSV, herpes simplex virus; HUS, hemolytic uremic syndrome;

I&D, incision and drainage; IDSA, Infectious Diseases Society of America; IM, intramuscular; INH, isoniazid; IV, intravenous; IVIG, intravenous immune globulin; LFT, liver function test; LP, lumbar puncture; MRSA, methicillin-resistant *Staphylococcus aureus;* MRSE, methicillin-resistant *Staphylococcus epidermidis;* MSSA, methicillin-susceptible *S aureus;* MSSE, methicillin-sensitive *S epidermidis;* NIH, National Institutes of Health; ophth, ophthalmic; PCR, polymerase chain reaction; PCV13, Prevnar 13-valent pneumococcal conjugate vaccine; pen-R, penicillin-resistant; pen-S, penicillin-susceptible; PIDS, Pediatric Infectious Diseases Society; pip/tazo, piperacillin/tazobactam; PO, oral; PPD, purified protein derivative; PZA, pyrazinamide; qd, once daily; qid, 4 times daily; qod, every other day; RSV, respiratory syncytial virus; SPAG-2, small particle aerosol generator-2; spp, species; STEC, Shiga toxin–producing *E coli;* STI, sexually transmitted infection; TB, tuberculosis; Td, tetanus-diphtheria; Tdap, tetanus-diphtheria-acellular pertussis; ticar/clav, ticarcillin/clavulanate; tid, 3 times daily; TIG, tetanus immune globulin; TMP/SMX, trimethoprim/sulfamethoxazole; ULN, upper limit of normal; UTI, urinary tract infection; VDRL, Venereal Disease Research Laboratories; WBC, white blood cell.

A. SKIN AND SOFT TISSUE INFECTIONS

Clinical Diagnosis	Therapy (evidence grade)	Comments
NOTE: CA-MRSA (see Chapter 4) is increasingly prevalent in most areas of the world. Recommendations are given for 2 scenarios: standard and CA-MRSA. Antibiotic recommendations for CA-MRSA should be used for empiric therapy in regions with greater than 5% to 10% of serious staphylococcal infections caused by MRSA, in situations where CA-MRSA is suspected, and for documented CA-MRSA infections, while standard recommendations refer to treatment of MSSA. During the past few years, clindamycin resistance in MRSA has increased to 40% in some areas but remained stable at 5% in others, although this increase may be an artifact of changes in reporting, with many laboratories now reporting all clindamycin-susceptible but D-test–positive strains as resistant. Please check your local susceptibility data for *S aureus* before using clindamycin for empiric therapy. For MSSA, oxacillin/nafcillin are considered equivalent agents.		
Adenitis, acute bacterial[1–7] (*S aureus,* including CA-MRSA, and group A streptococcus; consider *Bartonella* [CSD] for subacute adenitis)[8]	Empiric therapy: Standard: oxacillin/nafcillin 150 mg/kg/day IV div q6h OR cefazolin 100 mg/kg/day IV div q8h (AI), OR cephalexin 50–75 mg/kg/day PO div tid CA-MRSA: clindamycin 30 mg/kg/day IV or PO div q8h OR vancomycin 40 mg/kg/day IV q8h (BII) CSD: azithromycin 12 mg/kg once daily (max 500 mg) for 5 days (BIII)	May need surgical drainage for staph/strep infection; not usually needed for CSD. Following drainage of mild to moderate suppurative adenitis caused by staph or strep, additional antibiotics may not be required. For oral therapy for MSSA: cephalexin or amox/clav; for CA-MRSA: clindamycin, TMP/SMX, or linezolid. For oral therapy of group A strep: amoxicillin or penicillin V. Total IV plus PO therapy for 7–10 days. For CSD: this is the same high dose of azithromycin that is recommended routinely for strep pharyngitis.
Adenitis, nontuberculous (atypical) mycobacterial[9–12]	Excision usually curative (BII); azithromycin PO OR clarithromycin PO for 6–12 wk (with or without rifampin) if susceptible (BII)	Antibiotic susceptibility patterns are quite variable; cultures should guide therapy; medical therapy 60%–70% effective. Newer data suggest toxicity of antimicrobials may not be worth the small clinical benefit of medical therapy over surgery.
Adenitis, tuberculous[13,14] (*M tuberculosis* and *M bovis*)	INH 10–15 mg/kg/day (max 300 mg) PO qd, IV for 6 mo AND rifampin 10–20 mg/kg/day (max 600 mg) PO qd, IV for 6 mo AND PZA 20–40 mg/kg/day PO qd for first 2 mo therapy (BI); if suspected multidrug resistance, add ethambutol 20 mg/kg/day PO qd.	Surgical excision usually not indicated because organisms are treatable. Adenitis caused by *Mycobacterium bovis* (unpasteurized dairy product ingestion) is uniformly resistant to PZA. Treat 9–12 mo with INH and rifampin, if susceptible (BII).

A. SKIN AND SOFT TISSUE INFECTIONS (cont)

Clinical Diagnosis	Therapy (evidence grade)	Comments
Anthrax, cutaneous[15]	Empiric therapy: ciprofloxacin 20–30 mg/kg/day PO div bid OR doxycycline 4 mg/kg/day (max 200 mg) PO div bid (regardless of age) (AIII)	If susceptible, amoxicillin or clindamycin (BIII). Ciprofloxacin and levofloxacin are FDA approved for inhalation anthrax (BIII).
Bites, animal and human[1,16–19] *Pasteurella multocida* (animal), *Eikenella corrodens* (human), *Staphylococcus* spp, and *Streptococcus* spp	Amox/clav 45 mg/kg/day PO div tid (amox/clav 7:1; see Chapter 1, Aminopenicillins) for 5–10 days (AII); for hospitalized children, use ticar/clav 200 mg ticarcillin/kg/day div q6h OR ampicillin and clindamycin (BII). For penicillin allergy, ciprofloxacin (for *Pasteurella*) plus clindamycin (BIII).	Consider rabies prophylaxis[20] for bites from at-risk animals (observe animal for 10 days, if possible) (AI); consider tetanus prophylaxis. Human bites have a very high rate of infection (do not close open wounds). *S aureus* (MSSA) coverage is only fair with amox/clav, ticar/clav; no MRSA coverage. For penicillin allergy, ciprofloxacin (for *Pasteurella*) plus clindamycin (BIII).
Bullous impetigo[1–3,5–7] (usually *S aureus,* including CA-MRSA)	Standard: cephalexin 50–75 mg/kg/day PO div tid OR amox/clav 45 mg/kg/day PO div tid (CII) CA-MRSA: clindamycin 30 mg/kg/day PO div tid OR TMP/SMX 8 mg/kg/day of TMP PO div bid; for 5–7 days (CI)	For topical therapy if mild infection: mupirocin or retapamulin ointment
Cellulitis of unknown etiology (usually *S aureus,* including CA-MRSA, or group A streptococcus)[1–7,21]	Empiric IV therapy: Standard: oxacillin/nafcillin 150 mg/kg/day IV div q6h OR cefazolin 100 mg/kg/day IV div q8h (BII) CA-MRSA: clindamycin 30 mg/kg/day IV div q8h OR vancomycin 40 mg/kg/day IV q8h (BII) For oral therapy for MSSA: cephalexin (AII) OR amox/clav 45 mg/kg/day PO div tid (BII); for CA-MRSA: clindamycin (BII), TMP/SMX (CIII), or linezolid (BII)	For periorbital or buccal cellulitis, also consider *Streptococcus pneumoniae* or *Haemophilus influenzae* type b in unimmunized infants. Total IV plus PO therapy for 7–10 days.

Cellulitis, buccal (for unimmunized infants and preschool-aged children, *H influenzae* type b)[22]	Cefotaxime 100–150 mg/kg/day IV div q8h OR ceftriaxone 50 mg/kg/day (AI) IV, IM q24h; for 2–7 days parenteral therapy before switch to oral (BII)	Rule out meningitis (larger dosages may be needed). For penicillin allergy, levofloxacin IV/PO covers pathogens, but no clinical data available; safer than chloramphenicol. Oral therapy: amoxicillin if beta-lactamase negative; amox/clav or oral 2nd- or 3rd-generation cephalosporin if beta-lactamase positive.
Cellulitis, erysipelas (streptococcal)[1,2,7]	Penicillin G 100,000–200,000 U/kg/day IV div q4–6h (BII) initially then penicillin V 100 mg/kg/day PO div qid or tid OR amoxicillin 50 mg/kg/day PO div tid for 10 days	These dosages may be unnecessarily large, but there is little clinical experience with smaller dosages.
Gas gangrene (See Necrotizing fasciitis.)		
Impetigo (*S aureus,* including CA-MRSA; occasionally group A streptococcus)[1,2,6,7,23,24]	Mupirocin OR retapamulin topically (BII) to lesions tid; OR for more extensive lesions, oral therapy: Standard: cephalexin 50–75 mg/kg/day PO div tid OR amox/clav 45 mg/kg/day PO div tid (AII) CA-MRSA: clindamycin 30 mg/kg/day (CII) PO div tid OR TMP/SMX 8 mg/kg/day TMP PO div bid (CI); for 5–7 days	Cleanse infected area with soap and water.
Ludwig angina[25]	Penicillin G 200,000–250,000 U/kg/day IV div q6h AND clindamycin 40 mg/kg/day IV div q8h (CIII)	Alternatives: meropenem, imipenem, ticar/clav, pip/tazo if gram-negative aerobic bacilli also suspected (CIII); high risk of respiratory tract obstruction from inflammatory edema
Lymphadenitis (See Adenitis, acute bacterial.)		
Lymphangitis, blistering dactylitis (usually group A streptococcus)[1,2,7]	Penicillin G 200,000 U/kg/day IV div q6h (BII) initially then penicillin V 100 mg/kg/day PO div qid OR amoxicillin 50 mg/kg/day PO div tid for 10 days	For mild disease, penicillin V 50 mg/kg/day PO div qid for 10 days Some recent reports of *S aureus* as a cause

A. SKIN AND SOFT TISSUE INFECTIONS (cont)

Clinical Diagnosis	Therapy (evidence grade)	Comments
Myositis, suppurative[26] (*S aureus,* including CA-MRSA; synonyms: tropical myositis, pyomyositis)	Standard: oxacillin/nafcillin 150 mg/kg/day IV div q6h OR cefazolin 100 mg/kg/day IV div q8h (CII) CA-MRSA: clindamycin 40 mg/kg/day IV div q8h OR vancomycin 40 mg/kg/day IV q8h (CIII)	Aggressive, emergent debridement; use clindamycin to help decrease toxin production; consider IVIG to bind bacterial toxins for life-threatening disease; abscesses may develop with CA-MRSA while on therapy.
Necrotizing fasciitis (Pathogens vary depending on the age of the child and location of infection. Single pathogen: group A streptococcus; *Clostridia* spp, *S aureus* [including CA-MRSA], *Pseudomonas aeruginosa, Vibrio* spp, *Aeromonas;* multiple pathogen, mixed aerobic/anaerobic synergistic fasciitis: any organism[s] above, plus gram-negative bacilli, plus *Bacteroides* spp, and other anaerobes.)[1,27–30]	Empiric therapy: ceftazidime 150 mg/kg/day IV div q8h, or cefepime 150 mg/kg/day IV div q8h or cefotaxime 200 mg/kg/day IV div q6h AND clindamycin 40 mg/kg/day IV div q8h (BIII); OR meropenem 60 mg/kg/day IV div q8h; OR pip/tazo 400 mg/kg/day pip component IV div q6h (AIII). ADD vancomycin for suspect CA-MRSA, pending culture results (AIII). Group A streptococcal: penicillin G 200,000–250,000 U/kg/day div q6h AND clindamycin 40 mg/kg/day div q8h (AIII). Mixed aerobic/anaerobic/gram-negative: meropenem or pip/tazo AND clindamycin (AIII).	Aggressive emergent wound debridement (AII). Add clindamycin to inhibit synthesis of toxins during the first few days of therapy (AIII). If CA-MRSA identified and susceptible to clindamycin, additional vancomycin is not required. Consider IVIG to bind bacterial toxins for life-threatening disease (BIII). Value of hyperbaric oxygen is not established (CIII). Focus definitive antimicrobial therapy based on culture results.
Pyoderma, cutaneous abscesses (*S aureus,* including CA-MRSA; group A streptococcus)[2,5–7,31–33]	Standard: cephalexin 50–75 mg/kg/day PO div tid OR amox/clav 45 mg/kg/day PO div tid (BII) CA-MRSA: clindamycin 30 mg/kg/day PO div tid (BII) OR TMP/SMX 8 mg/kg/day of TMP PO div bid (CI)	I&D when indicated; IV for serious infections. For prevention of recurrent CA-MRSA infection, use bleach baths daily (½ cup of bleach per full bathtub) (BII), OR bathe with chlorhexidine soap daily or qod. Decolonization with mupirocin may also be helpful.
Rat-bite fever (*Streptobacillus moniliformis, Spirillum minus*)[34]	Penicillin G 100,000–200,000 U/kg/day IV div q6h (BII) for 7–10 days; for endocarditis, ADD gentamicin for 4–6 wk (CIII). For mild disease, oral therapy with amox/clav (CIII).	Organisms are normal oral flora for rodents. High rate of associated endocarditis. Alternatives: doxycycline; 2nd- and 3rd-generation cephalosporins (CIII).
Staphylococcal scalded skin syndrome[6,35]	Standard: oxacillin 150 mg/kg/day IV div q6h OR cefazolin 100 mg/kg/day IV div q8h (CII) CA-MRSA: clindamycin 30 mg/kg/day IV div q8h (CIII) OR vancomycin 40 mg/kg/day IV q8h (CIII)	Burow or Zephiran compresses for oozing skin and intertriginous areas. Corticosteroids are contraindicated.

B. SKELETAL INFECTIONS

Clinical Diagnosis	Therapy (evidence grade)	Comments
NOTE: CA-MRSA (see Chapter 4) is increasingly prevalent in most areas of the world. Recommendations are given for CA-MRSA and MSSA. Antibiotic recommendations for empiric therapy should include CA-MRSA when it is suspected or documented, while treatment for MSSA with beta-lactam antibiotics (eg, cephalexin) is preferred over clindamycin. During the past few years, clindamycin resistance in MRSA has increased to 40% in some areas but remained stable at 5% in others, although this increase may be an artifact of changes in reporting, with many laboratories now reporting all clindamycin-susceptible but D-test–positive strains as resistant. Please check your local susceptibility data for *S aureus* before using clindamycin for empiric therapy. For MSSA, oxacillin/nafcillin are considered equivalent agents. The first pediatric-specific PIDS/IDSA guidelines for bacterial osteomyelitis and bacterial arthritis are currently being written.		
Arthritis, bacterial[36–40]	Switch to appropriate high-dose oral therapy when clinically improved, CRP decreasing (see Chapter 13).[41]	
– Newborns	See Chapter 5.	
– Infants (*S aureus,* including CA-MRSA; group A streptococcus; *Kingella kingae;* in unimmunized or immunocompromised children: pneumococcus, *H influenzae* type b) – Children (*S aureus,* including CA-MRSA; group A streptococcus; *K kingae*)	Empiric therapy: clindamycin (to cover CA-MRSA unless clindamycin resistance locally is >10%, then use vancomycin). For serious infections, ADD cefazolin to provide better MSSA coverage and add *Kingella* coverage. For CA-MRSA: clindamycin 30 mg/kg/day IV div q8h OR vancomycin 40 mg/kg/day IV q8h. For MSSA: oxacillin/nafcillin 150 mg/kg/day IV div q6h OR cefazolin 100 mg/kg/day IV div q8h. For *Kingella:* cefazolin 100 mg/kg/day IV div q8h OR ampicillin 150 mg/kg/day IV div q6h, OR ceftriaxone 50 mg/kg/day IV, IM q24h. For pen-S pneumococci or group A streptococcus: penicillin G 200,000 U/kg/day IV div q6h. For pen-R pneumococci or *Haemophilus:* ceftriaxone 50–75 mg/kg/day IV, IM q24h, OR cefotaxime (BII). Total therapy (IV plus PO) for up to 21 days with normal ESR; low-risk, non-hip MSSA arthritis may respond to a 10-day course.[37,38]	Oral therapy options: For CA-MRSA: clindamycin OR linezolid[40] For MSSA: cephalexin OR cloxacillin caps for older children For *Kingella,* most penicillins or cephalosporins (but not clindamycin)

B. SKELETAL INFECTIONS (cont)

Clinical Diagnosis	Therapy (evidence grade)	Comments
– Gonococcal arthritis or tenosynovitis[42,43]	Ceftriaxone 50 mg/kg IV, IM q24h (BII); for 7 days	Cefixime 8 mg/kg/day PO as a single daily dose has not yet been studied in children but is recommended as step-down therapy in adults, to complete a 7-day treatment course.
– Other bacteria	See Chapter 7 for preferred antibiotics.	
Osteomyelitis[36,39,40,44–49]	Step down to appropriate high-dose oral therapy when clinically improved (See Chapter 13.)[40,47]	
– Newborn	See Chapter 5.	
– Infants and children, acute infection (usually *S aureus,* including CA-MRSA; group A streptococcus; *K kingae*)	Empiric therapy: clindamycin (for coverage of MSSA and MRSA in most locations). For serious infections, ADD cefazolin to provide better MSSA coverage and add *Kingella* coverage (CIII). For CA-MRSA: clindamycin 30 mg/kg/day IV div q8h or vancomycin 40 mg/kg/day IV q8h (BII). For MSSA: oxacillin/nafcillin 150 mg/kg/day IV div q6h OR cefazolin 100 mg/kg/day IV div q8h (AII). For *Kingella:* cefazolin 100 mg/kg/day IV div q8h OR ampicillin 150 mg/kg/day IV div q6h, OR ceftriaxone 50 mg/kg/day IV, IM q24h (BIII). Total therapy (IV plus PO) usually 4–6 wk for MSSA (with end-of-therapy normal ESR, radiograph to document healing) but may be as short as 3 wk for mild infection. May need longer than 4–6 wk for CA-MRSA (BII). Follow closely for clinical response to empiric therapy.	In children with open fractures secondary to trauma, add ceftazidime for extended aerobic gram-negative bacilli activity. *Kingella* is often resistant to clindamycin and vancomycin. For MSSA (BI) and *Kingella* (BIII), step-down oral therapy with cephalexin 100 mg/kg/day PO div tid. Oral step-down therapy alternatives for CA-MRSA include clindamycin and linezolid,[50] with insufficient data to recommend TMP/SMX.

– Acute, other organisms	See Chapter 7 for preferred antibiotics.	
– Chronic (staphylococcal)[48]	For MSSA: cephalexin 100 mg/kg/day PO div tid OR dicloxacillin caps 75–100 mg/kg/day PO div qid for 3–6 mo or longer (CIII) For CA-MRSA: clindamycin or linezolid (CIII)	Surgery to debride sequestrum is usually required for cure. For prosthetic joint infection caused by staphylococci, add rifampin (CIII). Watch for beta-lactam–associated neutropenia with high-dose, long-term therapy, and linezolid-associated neutropenia/thrombocytopenia with long-term (>2 wk) therapy.
Osteomyelitis of the foot[51] (osteochondritis after a puncture wound) *P aeruginosa* (occasionally *S aureus*, including CA-MRSA)	Ceftazidime 150 mg/kg/day IV, IM div q8h AND tobramycin 6–7.5 mg/kg/day IM, IV div q8h (BIII); OR cefepime 150 mg/kg/day IV div q8h (BIII); OR meropenem 60 mg/kg/day IV div q8h (BIII); ADD vancomycin 40 mg/kg/day IV q8h for serious infection (for CA-MRSA), pending culture results	Thorough surgical debridement required (2nd drainage procedure needed in at least 20% of children); oral convalescent therapy with ciprofloxacin (BIII)[52] Treatment course 7–10 days after surgery

C. EYE INFECTIONS

Clinical Diagnosis	Therapy (evidence grade)	Comments
Cellulitis, orbital[53–55] (usually secondary to sinus infection; caused by respiratory tract flora and *S aureus*, including CA-MRSA)	Cefotaxime 150 mg/kg/day div q8h or ceftriaxone 50 mg/kg/day q24h; ADD (for *S aureus*, including CA-MRSA) clindamycin 30 mg/kg/day IV div q8h OR vancomycin 40 mg/kg/day IV q8h (AIII). If MSSA isolated, use oxacillin/nafcillin IV OR cefazolin IV.	Surgical drainage of larger collections of pus, if present by CT scan in orbit or subperiosteal tissue. Try medical therapy alone for small abscess (BIII).[56] Treatment course for 10–14 days after surgical drainage, up to 21 days. CT scan to confirm cure (BIII).
Cellulitis, periorbital[57] (preseptal infection)		
– Associated with entry site lesion on skin (*S aureus*, including CA-MRSA, group A streptococcus) in the fully immunized child	Standard: oxacillin/nafcillin 150 mg/kg/day IV div q6h OR cefazolin 100 mg/kg/day IV div q8h (BII) CA-MRSA: clindamycin 30 mg/kg/day IV div q8h or vancomycin 40 mg/kg/day IV q8h (BIII)	Oral antistaphylococcal antibiotic for less severe infection; treatment course for 7–10 days

C. EYE INFECTIONS (cont)

Clinical Diagnosis	Therapy (evidence grade)	Comments
– No associated entry site (in febrile, unimmunized infants): pneumococcal or *H influenzae* type b	Ceftriaxone 50 mg/kg/day q24h OR cefotaxime 100–150 mg/kg/day IV, IM div q8h OR cefuroxime 150 mg/kg/day IV div q8h (AII)	Treatment course for 7–10 days; rule out meningitis; alternative: other 2nd-, 3rd-, or 4th-generation cephalosporins or chloramphenicol.
– Periorbital, non-tender erythematous swelling (not true cellulitis, usually associated with sinusitis); sinus pathogens rarely may erode anteriorly, causing cellulitis.	Ceftriaxone 50 mg/kg/day q24h OR cefotaxime 100–150 mg/kg/day IV, IM div q8h OR cefuroxime 150 mg/kg/day IV div q8h (BIII) ADD clindamycin 30 mg/kg/day IV div q8h for more severe infection with suspect *S aureus* including CA-MRSA or for chronic sinusitis (covers anaerobes) (AIII)	For oral convalescent antibiotic therapy, see Sinusitis, acute; total treatment course of 14–21 days or 7 days after resolution of symptoms.
Conjunctivitis, acute (*Haemophilus* and pneumococcus predominantly)[58–60]	Polymyxin/trimethoprim ophth solution OR polymyxin/bacitracin ophth ointment OR ciprofloxacin ophth solution (BII), for 7–10 days. For neonatal infection, see Chapter 5. Steroid-containing therapy only if HSV ruled out.	Other topical antibiotics (gentamicin, tobramycin ophth solution erythromycin, besifloxacin, moxifloxacin, norfloxacin, ofloxacin, levofloxacin) may offer advantages for particular pathogens (CII). High rates of resistance to sulfacetamide.
Conjunctivitis, herpetic[61–63]	1% trifluridine, 0.1% iododeoxyuridine, or 0.15% ganciclovir ophthalmic gel (AII) AND acyclovir PO (80 mg/kg/day div qid; max daily dose: 3,200 mg/day) has been effective in limited studies (BIII).	Refer to ophthalmologist. Recurrences common; corneal scars may form. Topical steroids for keratitis concurrent with topical antiviral solution. Long-term prophylaxis for suppression of recurrent infection with oral acyclovir 300 mg/m^2/dose PO tid (max 400 mg/dose) (little long-term safety data in children). Assess for neutropenia on long-term therapy; potential risks must balance potential benefits to vision (BIII).
Dacryocystitis	No antibiotic usually needed; oral therapy for more symptomatic infection, based on Gram stain and culture of pus; topical therapy as for conjunctivitis may be helpful.	Warm compresses; may require surgical probing of nasolacrimal duct

Endophthalmitis[64,65]		
NOTE: Subconjunctival/sub-Tenon antibiotics are likely to be required (vancomycin/ceftazidime or clindamycin/gentamicin); steroids commonly used; requires anterior chamber or vitreous tap for microbiological diagnosis. Listed systemic antibiotics to be used in addition to ocular injections.		Refer to ophthalmologist; vitrectomy may be necessary for advanced endophthalmitis.
– Empiric therapy following open globe injury	Vancomycin 40 mg/kg/day IV div q8h AND cefepime 150 mg/kg/day IV div q8h (AIII)	
– Staphylococcal	Vancomycin 40 mg/kg/day IV div q8h pending susceptibility testing; oxacillin/nafcillin 150 mg/kg/day IV div q6h if susceptible (AIII)	
– Pneumococcal, meningococcal, *Haemophilus*	Ceftriaxone 100 mg/kg/day IV q24h; penicillin G 250,000 U/kg/day IV div q4h if susceptible (AIII)	Rule out meningitis; treatment course for 10–14 days.
– Gonococcal	Ceftriaxone 50 mg/kg q24h IV, IM (AIII)	Treatment course 7 days or longer
– *Pseudomonas*	Cefepime 150 mg/kg/day IV div q8h for 10–14 days (AIII)	Cefepime is preferred over ceftazidime for *Pseudomonas* based on decreased risk of development of resistance on therapy; meropenem IV or imipenem IV are alternatives (no clinical data). Very poor outcomes.
– *Candida*	Intravitreal amphotericin AND fluconazole 12 mg/kg/day IV (AIII)	Echinocandins may not be able to achieve antifungal activity in the eye.[66]
Hordeolum (sty) or chalazion	None (topical antibiotic not necessary)	Warm compresses; I&D when necessary
Retinitis		
– CMV[67–69] For neonatal: See Chapter 5. For HIV-infected children, visit NIH Web site at http://aidsinfo.nih.gov/guidelines/html/5/pediatric-oi-prevention-and-treatment-guidelines/0.	Ganciclovir 10 mg/kg/day IV div q12h for 2 wk (BIII); if needed, continue at 5 mg/kg/day q24h to complete 6 wk total (BIII)	Neutropenia risk increases with duration of therapy. Foscarnet IV and cidofovir IV are alternatives but demonstrate significant toxicities. Oral valganciclovir has not been evaluated in HIV-infected children with CMV retinitis but is an option primarily for older children who weigh enough to receive the adult dose of valganciclovir (CIII). Intravitreal ganciclovir and combination therapy for non-responding, immunocompromised hosts.

D. EAR AND SINUS INFECTIONS

Clinical Diagnosis	Therapy (evidence grade)	Comments
Bullous myringitis (See Otitis media, acute.)	Believed to be a clinical presentation of acute bacterial otitis media	
Mastoiditis, acute (pneumococcus, *S aureus,* including CA-MRSA; group A streptococcus; increasing *Pseudomonas* in adolescents, *Haemophilus* rare)[84–86]	Cefotaxime 150 mg/kg/day IV div q8h or ceftriaxone 50 mg/kg/day q24h AND clindamycin 40 mg/kg/day IV div q8h (BIII) For adolescents: ceftazidime 150 mg/kg/day IV div q8h AND clindamycin 40 mg/kg/day IV div q8h (BIII)	Rule out meningitis; surgery as needed for mastoid and middle ear drainage. Change to appropriate oral therapy after clinical improvement.
Mastoiditis, chronic (See also Otitis, chronic suppurative.) (anaerobes, *Pseudomonas, S aureus* [including CA-MRSA])[85]	Antibiotics only for acute superinfections (according to culture of drainage); for *Pseudomonas:* meropenem 60 mg/kg/day IV div q8h, OR pip/tazo 240 mg/kg/day IV div q4–6h for 1 wk after drainage stops (BIII)	Daily cleansing of ear important; if no response to antibiotics, surgery. Alternatives: cefepime IV or ceftazidime IV (poor anaerobic coverage). Be alert for CA-MRSA.
Otitis externa		
Bacterial, swimmer's ear (*P aeruginosa, S aureus,* including CA-MRSA)[70–73]	Topical antibiotics: fluoroquinolone (ciprofloxacin or ofloxacin) with steroid, OR neomycin/polymyxin B/hydrocortisone (BII) Irrigation and cleaning canal of detritus important	Wick moistened with Burow solution, used for marked swelling of canal; to prevent swimmer's ear, 2% acetic acid to canal after water exposure will restore acid pH.
– Bacterial, malignant otitis externa (*P aeruginosa*)[72]	Cefepime 150 mg/kg/day IV div q8h (AIII)	Other antipseudomonal antibiotics should also be effective: ceftazidime IV AND tobramycin IV, OR meropenem IV or imipenem IV, pip/tazo IV. For more mild infection, ciprofloxacin PO.
– Bacterial furuncle of canal (*S aureus,* including CA-MRSA)	Standard: oxacillin/nafcillin 150 mg/kg/day IV div q6h OR cefazolin 100 mg/kg/day IV div q8h (BIII) CA-MRSA: clindamycin 30 mg/kg/day IV div q8h or vancomycin 40 mg/kg/day IV q8h (BIII)	I&D; antibiotics for cellulitis Oral therapy for mild disease, convalescent therapy: for MSSA: cephalexin; for CA-MRSA: clindamycin, TMP/SMX, OR linezolid (BIII)
– *Candida*	Fluconazole 6–12 mg/kg/day PO qd for 5–7 days (CIII)	May occur following antibiotic therapy of bacterial external otitis; debride canal

Otitis media, acute

A note on AOM: The natural history of AOM in different age groups by specific pathogens has not been well defined; therefore, the actual contribution of antibiotic therapy on resolution of disease has also been poorly defined until 2 recent amox/clav vs placebo, blinded, prospective studies were published,[74,75] although neither study required tympanocentesis to define a pathogen. The benefits and risks (including development of antibiotic resistance) of antibiotic therapy for AOM need to be further evaluated before the most accurate advice on the "best" antibiotic can be provided. However, based on available data, for most children, amoxicillin or amox/clav can be used initially. Considerations for the need for extended antimicrobial activity of amox/clav include severity of disease, age of child, previous antibiotics, child care attendance, in vitro antibacterial spectrum of antibiotic, and palatability of suspensions. With universal PCV13 immunization, preliminary data suggest that the risk of antibiotic-resistant pneumococcal otitis has decreased and the percent of *Haemophilus* responsible for AOM has increased, which may soon result in a recommendation for the use of amox/clav as first-line therapy for well-documented AOM. The most current AAP guidelines[76] and meta-analyses[77] suggest the greatest benefit with therapy occurs in children with bilateral AOM who are younger than 2 years; for other children, close observation is also an option. AAP guidelines provide an option to treatment in non-severe cases, particularly unilateral disease and disease in older children, to provide a prescription to parents but have them only fill the prescription if the child deteriorates.[76] Although prophylaxis is only rarely indicated, amoxicillin or other antibiotics can be used in half the therapeutic dose once or twice daily to prevent infections if the benefits outweigh the risks of development of resistant organisms for that child.[78]

– Newborns	See Chapter 5.

D. EAR AND SINUS INFECTIONS (cont)

Clinical Diagnosis	Therapy (evidence grade)	Comments
– Infants and children (pneumococcus, *H influenzae* non–type b, *Moraxella* most common)[78–80]	Usual therapy: amoxicillin 90 mg/kg/day PO div bid, with or without clavulanate; failures will be caused by highly pen-R pneumococcus or, if amoxicillin is used alone, by beta-lactamase–producing *Haemophilus* (or *Moraxella*). a) For *Haemophilus* strains that are beta-lactamase positive, the following oral antibiotics offer better in vitro activity than amoxicillin: amox/clav, cefdinir, cefpodoxime, cefuroxime, ceftriaxone IM, levofloxacin. b) For pen-R pneumococci: high-dosage amoxicillin achieves greater middle ear activity than oral cephalosporins. Options include ceftriaxone IM 50 mg/kg/day q24h for 1–3 doses; OR levofloxacin 20 mg/kg/day PO div bid for children ≤5 y and 10 mg/kg PO qd for children >5 y; OR a macrolide-class antibiotic*: azithromycin PO at 1 of 3 dosages: (1) 10 mg/kg on day 1, followed by 5 mg/kg qd on days 2–5; (2) 10 mg/kg qd for 3 days; or (3) 30 mg/kg once. *Caution: Up to 40% of pen-R pneumococci are also macrolide resistant.	See Chapter 11 for dosages. Until published data document the lack of penicillin resistance in pneumococci isolated from infants with AOM,[79] high-dosage amoxicillin (90 mg/kg/day) should be used for empiric therapy. The high serum and middle ear fluid concentrations achieved with 45 mg/kg/dose of amoxicillin, combined with a long half-life in middle ear fluid, allow for a therapeutic antibiotic exposure in the middle ear with only twice-daily dosing; high-dose amoxicillin (90 mg/kg/day) with clavulanate (Augmentin ES) is also available. As published data document decreasing resistance to amoxicillin, standard dosage (45 mg/kg/day) can again be recommended. Tympanocentesis should be performed in children who fail second-line therapy.
Otitis, chronic suppurative (*P aeruginosa, S aureus,* including CA-MRSA, and other respiratory tract/skin flora)[81,82]	Topical antibiotics: fluoroquinolone (ciprofloxacin, ofloxacin, besifloxacin) with or without steroid (BIII) Cleaning of canal, view of tympanic membrane, for patency; cultures important	Presumed middle ear drainage through open tympanic membrane; possible aminoglycoside toxicity if neomycin-containing topical therapy used[83] Other topical fluoroquinolones with/without steroids available

Sinusitis, acute (*H influenzae* non–type b, pneumococcus, group A streptococcus, *Moraxella*)[87–90]	Same antibiotic therapy as for AOM as pathogens similar: amoxicillin 90 mg/kg/day PO div bid, OR for children at higher risk of *Haemophilus,* amox/clav 14:1 ratio, with amoxicillin component at 90 mg/kg/day PO div bid (BIII). Therapy of 14 days may be necessary while mucosal swelling resolves and ventilation is restored.	IDSA sinusitis guidelines recommend amox/clav as first-line therapy,[90] while AAP guidelines (same pediatric authors) recommend amoxicillin.[88] Lack of data prevents a definitive evidence-based recommendation. Sinus irrigations for severe disease or failure to respond.

E. OROPHARYNGEAL INFECTIONS

Clinical Diagnosis	Therapy (evidence grade)	Comments
Dental abscess[91,92]	Clindamycin 30 mg/kg/day PO, IV, IM div q6–8h OR penicillin G 100–200,000 U/kg/day IV div q6h (AIII)	Amox/clav PO; amoxicillin PO; ampicillin AND metronidazole IV are other options. Tooth extraction usually necessary. Erosion of abscess may occur into facial, sinusitis, deep head, and neck compartments.
Diphtheria[93]	Erythromycin 40–50 mg/kg/day PO div qid for 14 days OR penicillin G 150,000 U/kg/day IV div q6h; PLUS antitoxin (AIII)	DAT, a horse antisera, is investigational and only available from CDC Emergency Operations Center at 770/488-7100. The investigational protocol and dosages of DAT are provided on the CDC Web site at www.cdc.gov/diphtheria/downloads/protocol.pdf (protocol version 3/26/14; accessed October 10, 2014).
Epiglottitis (aryepiglottitis, supraglottitis; *H influenzae* type b in an unimmunized child; rarely pneumococcus, *S aureus*)[94,95]	Ceftriaxone 50 mg/kg/day IV, IM q24h OR cefotaxime 150 mg/kg/day IV div q8h for 7–10 days	Emergency: provide airway. For *S aureus* (causes only 5% of epiglottitis), consider adding clindamycin 40 mg/kg/day IV div q8h.

E. OROPHARYNGEAL INFECTIONS (cont)

Clinical Diagnosis	Therapy (evidence grade)	Comments
Gingivostomatitis, herpetic[96–98]	Acyclovir 80 mg/kg/day PO div qid for 7 days (for severe disease, use IV therapy at 30 mg/kg/day div q8h) (BIII); OR for infants ≥3 mo of age, valacyclovir 20 mg/kg/dose PO bid (instructions for preparing liquid formulation with 28-day shelf life included in package insert) (CIII)[98]	Early treatment is likely to be the most effective. Start treatment as soon as oral intake is compromised. This oral acyclovir dose is safe and effective for varicella; 75 mg/kg/day div into 5 equal doses has been studied for HSV.[97] Limited pediatric valacyclovir pharmacokinetics and preparation of an extemporaneous suspension are included in the valacyclovir FDA-approved package label. Consider adding amox/clav or clindamycin for severe disease with oral flora superinfection.
Lemierre syndrome (*Fusobacterium necrophorum*)[99,100] (pharyngitis with internal jugular vein septic thrombosis, postanginal sepsis, necrobacillosis)	Empiric: meropenem 60 mg/kg/day div q8h (or 120 mg/kg/day div q8h for CNS metastatic foci) (AIII) OR ceftriaxone 100 mg/kg/day q24h AND metronidazole 40 mg/kg/day div q8h or clindamycin 40 mg/kg/day div q6h (BIII)	Anecdotal reports suggest metronidazole may be effective for apparent failures with other agents. Often requires anticoagulation. Metastatic and recurrent abscesses often develop while on active, appropriate therapy, requiring multiple debridements and prolonged antibiotic therapy. Treat until CRP and ESR are normal (AIII).
Peritonsillar cellulitis or abscess (group A streptococcus with mixed oral flora, including anaerobes)[101]	Clindamycin 30 mg/kg/day PO, IV, IM div q8h AND cefotaxime 150 mg/kg/day IV div q8h or ceftriaxone 50 mg/kg/day IV q24h (BIII)	Consider incision and drainage for abscess. Alternatives: meropenem or imipenem; pip/tazo; amox/clav for convalescent oral therapy (BIII). No useful data on benefits of steroids.

Pharyngitis (group A streptococcus) (tonsillopharyngitis)[7,102–104]	Amoxicillin 50–75 mg/kg/day PO, either qd, bid, or tid for 10 days OR penicillin V 50–75 mg/kg/day PO div bid or tid, OR benzathine penicillin 600,000 units IM for children <27 kg, 1.2 million units IM if >27 kg, as a single dose (AII) For penicillin-allergic children: erythromycin (estolate at 20–40 mg/kg/day PO div bid to qid; or ethylsuccinate at 40 mg/kg/day PO div bid to qid) for 10 days; or azithromycin 12 mg/kg qd for 5 days (AII)	Amoxicillin displays better GI absorption than oral penicillin V; the suspension is better tolerated. These advantages should be balanced by the unnecessary increased spectrum of activity. Once-daily amoxicillin dosage: for children 50 mg/kg (max 1,000–1,200 mg).[7] Meta-analysis suggests that oral cephalosporins are more effective than penicillin for treatment of strep.[105] Clindamycin is also effective. A 5-day treatment course is FDA approved for some oral cephalosporins (cefdinir, cefpodoxime), but longer follow-up for rheumatic fever is important before short-course therapy can be recommended for all streptococcal pharyngitis (CIII).[106]
Retropharyngeal, parapharyngeal, or lateral pharyngeal cellulitis or abscess (mixed aerobic/anaerobic flora, now including CA-MRSA)[101,107,108]	Clindamycin 40 mg/kg/day IV div q8h AND cefotaxime 150 mg/kg/day IV div q8h or ceftriaxone 50 mg/kg/day IV q24h	Consider I&D; possible airway compromise, mediastinitis. Alternatives: meropenem or imipenem (BIII); pip/tazo; amox/clav for convalescent oral therapy (BIII).
Tracheitis, bacterial (*S aureus*, including CA-MRSA; group A streptococcus; pneumococcus; *H influenzae* type b, rarely *Pseudomonas*)[109,110]	Vancomycin 40 mg/kg/day IV div q8h or clindamycin 40 mg/kg/day IV div q8h AND ceftriaxone 50 mg/kg/day q24h or cefotaxime 150 mg/kg/day div q8h	For susceptible *S aureus*, oxacillin/nafcillin or cefazolin May represent bacterial superinfection of viral laryngotracheobronchitis, including influenza

F. LOWER RESPIRATORY TRACT INFECTIONS

Clinical Diagnosis	Therapy (evidence grade)	Comments
Abscess, lung		
– Primary (severe, necrotizing community-acquired pneumonia caused by pneumococcus, *S aureus,* including CA-MRSA, group A streptococcus)[111,112]	Empiric therapy with ceftriaxone 50–75 mg/kg/day q24h or cefotaxime 150 mg/kg/day div q8h AND clindamycin 40 mg/kg/day div q8h or vancomycin 45 mg/kg/day IV div q8h for 14–21 days or longer (AIII)	For severe CA-MRSA infections, see Chapter 4. Bronchoscopy may be necessary if abscess fails to drain; surgical excision rarely necessary for pneumococcus but more important for CA-MRSA and MSSA. Focus antibiotic coverage based on culture results. For susceptible staph: oxacillin/nafcillin or cefazolin.
– Primary, putrid (ie, foul-smelling; polymicrobial infection with oral aerobes and anaerobes)[113]	Clindamycin 40 mg/kg/day IV div q8h or meropenem 60 mg/kg/day IV div q8h for 10 days or longer (AIII)	Alternatives: imipenem IV or pip/tazo IV or ticar/clav IV (BIII) Oral step-down therapy with clindamycin or amox/clav (BIII)
Allergic bronchopulmonary aspergillosis[114]	Prednisone 0.5 mg/kg qod (BII) AND voriconazole 18 mg/kg/day div q12h load followed by 16 mg/kg/day div q12h (AIII) OR itraconazole 10 mg/kg/day div q12h (BII)	Larger steroid dosages may lead to tissue invasion by *Aspergillus.* Voriconazole not yet studied in allergic bronchopulmonary aspergillosis but is more active than itraconazole. Voriconazole or itraconazole requires trough concentration monitoring.
Aspiration pneumonia (polymicrobial infection with oral aerobes and anaerobes)[113]	Clindamycin 40 mg/kg/day IV div q8h; ADD ceftriaxone 50–75 mg/kg/day q24h or cefotaxime 150 mg/kg/day div q8h for additional *Haemophilus* activity OR meropenem 60 mg/kg/day IV div q8h; for 10 days or longer (BIII)	Alternatives: imipenem IV or pip/tazo IV or ticar/clav IV (BIII) Oral step-down therapy with clindamycin or amox/clav (BIII)
Atypical pneumonia (see *M pneumoniae*, Legionnaires disease)		

Clinical Diagnosis	Therapy	Comments
Bronchitis (bronchiolitis), acute[115]	For bronchitis/bronchiolitis in children, no antibiotic needed for most cases, as disease is usually viral	
Community-acquired pneumonia (See Pneumonia: Community-acquired, bronchopneumonia; Pneumonia: Community-acquired, lobar consolidation.)		
Cystic fibrosis: Seek advice from those expert in acute and chronic management.		
– Acute exacerbation (*P aeruginosa* primarily; also *Burkholderia cepacia, Stenotrophomonas maltophilia, S aureus,* including CA-MRSA, nontuberculous mycobacteria)[116–119]	Ceftazidime 150–200 mg/kg/day div q6–8h or meropenem 120 mg/kg/day div q6h[120] AND tobramycin 6–10 mg/kg/day IM, IV div q6–8h for treatment of acute infection (AII); alternatives: imipenem, cefepime, or ciprofloxacin 30 mg/kg/day PO, IV div tid Duration of therapy not well defined: 10–14 days (BIII)[117]	Larger than normal dosages of antibiotics required in most patients with cystic fibrosis; monitor peak serum concentrations of aminoglycosides. Insufficient evidence to recommend routine use of inhaled antibiotics for acute exascerbations.[121] Cultures with susceptibility testing and synergy testing will help select antibiotics, as multidrug resistance is common.[122,123] Combination therapy may provide synergistic killing and delay the emergence of resistance (BIII). Attempt at early eradication of new onset *Pseudomonas* may decrease progression of disease.[119]
– Chronic inflammation (minimize long-term damage to lung)	Inhaled tobramycin 300 mg bid, cycling 28 days on therapy, 28 days off therapy, is effective adjunctive therapy between exacerbation[116,124] (AI). Inhaled aztreonam[125] provides an alternative to inhaled tobramycin (AI). Azithromycin adjunctive chronic therapy, greatest benefit for those colonized with *Pseudomonas* (AII).[116,126,127]	Alternative inhaled antibiotics: aztreonam[127]; colistin[121,128] (BIII) Two new powder preparations of inhaled tobramycin now available

F. LOWER RESPIRATORY TRACT INFECTIONS (cont)

Clinical Diagnosis	Therapy (evidence grade)	Comments
Pertussis[129,130]	Azithromycin 10 mg/kg/day for 5 days, or clarithromycin 15 mg/kg/day div bid for 7 days, or erythromycin (estolate preferable) 40 mg/kg/day PO div qid; for 7–10 days (AII) Alternative: TMP/SMX 8 mg/kg/day TMP div bid for 10 days (BIII)	Azithromycin and clarithromycin are better tolerated than erythromycin; azithromycin is preferred in young infants to reduce pyloric stenosis risk (see Chapter 5). The azithromycin dosage that is recommended for very young neonates <1 mo (12 mg/kg/day for 5 days) with the highest risk of mortality is FDA approved for streptococcal pharyngitis and is well tolerated and safe for older children. Alternatively, 10 mg/kg on day 1, followed by 5 mg/kg on days 2–5 should also be effective.[129] Provide prophylaxis to family members.
Pneumonia: Community-acquired, bronchopneumonia		
– Mild to moderate illness (overwhelmingly viral, especially in preschool children)[131]	No antibiotic therapy unless epidemiologic, clinical, or laboratory reasons to suspect bacteria or *Mycoplasma*	Broad-spectrum antibiotics may increase risk of subsequent infection with antibiotic-resistant pathogens.
– Moderate to severe illness (pneumococcus; group A streptococcus; *S aureus*, including CA-MRSA; or *Mycoplasma pneumoniae*[111,112,132–134]; and for those with aspiration due to underlying comorbidities, *Haemophilus influenzae*, non-typable)	Empiric therapy: For regions with high PCV13 vaccine use or low pneumococcal resistance to penicillin: ampicillin 200 mg/kg/day div q6h. For regions with low rates of PCV13 use or high pneumococcal resistance to penicillin: ceftriaxone 50–75 mg/kg/day q24h or cefotaxime 150 mg/kg/day div q8h (AI). For suspected CA-MRSA, use vancomycin 40–60 mg/kg/day (AIII).[2] For suspect *Mycoplasma*/atypical pneumonia agents, particularly in school-aged children, ADD azithromycin 10 mg/kg IV, PO on day 1, then 5 mg/kg qd for days 2–5 of treatment (AII).	Tracheal aspirate or bronchoalveolar lavage for Gram stain/culture for severe infection in intubated children. Check vancomycin serum concentrations and renal function, particularly at the higher dosage for CA-MRSA. Alternatives to azithromycin for atypical pneumonia include erythromycin IV, PO, or clarithromycin PO, or doxycycline IV, PO for children >7 y, or levofloxacin for postpubertal older children. New data suggest that combination empiric therapy with a beta-lactam and a macrolide result in shorter hospitalization compared with a beta-lactam alone, but we are not ready to recommend routine empiric combination therapy yet.[135]

Pneumonia: Community-acquired, lobar consolidation		
Pneumococcus (Even if immunized; *S aureus,* including CA-MRSA [can cause necrotizing pneumonia] and group A streptococcus.[111,112,132–134] Consider *H influenzae* type b in the unimmunized child. *M pneumoniae* may cause lobar pneumonia.)	Empiric therapy: For regions with high PCV13 vaccine use or low pneumococcal resistance to penicillin: ampicillin 200 mg/kg/day div q6h. For regions with low rates of PCV13 use or high pneumococcal resistance to penicillin: ceftriaxone 50–75 mg/kg/day q24h or cefotaxime 150 mg/kg/day div q8h (AI); for more severe disease ADD clindamycin 40 mg/kg/day div q8h or vancomycin 40–60 mg/kg/day div q8h for *S aureus* (AIII).[2] For suspect *Mycoplasma*/atypical pneumonia agents, particularly in school-aged children, ADD azithromycin 10 mg/kg IV, PO on day 1, then 5 mg/kg qd for days 2–5 of treatment (AII). Empiric oral outpatient therapy for less severe illness: high-dosage amoxicillin 80–100 mg/kg/day PO div q8h (NOT q12h); for *Mycoplasma,* ADD a macrolide as above (BIII).	Change to PO after improvement (decreased fever, no oxygen needed); treat until clinically asymptomatic and chest radiography significantly improved (7–21 days) (BIII). No reported failures of ceftriaxone/cefotaxime for pen-R pneumococcus; no need to add empiric vancomycin for this reason (CIII). Oral therapy for pneumococcus and *Haemophilus* may also be successful with amox/clav, cefdinir, cefixime, cefpodoxime, or cefuroxime. Levofloxacin is an alternative, particularly for those with severe allergy to beta-lactam antibiotics (BI)[136] but, due to theoretical cartilage toxicity concerns, should not be first-line therapy.
– Pneumococcal, pen-S	Penicillin G 250,000–400,000 U/kg/day IV div q4–6h for 10 days (BII) or ampicillin 200 mg/kg/day IV divided q6h	After improvement, change to PO amoxicillin 50–75 mg/kg/day PO div tid, or penicillin V 50–75 mg/kg/day div qid.
– Pneumococcal, pen-R	Ceftriaxone 75 mg/kg/day q24h, or cefotaxime 150 mg/kg/day div q8h for 10–14 days (BIII)	Addition of vancomycin has not been required for eradication of pen-R strains. For oral convalescent therapy, high-dosage amoxicillin (100–150 mg/kg/day PO div tid), or clindamycin (30 mg/kg/day PO div tid), or linezolid (30 mg/kg/day PO div tid).

F. LOWER RESPIRATORY TRACT INFECTIONS (cont)

Clinical Diagnosis	Therapy (evidence grade)	Comments
S aureus (including CA-MRSA)[2,6,111,132,137]	For MSSA: oxacillin/nafcillin 150 mg/kg/day IV div q6h or cefazolin 100 mg/kg/day IV div q8h (AII) For CA-MRSA: vancomycin 60 mg/kg/day; may need addition of rifampin, clindamycin, or gentamicin (AIII) (See Chapter 4.)	Check vancomycin serum concentrations and renal function, particularly at the higher dosage designed to attain an AUC:MIC of 400, or serum trough concentrations of 15 µg/mL for invasive CA-MRSA disease. For life-threatening disease, optimal therapy of CA-MRSA is not defined: add gentamicin and/or rifampin. Linezolid 30 mg/kg/day IV, PO div q8h is another option, more effective in adults than vancomycin for MRSA nosocomial pneumonia[138] (follow platelets and WBC weekly).
Pneumonia: Immunosuppressed, neutropenic host[143] (*P aeruginosa,* other community-associated or nosocomial gram-negative bacilli, *S aureus,* fungi, AFB, *Pneumocystis,* viral [adenovirus, CMV, EBV, influenza, RSV, others])	Cefepime 150 mg/kg/day IV div q8h and tobramycin 6.0–7.5 mg/kg/day IM, IV div q8h (AII), OR meropenem 60 mg/kg/day div q8h (AII) ± tobramycin (BIII); AND if *S aureus* (including MRSA) is suspected clinically, ADD vancomycin 40–60 mg/kg/day IV div q8h (AIII).	Biopsy or bronchoalveolar lavage usually needed to determine need for antifungal, antiviral, antimycobacterial treatment. Antifungal therapy usually started if no response to antibiotics in 48–72 h (AmB, voriconazole, or caspofungin/micafungin—see Chapter 8). Amikacin 15–22.5 mg/kg/day is an alternative aminoglycoside. Use 2 active agents for definitive therapy based on possible antibacterial synergy and decreased risk of emergence of resistance (BIII).
– Pneumonia: Interstitial pneumonia syndrome of early infancy	If *Chlamydia trachomatis* suspected, azithromycin 10 mg/kg on day 1, followed by 5 mg/kg/day qd days 2–5 OR erythromycin 40 mg/kg/day PO div qid for 14 days (BII)	Most often respiratory viral pathogens, CMV, or chlamydial; role of *Ureaplasma* uncertain

– **Pneumonia, nosocomial (health care–associated/ ventilator-associated)** (*P aeruginosa,* gram-negative enteric bacilli [*Enterobacter, Klebsiella, Serratia, Escherichia coli*], *Acinetobacter, Stenotrophomonas,* and gram-positive organisms including CA-MRSA and *Enterococcus*)[144–147]	Commonly used regimens: Meropenem 60 mg/kg/day div q8h, OR pip/tazo 240–300 mg/kg/day div q6–8h, OR cefepime 150 mg/kg/day div q8h; ± gentamicin 6.0–7.5 mg/kg/day div q8h (AIII); ADD vancomycin 40–60 mg/kg/day div q8h for suspect CA-MRSA (AIII).	For multidrug-resistant gram-negative bacilli, colistin IV may be required. Empiric therapy should be institution specific, based on your hospital's nosocomial pathogens and susceptibilities. Pathogens that cause nosocomial pneumonia often have multidrug resistance. Cultures are critical. Empiric therapy also based on child's prior colonization/infection. Aminoglycosides may not achieve therapeutic concentrations in ELF.[147] Aerosol delivery of antibiotics may be required for multidrug-resistant pathogens.[148]
Pneumonia: With pleural fluid/empyema (same pathogens as for community-associated bronchopneumonia) (Based on extent of fluid and symptoms, may benefit from chest tube drainage with fibrinolysis or video-assisted thoracoscopic surgery[132,139–142])	Empiric therapy: ceftriaxone 50–75 mg/kg/day q24h or cefotaxime 150 mg/kg/day div q8h AND vancomycin 40–60 mg/kg/day IV div q8h (BIII)	Initial therapy based on Gram stain of empyema fluid; typically clinical improvement is slow, with persisting but decreasing "spiking" fever for 2–3 wk.
– Group A streptococcal	Penicillin G 250,000 U/kg/day IV div q4–6h for 10 days (BII)	Change to PO amoxicillin 75 mg/kg/day div tid or penicillin V 50–75 mg/kg/day div qid to tid after clinical improvement (BIII).
– Pneumococcal	(See Pneumonia: Community-acquired, lobar consolidation, Pneumococcal.)	
– *S aureus* (including CA-MRSA)[2,6,111,137]	For MSSA: oxacillin/nafcillin or cefazolin (AII). For CA-MRSA: use vancomycin 60 mg/kg/day (AIII) (designed to attain an AUC:MIC of 400, or serum trough concentrations of 15 µg/mL); follow serum concentrations and renal function; may need additional antibiotics (see Chapter 4).	For life-threatening disease, optimal therapy of CA-MRSA is not defined: add gentamicin and/or rifampin. Oral convalescent therapy for MSSA: cephalexin PO; for CA-MRSA: clindamycin PO. Total course for 21 days or longer (AIII). Linezolid 30 mg/kg/day IV, PO div q8h is another option (follow platelets and WBC weekly).

F. LOWER RESPIRATORY TRACT INFECTIONS (cont)

Clinical Diagnosis	Therapy (evidence grade)	Comments
Pneumonias of other established etiologies (See Chapter 7 for treatment by pathogen.)		
– *Chlamydophila*[149] (formerly *Chlamydia*) *pneumoniae, C psittaci,* or *C trachomatis*[149]	Azithromycin 10 mg/kg on day 1, followed by 5 mg/kg/day qd days 2–5 or erythromycin 40 mg/kg/day PO div qid; for 14 days	Doxycycline (patients >7 y)
– CMV (immunocompromised host)[150, 151] (See chapters 5 and 9 for CMV infection in newborns.)	Ganciclovir IV 10 mg/kg/day IV div q12h for 2 wk (BIII); if needed, continue at 5 mg/kg/day q24h to complete 4–6 wk total (BIII).	Add IVIG or CMV immune globulin to provide a small incremental benefit in bone marrow transplant patients (BII). For older children, oral valganciclovir may be used for convalescent therapy (BIII).
– *E coli*	Ceftriaxone 50–75 mg/kg/day q24h or cefotaxime 150 mg/kg/day div q8h (AII)	For cephalosporin-resistant strains (ESBL producers), use meropenem, imipenem, or ertapenem (AIII).
– *Enterobacter* spp	Cefepime 100 mg/kg/day div q12h or meropenem 60 mg/kg/day div q8h; OR ceftriaxone 50–75 mg/kg/day q24h or cefotaxime 150 mg/kg/day div q8h AND gentamicin 6.0–7.5 mg/kg/day IM, IV div q8h (AIII)	Addition of aminoglycoside to 3rd-generation cephalosporins may retard the emergence of ampC-mediated constitutive high-level resistance, but concern exists for inadequate aminoglycoside concentration in airways[147]; not needed with cefepime, meropenem, or imipenem.
– *Francisella tularensis*[152]	Gentamicin 6.0–7.5 mg/kg/day IM, IV div q8h for 10 days or longer for more severe disease (AIII); for less severe disease, doxycycline PO for 14–21 days (AIII)	Alternatives for oral therapy of mild disease: ciprofloxacin or levofloxacin (BIII)

– Fungi (See Chapter 8.) – Community-associated pathogens, vary by region (eg, *Coccidioides*,[153,154] *Histoplasma*[155,156]) – *Aspergillus*, mucormycosis, other mold infections in immunocompromised hosts[143]	For pathogen-specific recommendations, see Chapter 8. For suspected endemic fungi or mucormycosis in immunocompromised host, treat empirically with a lipid AmB and not voriconazole; biopsy needed to guide therapy. For suspected invasive aspergillosis, treat with voriconazole (AI) (load 18 mg/kg/day div q12h on day 1, then continue 16 mg/kg/day div q12h).	For normal hosts, triazoles (fluconazole, itraconazole, voriconazole, posaconazole) are better tolerated than AmB and equally effective for many community-associated pathogens (see Chapter 2). For dosage, see Chapter 8. Check voriconazole trough concentrations; need to be at least >1 µg/mL. For refractory *Coccidioides* infection, combination therapy with voriconazole and caspofungin may be effective[153] (AIII).
– Influenza virus[157,158] – Recent seasonal influenza A and influenza B strains continue to be resistant to adamantanes.	Empiric therapy, or documented influenza A or influenza B: Oseltamivir[158,159] (AII): <12 mo: Term infants 0–8 mo: 3 mg/kg/dose bid 9–11 mo: 3.5 mg/kg/dose bid ≥12 mo: ≤15 kg: 30 mg PO bid >15–23 kg: 45 mg PO bid >23–40 kg: 60 mg PO bid >40 kg: 75 mg PO bid Zanamivir inhaled (AII): for those ≥7 y 10 mg (two 5-mg inhalations) bid	Check for antiviral susceptibility each season at www.cdc.gov/flu/professionals/antivirals/index.htm (accessed October 10, 2014). For children 12–23 mo, the unit dose of 30 mg/dose may provide inadequate drug exposure. 3.5 mg/kg/dose PO bid has been studied, but sample sizes have been inadequate to recommend weight-based dosing at this time. Adamantanes are amantadine and rimantadine. Influenza B is intrinsically resistant to adamantanes. Limited data for premature neonates[158]: <38 wk postmenstrual age (gestational plus chronologic age): 1.0 mg/kg/dose, PO bid 38–40 wk postmenstrual age: 1.5 mg/kg/dose, PO bid
– *Klebsiella pneumoniae*[160,161]	Ceftriaxone 50–75 mg/kg/day IV, IM q24h OR cefotaxime 150 mg/kg/day IV, IM div q8h (AIII); for ceftriaxone-resistant strains (ESBL strains), use meropenem 60 mg/kg/day IV div q8h (AIII) or other carbapenem.	For *K pneumoniae* carbapenemase-producing strains: alternatives include fluoroquinolones or colistin (BIII).
– Legionnaires disease (*Legionella pneumophila*)	Azithromycin 10 mg/kg IV, PO q24h for 5 days (AIII)	Alternatives: clarithromycin, erythromycin, ciprofloxacin, levofloxacin, doxycycline

F. LOWER RESPIRATORY TRACT INFECTIONS (cont)

Clinical Diagnosis	Therapy (evidence grade)	Comments
– Mycobacteria, nontuberculous (*M avium* complex most common)[11]	In a normal host: azithromycin PO or clarithromycin PO for 6–12 wk if susceptible For more extensive disease: a macrolide AND rifampin AND ethambutol; ± amikacin or streptomycin (AIII)	Highly variable susceptibilities of different nontuberculous mycobacterial species Check if immunocompromised: HIV or gamma-interferon receptor deficiency
– *Mycobacterium tuberculosis* (See Tuberculosis.)		
– *M pneumoniae*[132,162]	Azithromycin 10 mg/kg on day 1, followed by 5 mg/kg/day qd days 2–5, or clarithromycin 15 mg/kg/day div bid for 7–14 days, or erythromycin 40 mg/kg/day PO div qid for 14 days	*Mycoplasma* often causes self-limited infection and does not require treatment (AIII). For children, doxycycline. Macrolide-resistant strains have recently appeared worldwide.[163]
– *Paragonimus westermani*	See Chapter 10.	
– *Pneumocystis jiroveci* (formerly *Pneumocystis carinii*)[164]	Severe disease: preferred regimen is TMP/SMX, 15–20 mg TMP component/kg/day IV div q8h for 3 wk (AI). Mild-moderate disease: may start with IV therapy, then after acute pneumonitis is resolving, TMP/SMX 20 mg of TMP/kg/day PO div qid for 21 days (AII). Use steroid adjunctive treatment for more severe disease (AII).	Alternatives for TMP/SMX intolerant, or clinical failure: pentamidine 3–4 mg IV qd, infused over 60–90 min (AII); TMP AND dapsone; OR primaquine AND clindamycin; OR atovaquone. Prophylaxis: TMP/SMX as 5 mg TMP/kg/day PO, divided in 2 doses, q12h, daily or 3 times/wk on consecutive days (AI); OR TMP/SMX 5 mg TMP/kg/day PO as a single dose, once daily, given 3 times/wk on consecutive days (AI); once-weekly regimens have also been successful[165]; OR dapsone 2 mg/kg (max 100 mg) PO once daily, or 4 mg/kg (max 200 mg) once weekly; OR atovaquone: 30 mg/kg/day for infants 1–3 mo; 45 mg/kg/day for infants 4–24 mo; and 30 mg/kg/day for infants >24 mo.

– *P aeruginosa*[144,147,166,167]	Cefepime 150 mg/kg/day IV div q8h ± tobramycin 6.0–7.5 mg/kg/day IM, IV div q8h (AII). Alternatives: meropenem 60 mg/kg/day div q8h, OR pip/tazo 240–300 mg/kg/day div q6–8h (AII) ± tobramycin (BIII).	Ciprofloxacin IV, or colistin IV for multidrug-resistant strains
– RSV infection (bronchiolitis, pneumonia)[168]	For immunocompromised hosts, the only FDA-approved treatment is ribavirin aerosol: 6-g vial (20 mg/mL in sterile water), by SPAG-2 generator, over 18–20 h daily for 3–5 days. Two antivirals are currently under investigation in children.	Treat only for severe disease, immunocompromised, severe underlying cardiopulmonary disease, as aerosol ribavirin only provides a small benefit. Airway reactivity with inhalation precludes routine use. Ribavirin may also be given systemically (PO or IV) but has not been systemically evaluated for RSV. Palivizumab (Synagis) is not effective for treatment of an active RSV infection, only effective for prevention of hospitalization in high-risk patients.
Tuberculosis		
– Primary pulmonary disease[13,14]	INH 10–15 mg/kg/day (max 300 mg) PO qd for 6 mo AND rifampin 10–20 mg/kg/day (max 600 mg) PO qd for 6 mo AND PZA 20–40 mg/kg/day PO qd for first 2 mo therapy only (AII). If risk factors present for multidrug resistance, ADD ethambutol 20 mg/kg/day PO qd OR streptomycin 30 mg/kg/day IV, IM div q12h initially.	Contact TB specialist for therapy of drug-resistant TB. Fluoroquinolones may play a role in treating multidrug-resistant strains. Bedaquiline, in a new drug class for TB therapy, was recently approved for adults with multidrug-resistant TB, when used in combination therapy. Toxicities and lack of pediatric data preclude routine use in children. Directly observed therapy preferred; after 2 wk of daily therapy, can change to twice-weekly dosing double dosage of INH (max 900 mg), PZA (max 2 g), and ethambutol (max 2.5 g); rifampin remains same dosage (10–20 mg/kg/day, max 600 mg) (AII). LP ± CT of head for children ≤2 y to rule out occult, concurrent CNS infection; consider testing for HIV infection (AIII).

F. LOWER RESPIRATORY TRACT INFECTIONS (cont)

Clinical Diagnosis	Therapy (evidence grade)	Comments
– Latent TB infection (skin test conversion)	INH 10–15 mg/kg/day (max 300 mg) PO daily for 9 mo (12 mo for immunocompromised patients) (AIII); treatment with INH at 20–30 mg/kg twice weekly for 9 mo is also effective (AIII). Alternative[169] (BII): For children ≥12 y, once-weekly DOT for 12 weeks: INH (15 mg/kg/dose, max 900 mg), AND rifapentine: 10.0–14.0 kg: 300 mg 14.1–25.0 kg: 450 mg 25.1–32.0 kg: 600 mg 32.1–49.9 kg: 750 mg ≥50.0 kg: 900 mg (max)	Obtain baseline LFTs. Consider monthly LFTs or as needed for symptoms. Stop INH-rifapentine if AST or ALT ≥5 times the ULN even in the absence of symptoms or ≥3 times the ULN in the presence of symptoms. For children ≥2–12 years, 12 wk of INH and rifapentine may be used, but less data on safety and efficacy. Insufficient data for children <2 y. For exposure to known INH-R but rifampin-S strains, use rifampin 6 mo (AIII).
– Exposed infant <4 y, or immunocompromised patient (high risk of dissemination)	INH 10–15 mg/kg PO daily for 2–3 mo after last exposure with repeat skin test or interferon-gamma release assay test negative (AIII)	If PPD remains negative at 2–3 mo and child well, consider stopping empiric therapy. PPD may not be reliable in immunocompromised patients. Not much data to assess reliability of interferon-gamma release assays in very young infants or immunocompromised hosts, but not likely to be much better than the PPD skin test.

G. CARDIOVASCULAR INFECTIONS

Clinical Diagnosis	Therapy (evidence grade)	Comments
Bacteremia		
– Occult bacteremia (late-onset neonatal sepsis; fever without focus), infants <2 mo (group B streptococcus, *E coli*, *Listeria*, pneumococcus, meningococcus)[170–174]	In general, hospitalization for late-onset neonatal sepsis, with cultures of blood, urine, and CSF; start ampicillin 200 mg/kg/day IV div q6h AND cefotaxime 150 mg/kg/day IV div q8h (AII); higher dosages if meningitis is documented.	For a nontoxic, febrile infant with good access to medical care: cultures may be obtained of blood, urine, and CSF, ceftriaxone 50 mg/kg IM (lacks *Listeria* activity) given with outpatient follow-up the next day (Boston criteria) (BII); alternative is home without antibiotics if evaluation is negative (Rochester; Philadelphia criteria)[170,174] (BI).
– Occult bacteremia (fever without focus) in ages 2–3 mo to 36 mo (*H influenzae*, pneumococcus, meningococcus; increasingly *S aureus*)[173–175]	Empiric therapy: If unimmunized, febrile, mild-moderate toxic: after blood culture: ceftriaxone 50 mg/kg IM (BII). If fully immunized (*Haemophilus* and *Pneumococcus*) and nontoxic, no routine antibiotic therapy recommended, but follow closely in case of vaccine failure or meningococcal bacteremia (BIII).	Oral convalescent therapy is selected by susceptibility of blood isolate, following response to IM/IV treatment, with CNS and other foci ruled out by examination ± laboratory tests ± imaging.
– *H influenzae* type b, non-CNS infections	Ceftriaxone IM/IV OR, if beta-lactamase negative, ampicillin IV, followed by oral convalescent therapy (AII)	If beta-lactamase negative: amoxicillin 75–100 mg/kg/day PO div tid (AII) If positive: high-dosage cefixime, ceftibuten, cefdinir PO, or levofloxacin PO (CIII)
– Meningococcus	Ceftriaxone IM/IV or penicillin G IV, followed by oral convalescent therapy (AII)	Amoxicillin 75–100 mg/kg/day PO div tid (AIII)
– Pneumococcus, non-CNS infections	Ceftriaxone IM/IV or penicillin G IV (if pen-S), followed by oral convalescent therapy (AII)	If pen-S: amoxicillin 75–100 mg/kg/day PO div tid (AII). If pen-R: continue ceftriaxone IM, or switch to clindamycin if susceptible (CIII); linezolid or levofloxacin may also be options (CIII).

G. CARDIOVASCULAR INFECTIONS (cont)

Clinical Diagnosis	Therapy (evidence grade)	Comments
– *S aureus*[2,6,176–179] usually associated with focal infection	MSSA: nafcillin or oxacillin/nafcillin IV 150–200 mg/kg/day div q6h ± gentamicin 6 mg/kg/day div q8h. MRSA: vancomycin 40–60 mg/kg/day IV div q8h ± gentamicin 6 mg/kg/day div q8h ± rifampin 20 mg/kg/day div q12h. Treat for 2 weeks (IV plus PO) from negative blood cultures unless endocarditis/endovascular thrombus present, which may require 6 wk of therapy.	For persisting bacteremia caused by MRSA, consider adding gentamicin, or switching vancomycin to daptomycin 6–8 mg/kg qd (but will not treat pneumonia) or ceftaroline, particularly for MRSA with vancomycin MIC of >2 µg/mL. For toxic shock syndrome, clindamycin should be added for the initial 48–72 h of therapy to decrease toxin production; IVIG may be added to bind circulating toxin (linezolid may also act in this way), no controlled data exist for these measures. Watch for the development of metastatic foci of infection, including endocarditis. If catheter-related, remove catheter.[179]
Endocarditis: Surgical indications: intractable heart failure; persistent infection; large mobile vegetations; peripheral embolism; and valve dehiscence, perforation, rupture or fistula, or a large perivalvular abscess[180–182]		
– **Native valve**[180,181]		
– Empiric therapy for presumed endocarditis	Ceftriaxone IV 100 mg/kg q24h AND gentamicin IV, IM 6 mg/kg/day div q8h (AII). For severe infection, ADD vancomycin 40–60 mg/kg/day IV div q8h to cover *S aureus* (AIII).	Combination (ceftriaxone + gentamicin) provides bactericidal activity against most strains of viridans streptococci, the most common pathogens in infective endocarditis. May administer gentamicin with a qd regimen (CIII). For beta-lactam allergy, use vancomycin 40 mg/kg/day IV div q8h AND gentamicin 6 mg/kg/day IV div q8h.
– Viridans streptococci: Follow echocardiogram for resolution of vegetation (BIII); for beta-lactam allergy: vancomycin.		
Fully susceptible to penicillin	Ceftriaxone 50 mg/kg IV, IM q24h for 4 wk OR penicillin G 200,000 U/kg/day IV div q4–6h for 4 wk (BII); OR penicillin G or ceftriaxone AND gentamicin 6 mg/kg/day IM, IV div q8h for 14 days (AII)	

Relatively resistant to penicillin	Penicillin G 300,000 U/kg/day IV div q4–6h for 4 wk, or ceftriaxone 100 mg/kg IV q24h for 4 wk; AND gentamicin 6 mg/kg/day IM, IV div q8h for 2 wk (AIII)	Gentamicin is used for the first 2 wk of a total of 4 wk of therapy for relatively resistant strains.
– Enterococcus (dosages for native or prosthetic valve infections)		
Ampicillin-susceptible (gentamicin-S)	Ampicillin 300 mg/kg/day IV, IM div q6h or penicillin G 300,000 U/kg/day IV div q4–6h; AND gentamicin 6.0 mg/kg/day IV div q8h; for 4–6 wk (AII)	Combined treatment with cell-wall active antibiotic plus aminoglycoside used to achieve bactericidal activity. For beta-lactam allergy: vancomycin. Little data exist in children. Linezolid and quinupristin/dalfopristin are alternatives. For gentamicin-R strains, use streptomycin if susceptible.
Ampicillin-resistant (gentamicin-S)	Vancomycin 40 mg/kg/day IV div q8h AND gentamicin 6.0 mg/kg/day IV div q8h; for 4–6 wk (AIII)	
Vancomycin-resistant (gentamicin-S)	Daptomycin 6–8 mg/kg/day q24h AND gentamicin 6.0 mg/kg/day IV div q8h; for 4–6 wk (AIII)	
– Staphylococci: *S aureus*, including CA-MRSA; *S epidermidis*.[6,177] Consider continuing therapy at end of 6 wk if vegetations persist on echocardiogram.	MSSA or MSSE: nafcillin or oxacillin/nafcillin 150–200 mg/kg/day IV div q6h for 6 wk AND gentamicin 6 mg/kg/day div q8h for 14 days CA-MRSA or MRSE: vancomycin 40–60 mg/kg/day IV div q8h AND gentamicin; ADD rifampin 20 mg/kg/day IV div q8–12h	Surgery may be necessary in acute phase; avoid cephalosporins (conflicting data on efficacy). For failures on therapy, consider daptomycin 6–8 mg/kg/day q24h AND gentamicin 6 mg/kg/day div q8h.
– Pneumococcus, gonococcus, group A streptococcus	Penicillin G 200,000 U/kg/day IV div q4–6h for 4 wk; alternatives: ceftriaxone or vancomycin	Ceftriaxone for gonococcus until susceptibilities known. For penicillin non-susceptible strains of pneumococcus, use high-dosage penicillin G 300,000 U/kg/day IV div q4–6h or high-dosage ceftriaxone 100 mg/kg IV q24h for 4 wk.

G. CARDIOVASCULAR INFECTIONS (cont)

Clinical Diagnosis	Therapy (evidence grade)	Comments
– **Prosthetic valve/material**[180,181]		
– Viridans streptococci		Follow echocardiogram for resolution of vegetation. For beta-lactam allergy: vancomycin.
Fully susceptible to penicillin	Ceftriaxone 100 mg/kg IV, IM q24h for 6 wk OR penicillin G 300,000 U/kg/day IV div q4–6h for 6 wk (AII); OR penicillin G or ceftriaxone AND gentamicin 6.0 mg/kg/day IM, IV div q8h for 14 days (AII)	Gentamicin is used for the first 2 wk of a total of 6 wk of therapy for prosthetic valve/material endocarditis.
Relatively resistant to penicillin	Penicillin G 300,000 U/kg/day IV div q4–6h for 6 wk, or ceftriaxone 100 mg/kg IV q24h for 6 wk; AND gentamicin 6.0 mg/kg/day IM, IV div q8h for 6 wk (AIII)	Gentamicin is used for all 6 wk of therapy for prosthetic valve/material endocarditis caused by relatively resistant strains.
– Enterococcus (See dosages under Native valve.)		
– Staphylococci: *S aureus,* including CA-MRSA; *S epidermidis* (See dosages under Native valve.)		
– *Candida*	Caspofungin 70 mg/m^2 load on day 1, then 50 mg/m^2/day OR micafungin 2–4 mg/kg/day (BIII)	Fluconazole is known to not sterile cardiac vegetations well, and AmB products are also not ideal; echinocandins preferred. Suspect *Candida* vegetations when lesions are large.

Endocarditis Prophylaxis[181,183,184]: Given that (1) endocarditis is rarely caused by dental/GI procedures and (2) prophylaxis for procedures prevents an exceedingly small number of cases, the risks of antibiotics outweigh the benefits. Highest risk conditions currently recommended for prophylaxis: (1) prosthetic heart valve (or prosthetic material used to repair a valve); (2) previous endocarditis; (3) cyanotic congenital heart disease that is unrepaired (or palliatively repaired with shunts and conduits); (4) congenital heart disease that is repaired but with defects at the site of repair adjacent to prosthetic material; (5) completely repaired congenital heart disease using prosthetic material, for the first 6 mo after repair; or (6) cardiac transplant patients with valvulopathy. Routine prophylaxis no longer is required for children with native valve abnormalities. Long-term assessment of new prophylaxis guidelines documents no significant increase in endocarditis.[181]

– In highest risk patients: dental procedures that involve manipulation of the gingival or periodontal region of teeth	Amoxicillin 50 mg/kg PO 60 min before procedure OR ampicillin or ceftriaxone or cefazolin, all at 50 mg/kg IM/IV 30–60 min before procedure	If penicillin allergy: clindamycin 20 mg/kg PO (60 min before) or IV (30 min before); OR azithromycin 15 mg/kg or clarithromycin 15 mg/kg, 60 min before
– Genitourinary and GI procedures	None	No longer recommended
Lemierre syndrome (*Fusobacterium necrophorum* primarily, new reports with MRSA)[99,100,185,186] postanginal sepsis, pharyngitis with internal jugular vein septic thrombosis	Empiric: meropenem 60 mg/kg/day div q8h (or 120 mg/kg/day div q8h for CNS metastatic foci) (AIII) OR ceftriaxone 100 mg/kg/day q24h AND metronidazole 40 mg/kg/day div q8h or clindamycin 40 mg/kg/day div q6h (BIII) ADD empiric vancomycin if MRSA suspected.	Anecdotal reports suggest metronidazole may be effective for apparent failures with other agents. Metastatic and recurrent abscesses often develop while on active, appropriate therapy, requiring multiple debridements and prolonged antibiotic therapy.
Purulent pericarditis		
– Empiric (acute, bacterial: *S aureus,* group A streptococcus, pneumococcus, meningococcus, *H influenzae* type b)[187,188]	Vancomycin 40 mg/kg/day IV div q8h AND ceftriaxone 50–75 mg/kg/day q24h (AIII). For presumed staphylococcal infection, ADD gentamicin (AIII).	Increasingly uncommon with immunization against pneumococcus and *H influenzae* type b.[187] Pericardiocentesis is essential to establish diagnosis. Surgical drainage of pus with pericardial window or pericardiectomy is important to prevent tamponade.
– *S aureus*	For MSSA: oxacillin/nafcillin 150–200 mg/kg/day IV div q6h OR cefazolin 100 mg/kg/day IV div q8h. Treat for 2–3 wk after drainage (BIII). For CA-MRSA: continue vancomycin. Treat for 3–4 wk after drainage (BIII).	Continue therapy with gentamicin; consider use of rifampin in severe cases.
– *H influenzae* type b in unimmunized children	Ceftriaxone 50 mg/kg/day q24h or cefotaxime 150 mg/kg/day div q8h; for 10–14 days (AIII)	Ampicillin for beta-lactamase–negative strains
– Pneumococcus, meningococcus, group A streptococcus	Penicillin G 200,000 U/kg/day IV, IM div q6h for 10–14 days OR ceftriaxone 50 mg/kg qd for 10–14 days (AIII)	Ceftriaxone or cefotaxime for penicillin non-susceptible pneumococci

G. CARDIOVASCULAR INFECTIONS (cont)

Clinical Diagnosis	Therapy (evidence grade)	Comments
– Coliform bacilli	Ceftriaxone 50–75 mg/kg/day q24h or cefotaxime 150 mg/kg/day div q8h for 3 wk or longer (AIII)	Alternative drugs depending on susceptibilities; for *Enterobacter, Serratia,* or *Citrobacter,* use cefepime or meropenem.
– Tuberculous[13]	INH 10–15 mg/kg/day (max 300 mg) PO qd, IV for 6 mo AND rifampin 10–20 mg/kg/day (max 600 mg) PO qd, IV for 6 mo. ADD PZA 20–40 mg/kg/day PO qd for first 2 mo therapy; if suspected multidrug resistance, also add ethambutol 20 mg/kg/day PO qd (AIII).	Corticosteroids improve survival in adults: prednisone 1 mg/kg/day for 4 wk, then 0.5 mg/kg/day for 4 wk, then 0.25 mg/kg/day for 2 wk, then 0.1 mg/kg/day for 1 wk (AIII).[13]

H. GASTROINTESTINAL INFECTIONS (See Chapter 10 for parasitic infections.)

Clinical Diagnosis	Therapy (evidence grade)	Comments
Diarrhea/Gastroenteritis		
Note on *E coli* and diarrheal disease: Antibiotic susceptibility of *E coli* varies considerably from region to region. For mild to moderate disease, TMP/SMX may be started as initial therapy, but for more severe disease and for locations with rates of TMP/SMX resistance greater than 10% to 20%, oral 3rd-generation cephalosporins (eg, cefixime, cefdinir, ceftibuten), azithromycin, or ciprofloxacin should be used (AIII). Cultures and antibiotic susceptibility testing are recommended for significant disease (AIII).		
– Empiric therapy of community-associated diarrhea in the United States (*E coli* [STEC, including O157:H7 strains, and ETEC], *Salmonella, Campylobacter,* and *Shigella* predominate; *Yersinia* and parasites causing <5%; however, viral pathogens are far more common, especially for children <3 y.)[189,190]	Azithromycin 10 mg/kg qd for 3 days (BII), OR cefixime 8 mg/kg/day PO qd (BII) for 5 days; OR ciprofloxacin 30 mg/kg/day PO div bid for 3 days	Alternatives: other oral 3rd-generation cephalosporins (eg, cefdinir, ceftibuten); or rifaximin 600 mg/day div tid for 3 days (for nonfebrile, non-bloody diarrhea for children >11 y). Controversy exists regarding treatment of O157:H7 strains, with retrospective data to support treatment or withholding treatment.[191–193]

– Traveler's diarrhea: empiric therapy (*E coli, Campylobacter, Salmonella, Shigella,* plus many other pathogens including protozoa)[194–201]	Azithromycin 10 mg/kg qd for 3 days (AII); OR rifaximin 600 mg/day div tid for 3 days (for nonfebrile, non-bloody diarrhea for children ≥12 y) (BII); OR cefixime 8–10 mg/kg qd for 5 days (CII); OR ciprofloxacin 30 mg/kg/day div bid for 3 days (CII)	Susceptibility patterns of *E coli, Campylobacter, Salmonella,* and *Shigella* vary widely by country; check country-specific data for departing or returning travelers. Azithromycin preferable to ciprofloxacin for travelers to Southeast Asia given high prevalence of quinolone-resistant *Campylobacter.* Rifaximin is less effective than ciprofloxacin for invasive bloody bacterial enteritis: rifaximin may also not be as effective for *Shigella*, *Salmonella,* and *Campylobacter* as other agents. Adjunctive therapy with loperamide (anti-motility) is not recommended for children <2 y and should be used only in nonfebrile, non-bloody diarrhea.[202,203] May shorten symptomatic illness by about 24 h.
– Traveler's diarrhea: prophylaxis[195,196]	– Prophylaxis: Early self-treatment with agents listed previously is preferred over long-term prophylaxis, but may use prophylaxis for a short-term (<14 days) visit to very high-risk region: rifaximin (for older children), azithromycin, or bismuth subsalicylate (BIII).	
– *Aeromonas hydrophila*[204]	Ciprofloxacin 30 mg/kg/day PO div bid for 5 days OR azithromycin 10 mg/kg qd for 3 days OR cefixime 8 mg/kg/day PO qd (BIII)	Not all strains produce enterotoxins and diarrhea; role in diarrhea questioned.[203] Resistance to TMP/SMX about 10%–15%. Choose most narrow spectrum agent based on in vitro susceptibilities.
– *Campylobacter jejuni*[205–207]	Azithromycin 10 mg/kg/day for 3 days (BII) or erythromycin 40 mg/kg/day PO div qid for 5 days (BII)	Alternatives: doxycycline or ciprofloxacin (high rate of fluoroquinolone resistance in Thailand and India). Single-dose azithromycin (1 g, once) is effective in adults.
– Cholera[200,208]	Azithromycin 20 mg/kg once; OR erythromycin 50 mg/kg/day PO div qid for 3 days; OR doxycycline 4 mg/kg/day (max 200 mg/day) PO div bid, for all ages	Ciprofloxacin or TMP/SMX (if susceptible)
– *Clostridium difficile* (antibiotic-associated colitis)[209,210]	Metronidazole 30 mg/kg/day PO div qid OR vancomycin 40 mg/kg/day PO div qid for 7 days; for relapsing *C difficile* enteritis, consider pulse therapy (1 wk on/1 wk off for 3–4 cycles) or prolonged tapering therapy.[209]	Vancomycin is more effective for severe infection.[211] Fidaxomicin approved for adults; pediatric studies underway. Many infants and children may have asymptomatic colonization with *C difficile.*[211] Higher risk of relapse in children with multiple comorbidities.

H. GASTROINTESTINAL INFECTIONS (cont) (See Chapter 10 for parasitic infections.)

Clinical Diagnosis	Therapy (evidence grade)	Comments
– *E coli*		
Enterotoxigenic (etiology of most traveler's diarrhea)[197,199,212]	Azithromycin 10 mg/kg qd for 3 days; OR cefixime 8 mg/kg/day PO qd for 3 days; OR ciprofloxacin 30 mg/kg/day PO div bid for 3 days	Most illnesses brief and self-limited Alternatives: rifaximin 600 mg/day div tid for 3 days (for nonfebrile, non-bloody diarrhea for children >11 y); OR TMP/SMX Resistance increasing worldwide[199]
Enterohemorrhagic (O157:H7; STEC, etiology of HUS)[191–193]	Controversy on whether treatment of O157:H7 diarrhea results in more or less toxin-mediated renal damage.[191–193] For severe infection, treat as for enterotoxigenic strains above.	Injury to colonic mucosa may lead to invasive bacterial colitis.
Enteropathogenic	Neomycin 100 mg/kg/day PO div q6–8h for 5 days	Most traditional "enteropathogenic" strains are not toxigenic or invasive. Postinfection diarrhea may be problematic.
– Gastritis, peptic ulcer disease (*Helicobacter pylori*)[213–216]	Triple agent therapy: clarithromycin 7.5 mg/kg/dose 2–3 times each day, AND amoxicillin 40 mg/kg/dose (max 1 g) PO bid AND omeprazole 0.5 mg/kg/dose PO bid 2 wk (BII)	Most data from studies in adults; of effective regimens, no one combination has been shown superior. New, current regimens use 4 drugs (with metronidazole) initially or with relapse, due to concerns for clarithromycin resistance.[213,215] Other regimens include bismuth, metronidazole instead of amoxicillin, and other proton pump inhibitors.
– Giardiasis (*Giardia lamblia*)	Metronidazole 30–40 mg/kg/day PO div tid for 7–10 days (BII); OR nitazoxanide PO (take with food), age 12–47 mo, 100 mg/dose bid for 7 days; age 4–11 y, 200 mg/dose bid for 7 days; age ≥12 y, 1 tab (500 mg)/dose bid for 7 days (BII); OR tinidazole 50 mg/kg/day (max 2 g) for 1 day (BII)	If therapy is inadequate, another course of the same agent is usually curative. Alternatives: furazolidone 6 mg/kg/day in 4 doses for 7–10 days; OR paromomycin 30 mg/kg/day div tid for 5–10 days; OR albendazole 10 mg/kg/day PO for 5 days (CII). Prolonged courses may be needed for immunocompromised conditions (eg, hypogammaglobulinemia). Treatment of asymptomatic carriers not usually recommended.

– Salmonellosis		
Non-typhoid strains[217,218]	Usually none for self-limited diarrhea (eg, diarrhea is much improved by the time culture results are available) For persisting symptomatic infection: azithromycin 10 mg/kg PO qd for 3 days (AII); OR ceftriaxone 75 mg/kg/day IV, IM q24h for 5 days (AII); OR cefixime 20–30 mg/kg/day PO for 5 days (BII); OR for susceptible strains: TMP/SMX 8 mg/kg/day of TMP PO div bid for 5 days (AI)	Alternatives: ciprofloxacin 30 mg/kg/day PO div bid for 5 days (AI). Carriage of strains is prolonged in treated children.
Typhoid fever[219–222]	Azithromycin 10 mg/kg qd for 5 days (AII); OR ceftriaxone 75 mg/kg/day IV, IM q24h for 5 days (AII); OR cefixime 20–30 mg/kg/day PO, div q12h for 14 days (BII); OR for susceptible strains: TMP/SMX 8 mg/kg/day of TMP PO div bid for 10 days (AI)	Increasing cephalosporin resistance. Watch for relapse if ceftriaxone used. Alternative: ciprofloxacin 30 mg/kg/day PO div bid for 5–7 days (AI).
– Shigellosis[223–225]	Cefixime 8 mg/kg/day PO qd for 5 days (AII); OR azithromycin 10 mg/kg/day PO for 3 days (AII); OR ciprofloxacin 30 mg/kg/day PO div bid for 3–5 days (BII)	Alternatives for susceptible strains: TMP/SMX 8 mg/kg/day of TMP PO div bid for 5 days; OR ampicillin (not amoxicillin). Ceftriaxone 50 mg/kg/day IM, IV if parenteral therapy necessary, for 2–5 days. Avoid antiperistaltic drugs. Treat to decrease communicability, even if symptoms resolving.
– *Yersinia enterocolitica*[226,227]	Antimicrobial therapy probably not of value for mild disease in normal hosts TMP/SMX PO, IV; OR ciprofloxacin PO, IV (BIII)	Alternatives: ceftriaxone or gentamicin. May mimic appendicitis. Limited clinical data exist on oral therapy.

H. GASTROINTESTINAL INFECTIONS (cont) (See Chapter 10 for parasitic infections.)

Clinical Diagnosis	Therapy (evidence grade)	Comments
Intra-abdominal Infection (abscess, peritonitis secondary to bowel/appendix contents)		
– Appendicitis; bowel-associated (enteric gram-negative bacilli, *Bacteroides* spp, *Enterococcus* spp, increasingly *Pseudomonas*)[228–233]	Meropenem 60 mg/kg/day IV div q8h or imipenem 60 mg/kg/day IV div q6h; OR pip/tazo 240 mg pip/kg/day div q6h; for 7–10 days or longer if suspicion of persisting intra-abdominal abscess (AII). Data support IV outpatient therapy[232] or oral step-down therapy[232] when clinically improved.	Many other regimens may be effective, including ampicillin 150 mg/kg/day div q8h AND gentamicin 6–7.5 mg/kg/day IV, IM div q8h AND metronidazole 40 mg/kg/day IV div q8h; OR ceftriaxone 50 mg/kg q24h AND metronidazole 40 mg/kg/day IV div q8h. Gentamicin demonstrates poor activity at low pH: surgical source control is critical to achieve cure.
– Tuberculosis, abdominal (*Mycobacterium bovis,* from unpasteurized dairy products)[13,14,234,235]	INH 10–15 mg/kg/day (max 300 mg) PO qd for 6 mo AND rifampin 10–20 mg/kg/day (max 600 mg) PO qd for 6 mo. *M bovis* is resistant to PZA. If risk factors are present for multidrug resistance (eg, poor adherence to previous therapy), add ethambutol 20 mg/kg/day PO qd OR a fluoroquinolone (moxifloxacin or levofloxacin).	Directly observed therapy preferred; after 2+ wk of daily therapy, can change to twice-weekly dosing double dosage of INH (max 900 mg); rifampin remains same dosage (10–20 mg/kg/day, max 600 mg) (AII). LP ± CT of head for children ≤2 y with active disease to rule out occult, concurrent CNS infection (AIII).
Perirectal abscess (*Bacteroides* spp other anaerobes, enteric bacilli, and *S aureus* predominate)[236]	Clindamycin 30–40 mg/kg/day IV div q8h AND cefotaxime or ceftriaxone or gentamicin (BIII)	Surgical drainage alone may be curative.
Peritonitis – Peritoneal dialysis indwelling catheter infection (staphylococcal; enteric gram-negatives; yeast)[237,238]	Antibiotic added to dialysate in concentrations approximating those attained in serum for systemic disease (eg, 4 µg/mL for gentamicin, 25 µg/mL for vancomycin, 125 µg/mL for cefazolin, 25 µg/mL for ciprofloxacin) after a larger loading dose (AII)[238]	Selection of antibiotic based on organism isolated from peritoneal fluid; systemic antibiotics if there is accompanying bacteremia/fungemia
– Primary (pneumococcus or group A streptococcus)[239]	Ceftriaxone 50 mg/kg/day q24h, or cefotaxime 150 mg/kg/day div q8h; if pen-S, then penicillin G 150,000 U/kg/day IV div q6h; for 7–10 days (AII)	Other antibiotics according to culture and susceptibility tests

I. GENITAL AND SEXUALLY TRANSMITTED INFECTIONS

Clinical Diagnosis	Therapy (evidence grade)	Comments
Consider testing for HIV and other STIs in a child with one documented STI; consider sexual abuse in prepubertal children. The most recent CDC STI treatment guidelines are posted online at www.cdc.gov/std/treatment.		
Chancroid (*Haemophilus ducreyi*)[42]	Azithromycin 1 g PO as single dose OR ceftriaxone 250 mg IM as single dose	Alternative: erythromycin 1.5 g/day PO div tid for 7 days OR ciprofloxacin 1,000 mg PO qd, div bid for 3 days
C trachomatis (cervicitis, urethritis)[42,240]	Azithromycin 20 mg/kg (max 1 g) PO for 1 dose; OR doxycycline (patients >7 y) 40 mg/kg/day (max 200 mg/day) PO div bid for 7 days	Alternatives: erythromycin 2 g/day PO div qid for 7 days; OR levofloxacin 500 mg PO q24h for 7 days
Epididymitis (associated with positive urine cultures and STIs)[42,241,242]	Ceftriaxone 50 mg/kg/day q24h for 7–10 days AND (for older children) doxycycline 200 mg/day div bid	Microbiology not well studied in children; in infants, also associated with urogenital tract anomalies. Treat infants for *S aureus* and *E coli;* may resolve spontaneously; in STI, caused by *Chlamydia* and gonococcus.
Gonorrhea		
– Newborns	See Chapter 5.	
– Genital infections (uncomplicated vulvovaginitis, cervicitis, urethritis, or proctitis)[42,240,243,244]	Ceftriaxone 250 mg IM for 1 dose (regardless of weight) AND azithromycin 1 g PO for 1 dose or doxycycline 200 mg/day div q12h for 7 days	Cefixime no longer recommended due to increasing cephalosporin resistance.[244] Fluoroquinolones are no longer recommended due to resistance.
– Pharyngitis[42,244,245]	Ceftriaxone 250 mg IM for 1 dose (regardless of weight) AND azithromycin 1 g PO for 1 dose or doxycycline 200 mg/day div q12h for 7 days	
– Disseminated gonococcal infection[42,244,245]	Ceftriaxone 50 mg/kg/day IM, IV q24h (max: 1 g); total course for 7 days	No studies in children: increase dosage for meningitis.
Granuloma inguinale (donovanosis, *Klebsiella granulomatis,* formerly *Calymmatobacterium*)[42]	Doxycycline 4 mg/kg/day div bid (max 200 mg/day), PO for 21 days until lesions completely healed	Primarily in tropical regions of India, Pacific, and Africa Option: azithromycin 1 g PO once weekly for 3 wk

I. GENITAL AND SEXUALLY TRANSMITTED INFECTIONS (cont)

Clinical Diagnosis	Therapy (evidence grade)	Comments
Herpes simplex virus, genital infection[42,246,247]	Acyclovir 20 mg/kg/dose (max 400 mg) PO tid for 7–10 days (first episode) (AI); OR valacyclovir 20 mg/kg/dose of extemporaneous suspension (directions on package label), max 1.0 g PO bid for 7–10 days (first episode) (AI); OR famciclovir 250 mg PO tid for 7–10 days (AI); for more severe infection: acyclovir 15 mg/kg/day IV div q8h as 1-h infusion for 7–10 days (AII) For recurrent episodes: treat as above with acyclovir PO, valacyclovir PO, or famciclovir PO, immediately when symptoms begin, for 5 days For suppression: acyclovir 20 mg/kg/dose (max 400 mg) PO bid; OR valacyclovir 20 mg/kg/dose PO qd (little long-term safety data in children; no efficacy data in children)	
Lymphogranuloma venereum (*C trachomatis*)[42]	Doxycycline 4 mg/kg/day (max 200 mg/day) PO (patients >7 y) div bid for 21 days; OR erythromycin 2 g/day PO div qid; for 21 days	Azithromycin 1 g PO once weekly for 3 wk
Pelvic inflammatory disease (*Chlamydia,* gonococcus, plus anaerobes)[42,248]	Cefoxitin 2 g IV q6h; AND doxycycline 200 mg/day PO or IV div bid; OR clindamycin 900 mg IV q8h and gentamicin 1.5 mg/kg IV, IM q8h for 14 days	Drugs given IV until clinical improvement for 24 h, followed by doxycycline 200 mg/day PO div bid AND clindamycin 1,800 mg/day PO div qid to complete 14 days of therapy Optional regimen: ceftriaxone 250 mg IM for 1 dose AND doxycycline 200 mg/day PO div bid; WITH/WITHOUT metronidazole 1 g/day PO div bid; for 14 days
Syphilis[42,249] (test for HIV)		
– Congenital	See Chapter 5.	

– Neurosyphilis (positive CSF VDRL or CSF pleocytosis with serologic diagnosis of syphilis)	Crystalline penicillin G 200–300,000 U/kg/day (max 24,000,000 U/day) div q6h for 10–14 days (AIII)	
– Primary, secondary	Benzathine penicillin G 50,000 U/kg (max 2,400,000 U) IM as a single dose (AIII); do not use benzathine-procaine penicillin mixtures.	Follow-up serologic tests at 6, 12, and 24 mo; 15% may remain seropositive despite adequate treatment. If allergy to penicillin: doxycycline (patients >7 y) 4 mg/kg/day (max 200 mg) PO div bid for 14 days. CSF examination should be obtained for children being treated for primary or secondary syphilis to rule out asymptomatic neurosyphilis. Test for HIV.
– Syphilis of <1 y duration, without clinical symptoms (early latent syphilis)	Benzathine penicillin G 50,000 U/kg (max 2,400,000 U) IM as a single dose (AIII)	Alternative if allergy to penicillin: doxycycline (patients >7 y) 4 mg/kg/day (max 200 mg/day) PO div bid for 14 days
– Syphilis of >1 y duration, without clinical symptoms (late latent syphilis) or syphilis of unknown duration	Benzathine penicillin G 50,000 U/kg (max 2,400,000 U) IM weekly for 3 doses (AIII)	Alternative if allergy to penicillin: doxycycline (patients >7 y) 4 mg/kg/day (max 200 mg/day) PO div bid for 28 days. Look for neurologic, eye, and aortic complications of tertiary syphilis.
Trichomoniasis[42]	Metronidazole 2 g PO as a single dose, OR 500 mg PO bid for 7 days	Tinidazole 50 mg/kg (max 2 g) PO for 1 dose twice daily for 7 days
Urethritis, nongonococcal (See page 79 for gonorrhea therapy.)[42]	Azithromycin 20 mg/kg (max 1 g) PO for 1 dose, OR doxycycline (patients >7 y) 40 mg/kg/day (max 200 mg/day) PO div bid for 7 days (AII)	Erythromycin, levofloxacin, or ofloxacin

I. GENITAL AND SEXUALLY TRANSMITTED INFECTIONS (cont)

Clinical Diagnosis	Therapy (evidence grade)	Comments
Vaginitis[42]		
– Bacterial vaginosis[250]	Metronidazole 500 mg PO twice daily for 7 days or metronidazole vaginal gel (0.75%) qd for 5 days	Alternative: tinidazole 1 g PO qd for 5 days, OR clindamycin 300 mg PO bid for 7 days or clindamycin vaginal cream for 7 days Relapse common Caused by synergy of *Gardnerella* with anaerobes
– Candidiasis, vulvovaginal[42,251]	Fluconazole 5 mg/kg PO (max 150 mg) for 1 dose; topical treatment with azole creams (see Comments).	Many topical vaginal azole agents are available without prescription (eg, butoconazole, clotrimazole, miconazole, tioconazole) and some require a prescription for unique agents or unique dosing regimens (terconazole, butoconazole).
– Prepubertal vaginitis[252]	No prospective studies	Cultures from symptomatic prepubertal girls are statistically more likely to yield *E coli*, enterococcus, coagulase negative staphylococci, and streptococci (viridans strep and group A strep), but these organisms may also be present in asymptomatic girls.
– *Shigella*[253]	Cefixime 8 mg/kg/day PO qd for 5 days OR ciprofloxacin 30 mg/kg/day PO div bid for 5 days	50% have bloody discharge; usually not associated with diarrhea.
– *Streptococcus*, group A[254]	Penicillin V 50–75 mg/kg/day PO div tid for 10 days	Amoxicillin 50–75 mg/kg/day PO div tid

J. CENTRAL NERVOUS SYSTEM INFECTIONS

Clinical Diagnosis	Therapy (evidence grade)	Comments
Abscess, brain (respiratory tract flora, skin flora, or bowel flora, depending on the pathogenesis of infection based on underlying comorbid disease and origin of bacteremia)[255,256]	Until etiology established, cover normal flora of respiratory tract, skin, and/or bowel, based on individual patient evaluation: meropenem 120 mg/kg/day div q8h (AIII); OR nafcillin 150–200 mg/kg/day IV div q6h AND cefotaxime 200–300 mg/kg/day IV div q6h or ceftriaxone 100 mg/kg/day IV q24h AND metronidazole 30 mg/kg/day IV div q8h (BIII); for 2–3 wk after successful drainage (depending on pathogen, size of abscess, and response to therapy); longer course if no surgery (3–6 wk) (BIII)	Surgery for abscesses ≥2 cm diameter. If CA-MRSA suspected, ADD vancomycin 60 mg/kg/day IV div q8h ± rifampin 20 mg/kg/day IV div q12h, pending culture results. If secondary to chronic otitis, include meropenem or cefepime in regimen for anti-*Pseudomonas* activity. Follow abscess size by CT.
Encephalitis[257,258]		
– Amebic (*Naegleria fowleri, Balamuthia mandrillaris,* and *Acanthamoeba*)	See Chapter 10, Amebiasis.	
– CMV[257]	Not studied in children. Consider ganciclovir 10–20 mg/kg/day IV div q12h; for severe immunocompromised, ADD foscarnet 180 mg/kg/day IV div q8h for 3 wk; follow quantitative PCR for CMV.	High-dose ganciclovir[259] IV 20 mg/kg/day div q12h not well studied. Reduce dose for renal insufficiency. Watch for neutropenia.
– Enterovirus	Supportive therapy; no antivirals currently FDA approved	Pocapavir PO is currently under investigation for enterovirus (poliovirus).
– EBV[260]	Not studied. Consider ganciclovir 10–20 mg/kg/day IV div q12h or acyclovir 60 mg/kg/day IV div q8h for 3 wk; follow quantitative PCR for EBV.	Efficacy and toxicity of high-dose ganciclovir and acyclovir are not well defined; some experts recommend against antiviral treatment.[257]

J. CENTRAL NERVOUS SYSTEM INFECTIONS (cont)

Clinical Diagnosis	Therapy (evidence grade)	Comments
– Herpes simplex virus[257,261]	Acyclovir 60 mg/kg/day IV as 1–2 h infusion div q8h; for 21 days for infants ≤4 mo. For older infants and children, 45–60 mg/kg/day IV for 21 days (AIII).	See Chapter 5 for neonatal infection. Safety of high-dose acyclovir (60 mg/kg/day) not well defined beyond the neonatal period; can be used, but monitor for neurotoxicity and nephrotoxicity; FDA has approved acyclovir at this dosage for encephalitis for children up to 12 y.
– *Toxoplasma*	See Chapter 10.	
– Arbovirus (flavivirus—West Nile, St Louis encephalitis, tick-borne encephalitis; togavirus—Western equine encephalitis, Eastern equine encephalitis; bunyavirus—La Crosse encephalitis, California encephalitis)[257,258]	Supportive therapy	Investigational only (antiviral, interferon, immune globulins)
Meningitis, bacterial, community-associated		

NOTES

- In areas where pen-R pneumococci exist (>5% of invasive strains), initial empiric therapy for suspect pneumococcal meningitis should be with vancomycin AND cefotaxime or ceftriaxone until susceptibility test results are available.
- Dexamethasone 0.6 mg/kg/day IV div q6h for 2 days as an adjunct to antibiotic therapy decreases hearing deficits and other neurologic sequelae in adults and children (for *Haemophilus* and pneumococcus; not studied in children for meningococcus or *E coli*). The first dose of dexamethasone is given before or concurrent with the first dose of antibiotic; probably little benefit if given ≥1 h after the antibiotic.[262,263]
- We hope to see more data on osmotic therapy before we recommend it, as early data suggesting benefits of oral glycerol have not yet been substantiated.[264,265]

Clinical Diagnosis	Therapy (evidence grade)	Comments
– Empiric therapy[266]	Cefotaxime 200–300 mg/kg/day IV div q6h, or ceftriaxone 100 mg/kg/day IV q24h; AND vancomycin 60 mg/kg/day IV div q8h (AII)	If Gram stain or cultures demonstrate a pathogen other than pneumococcus, vancomycin is not needed; vancomycin used empirically only for possible pen-R pneumococcus.

– *H influenzae* type b[266]	Cefotaxime 200–300 mg/kg/day IV div q6h, or ceftriaxone 100 mg/kg/day IV q24h; for 10 days (AI)	Alternative: ampicillin 200–400 mg/kg/day IV div q6h (for beta-lactamase–negative strains) OR chloramphenicol 100 mg/kg/day IV div q6h
– Meningococcus (*Neisseria meningitidis*)[266]	Penicillin G 250,000 U/kg/day IV div q4h; or ceftriaxone 100 mg/kg/day IV q24h, or cefotaxime 200 mg/kg/day IV div q6h; treatment course for 7 days (AI)	Meningococcal prophylaxis: rifampin 10 mg/kg PO q12h for 4 doses OR ceftriaxone 125–250 mg IM once OR ciprofloxacin 500 mg PO once (adolescents and adults)
– Neonatal	See Chapter 5.	
– Pneumococcus (*S pneumoniae*)[266]	For pen-S and cephalosporin-susceptible strains: penicillin G 250,000 U/kg/day IV div q4–6h, OR ceftriaxone 100 mg/kg/day IV q24h or cefotaxime 200–300 mg/kg/day IV div q6h; for 10 days (AI). For pen-R pneumococci: continue the combination of vancomycin and cephalosporin IV for total course (AIII).	Some pneumococci may be resistant to penicillin but susceptible to cefotaxime and ceftriaxone and may be treated with the cephalosporin alone. Test-of-cure LP helpful in those with pen-R pneumococci.
Meningitis, TB (*M tuberculosis; M bovis*)[13,14]	For non-immunocompromised children: INH 15 mg/kg/day PO, IV div q12–24h AND rifampin 15 mg/kg/day PO, IV, div q12–24h for 12 mo AND PZA 30 mg/kg/day PO div q12–24h for first 2 mo of therapy, AND streptomycin 30 mg/kg/day IV, IM div q12h for first 4–8 wk of therapy until susceptibility test results available. For recommendations for drug-resistant strains and treatment of TB in HIV-infected patients, visit the CDC Web site for TB: www.cdc.gov/tb.	Hyponatremia from inappropriate ADH secretion is common; ventricular drainage may be necessary for obstructive hydrocephalus. Corticosteroids (can use the same dexamethasone dose as for bacterial meningitis, 0.6 mg/kg/day IV div q6h) for 2–4 wk until neurologically stable, then taper dose for 1–3 mo to decrease neurologic complications and improve prognosis by decreasing the incidence of infarction.[267]

J. CENTRAL NERVOUS SYSTEM INFECTIONS (cont)

Clinical Diagnosis	Therapy (evidence grade)	Comments
Shunt infections: The use of antibiotic-impregnated shunts has decreased the frequency of this infection.[268] Shunt removal is usually necessary for cure.[269]		
– Empiric therapy pending Gram stain and culture[266,269]	Vancomycin 60 mg/kg/day IV div q8h, AND ceftriaxone 100 mg/kg/day IV q24h (AII)	If Gram stain shows only gram-positive cocci, can use vancomycin alone. Cefepime or meropenem should be used instead of ceftriaxone if *Pseudomonas* is suspected.
– *S epidermidis* or *S aureus*[266,269]	Vancomycin (for *S epidermidis* and CA-MRSA) 60 mg/kg/day IV div q8h; OR nafcillin (if organisms susceptible) 150–200 mg/kg/day AND (if severe infection or slow response) gentamicin or rifampin; for 10–14 days (AIII)	Shunt removal usually necessary; may need to treat with ventriculostomy until ventricular CSF cultures negative; obtain CSF cultures at time of shunt replacement, continue therapy an additional 48–72 h pending cultures. For children who cannot tolerate vancomycin, ceftaroline has anecdotally been successful.
– Gram-negative bacilli[266,269]	Empiric therapy with meropenem 120 mg/kg/day IV div q8h OR cefepime 150 mg/kg/day IV div q8h (AIII) For *E coli:* ceftriaxone 100 mg/kg/day IV q12h OR cefotaxime 200–300 mg/kg/day IV div q6h; ADD gentamicin 6–7.5 mg/kg/day IV until CSF sterile; for 21 days or longer	Remove shunt. Select appropriate therapy based on in vitro susceptibilities. Intrathecal therapy with aminoglycosides not routinely necessary with highly active beta-lactam therapy and shunt removal.

K. URINARY TRACT INFECTIONS

Clinical Diagnosis	Therapy (evidence grade)	Comments
NOTE: Antibiotic susceptibility profiles of *E coli,* the most common cause of UTI, vary considerably. For mild disease, TMP/SMX may be started as initial therapy if local susceptibility ≥80% and a 20% failure rate is acceptable. For moderate to severe disease (possible pyelonephritis), obtain cultures and begin oral 2nd- or 3rd-generation cephalosporins (cefuroxime, cefaclor, cefprozil, cefixime, ceftibuten, cefdinir, cefpodoxime), ciprofloxacin PO, or ceftriaxone IM. Antibiotic susceptibility testing will help direct your therapy to the most narrow spectrum agent.		
Cystitis, acute (*E coli*)[270,271]	For mild disease: TMP/SMX 8 mg/kg/day of TMP PO div bid for 3 days (See NOTE above about resistance to TMP/SMX.) For moderate to severe disease: cefixime 8 mg/kg/day PO qd; OR ceftriaxone 50 mg/kg IM q24h for 3–5 days (with normal anatomy) (BII); follow-up culture after 36–48 h treatment ONLY if still symptomatic	Alternative: amoxicillin 30 mg/kg/day PO div tid if susceptible (BII); ciprofloxacin 15–20 mg/kg/day PO div bid for otherwise resistant organisms
Nephronia, lobar *E coli* and other enteric rods (also called focal bacterial nephritis)[272,273]	Ceftriaxone 50 mg/kg/day IV, IM q24h. Duration depends on resolution of cellulitis vs development of abscess (10–21 days) (AIII).	Invasive, consolidative parenchymal infection; complication of pyelonephritis, can evolve into renal abscess. Step down therapy with oral cephalosporins once cellulitis/abscess has initially responded to therapy.
Pyelonephritis, acute (*E coli*)[270,271,274–276]	Ceftriaxone 50 mg/kg/day IV, IM q24h OR gentamicin 5–6 mg/kg/day IV, IM q24h. For documented or suspected ceftriaxone-resistant ESBL-positive strains, use meropenem IV, imipenem IV, or ertapenem IV; OR gentamicin IV, IM. Switch to oral therapy following clinical response (BII). If organism resistant to amoxicillin and TMP/SMX, use an oral 2nd- or 3rd-generation cephalosporin (BII); if cephalosporin-R, can use ciprofloxacin PO 30 mg/kg/day div q12h (BIII); for 7–10 days total (depending on response to therapy).	For mild to moderate infection, oral therapy is likely to be as effective as IV/IM therapy for susceptible strains, down to 3 mo of age. If bacteremia documented, and infant is <2–3 mo, rule out meningitis and treat 14 days IV + PO (AIII). Aminoglycosides at any dose are more nephrotoxic than beta-lactams (AI).
Recurrent urinary tract infection, prophylaxis[270,277–279]	Only for those with grade III–V reflux or with recurrent febrile UTI: TMP/SMX 2 mg/kg/dose of TMP PO qd OR nitrofurantoin 1–2 mg/kg PO qd at bedtime; more rapid resistance may develop using beta-lactams (BII).	Prophylaxis no longer recommended for patients with grade I–II reflux and no evidence of renal damage. Early treatment of new infections is recommended for these children. Resistance eventually develops to every antibiotic; follow resistance patterns for each patient.

L. MISCELLANEOUS SYSTEMIC INFECTIONS

Clinical Diagnosis	Therapy (evidence grade)	Comments
Actinomycosis[280,281]	Penicillin G 250,000 U/kg/day IV div q6h, or ampicillin 150 mg/kg/day IV div q8h until improved (often up to 6 wk); then long-term convalescent therapy with penicillin V 100 mg/kg/day (up to 4 g/day) PO for 6–12 mo (AII)	Surgery as indicated Alternatives: amoxicillin, clindamycin, erythromycin; ceftriaxone IM/IV, doxycycline for children >7 y
Anaplasmosis (human granulocytotropic anaplasmosis, *Anaplasma phagocytophilum*)	Doxycycline 4 mg/kg/day IV, PO (max 200 mg/day) div bid for 7–10 days (regardless of age) (AIII)	For mild disease, consider rifampin 20 mg/kg/day PO div bid for 7–10 days (BIII).
Anthrax, sepsis/pneumonia (inhalation, cutaneous, gastrointestinal)[15,282,283]	For bioterror-associated infection (regardless of age): ciprofloxacin 20–30 mg/kg/day IV div q12h, OR levofloxacin 16 mg/kg/day IV div q12h not to exceed 250 mg/dose (AIII); OR doxycycline 4 mg/kg/day PO (max 200 mg/day) div bid (regardless of age)	For oral step-down therapy, can use oral ciprofloxacin or doxycycline; if susceptible, can use penicillin, amoxicillin, or clindamycin. For community-associated anthrax infection, amoxicillin 75 mg/kg/day div q8h or doxycycline for children >7 y should be effective.
Appendicitis (See Peritonitis.)		
Brucellosis[284–287]	Doxycycline 4 mg/kg/day PO (max 200 mg/day) div bid (for children >7 y) AND rifampin (15–20 mg/kg/day div q12h) (BIII); OR for children <8 y: TMP/SMX 10 mg/kg/day TMP IV, PO div q12h AND rifampin 15–20 mg/kg/day div q12h (BIII); for 4–8 wk	Combination therapy with rifampin will decrease the risk of relapse. ADD gentamicin 6–7.5 mg/kg/day IV, IM div q8h for the first 1–2 wk of therapy to further decrease risk of relapse[286] (BIII), particularly for endocarditis, osteomyelitis, or meningitis. Prolonged treatment for 4–6 mo and surgical debridement may be necessary for deep infections (AIII).

Cat-scratch disease (*Bartonella henselae*)[288,289]	Supportive (incision and drainage of infected lymph node); azithromycin 12 mg/kg/day PO qd for 5 days shortens the duration of adenopathy (AIII).	This dosage of azithromycin has been documented to be safe and effective for streptococcal pharyngitis and may offer greater deep tissue exposure than the dosage studied by Bass et al[8] and used for otitis media. No prospective data exist for invasive infections: gentamicin (for 14 days) AND TMP/SMX AND rifampin for hepatosplenic disease and osteomyelitis (AIII). For CNS infection, use cefotaxime AND gentamicin ± TMP/SMX (AIII). Alternatives: ciprofloxacin, doxycycline.
Chickenpox/Shingles (varicella-zoster virus)[290,291]	Acyclovir 30 mg/kg/day IV as 1–2 h infusion div q8h; for 10 days (acyclovir doses of 45–60 mg/kg/day in 3 divided doses IV should be used for disseminated or CNS infection). Dosing can also be provided as 1,500 mg/m²/day IV div q8h. Duration in immunocompromised children: 7–14 days, based on clinical response (AI). For treatment in normal immunocompetent children, acyclovir 80 mg/kg/day PO div qid, for 5 days (AI). Valacyclovir pharmacokinetics have been assessed in an extemporaneously[291] compounded suspension of crushed tablets and simple syrup (60 mg/kg/day div tid) for children 3 mo to 12 y; instructions for preparation provided in package insert, and shelf life is 28 days.	See Chapter 9; therapy for 10 days in immunocompromised children. Famciclovir can be made into a suspension with 25-mg and 100-mg sprinkle capsules.[292] See Chapter 9 for dosages by body weight. No treatment data in children (CIII).
Ehrlichiosis (human monocytic ehrlichiosis, caused by *Ehrlichia chaffeensis,* and *Ehrlichia ewingii*)[293–296]	Doxycycline 4 mg/kg/day IV, PO div bid (max 100 mg/dose) for 7–10 days (regardless of age) (AIII)	For mild disease, consider rifampin 20 mg/kg/day PO div bid (max 300 mg/dose) for 7–10 days (BIII)

L. MISCELLANEOUS SYSTEMIC INFECTIONS (cont)

Clinical Diagnosis	Therapy (evidence grade)	Comments
Febrile neutropenic patient (empiric therapy of invasive infection: *Pseudomonas,* enteric gram-negative bacilli, staphylococci, streptococci, yeast, fungi)[297]	Cefepime 150 mg/kg/day div q8h (AI); or meropenem 60 mg/kg/day div q8h (AII); OR ceftazidime 150 mg/kg/day IV div q8h AND tobramycin 6 mg/kg/day IV q8h (AII). ADD vancomycin 40 mg/kg/day IV div q8h if MRSA or coagulation-negative staph suspected (eg, central catheter infection) (AIII). ADD metronidazole to ceftazidime or cefepime if colitis or other deep anaerobic infection suspected (AIII).	Alternatives: other anti-*Pseudomonas* beta-lactams (imipenem, pip/tazo) AND anti-staphylococcal antibiotics. If no response in 4–7 days and no alternative etiology demonstrated, begin additional empiric therapy with antifungals (BII); dosages and formulations outlined in Chapter 8. For low-risk patients with close follow-up, oral therapy with amox/clav and ciprofloxacin may be used.
Human immunodeficiency virus infection	See Chapter 9.	
Infant botulism[298]	Botulism immune globulin for infants (BabyBIG) 50 mg/kg IV for 1 dose (AI); BabyBIG can be obtained from the California Department of Public Health at www.infantbotulism.org.	www.infantbotulism.org provides information for physicians and parents. Web site organized by the California Department of Public Health (accessed October 10, 2014). Aminoglycosides should be avoided because they potentiate the neuromuscular effect of botulinum toxin.
Kawasaki syndrome[299–303]	No antibiotics; IVIG 2 g/kg as single dose (AI); may need to repeat dose in up to 15% of children for persisting fever that lasts 24 hours after completion of the IVIG infusion (AII). For subsequent relapse, consult an infectious disease physician or pediatric cardiologist.	Aspirin 80–100 mg/kg/day div qid in acute, febrile phase; once afebrile for 24–48 h, initiate low-dosage (3–5 mg/kg/day) aspirin therapy for 6–8 wk (assuming echocardiogram is normal). Role of corticosteroids,[300,301] infliximab,[302] and calcineurin inhibitors for IVIG-resistant Kawasaki syndrome under investigation but may improve outcome in severe cases.
Leprosy (Hansen disease)[304]	Dapsone 1 mg/kg/day PO qd AND rifampin 10 mg/kg/day PO qd; ADD (for multibacillary disease) clofazimine 1 mg/kg/day PO qd; for 12 mo for paucibacillary disease; for 24 mo for multibacillary disease (AII)	Consult Health Resources and Services Administration National Hansen's Disease (Leprosy) Program at www.hrsa.gov/hansensdisease (accessed October 10, 2014) for advice about treatment and free antibiotics: 800/642-2477.

Leptospirosis[305,306]	Penicillin G 250,000 U/kg/day IV, IM div q6h, or ceftriaxone 50 mg/kg/day q24h; for 7 days (BII) For mild disease, doxycycline (>7 y) 4 mg/kg/day (max 200 mg/day) PO div bid for 7–10 days and for those ≤7 y or intolerant of doxycycline, azithromycin 20 mg/kg on day 1, 10 mg/kg on days 2 and 3 (BII)	Alternative: amoxicillin for children ≤7 y of age with mild disease
Lyme disease (*Borrelia burgdorferi*)[295,307]	Neurologic evaluation, including LP, if there is clinical suspicion of CNS involvement	
– Early localized disease	>7 y of age: doxycycline 4 mg/kg/day (max 200 mg/day) PO div bid for 14–21 days (AII) ≤7 y of age: amoxicillin 50 mg/kg/day (max 1.5 g/day) PO div tid for 14–21 days (AII)	Alternative: erythromycin 30 mg/kg/day PO div tid
– Arthritis (no CNS disease)	Oral therapy as outlined previously; for 28 days (AIII)	Persistent or recurrent joint swelling after treatment: repeat a 4-wk course of oral antibiotics or give ceftriaxone 75–100 mg/kg IV q24h OR penicillin 300,000 U/kg/day IV div q4h; either for 14–28 days
– Erythema migrans	Oral therapy as outlined previously; for 21 days (AIII)	
– Isolated facial (Bell) palsy	Oral therapy as outlined previously; for 21–28 days (AIII)	LP is not routinely required unless CNS symptoms present. Treatment to prevent late sequelae; will not provide a quick response for palsy.
– Carditis	Ceftriaxone 75–100 mg/kg IV q24h IV OR penicillin 300,000 U/kg/day IV div q4h; for 14–21 days (AIII)	
– Neuroborreliosis	Ceftriaxone 75–100 mg/kg IV q24h, or penicillin G 300,000 U/kg/day IV div q4h; for 14–28 days (AIII)	
Melioidosis (*Burkholderia pseudomallei*)[308–310]	Acute sepsis: meropenem 75 mg/kg/day div q8h; OR ceftazidime 150 mg/kg/day IV div q8h; followed by TMP/SMX (10 mg/kg/day of TMP) PO div bid for 3–6 mo	Alternative convalescent therapy: amox/clav (90 mg/kg/day amox div tid, not bid) for children ≤7 y, or doxycycline for children >7 y; for 20 wk (AII)

L. MISCELLANEOUS SYSTEMIC INFECTIONS (cont)

Clinical Diagnosis	Therapy (evidence grade)	Comments
Mycobacteria, nontuberculous[8–12,311]		
– Adenitis in normal host (See Adenitis entries in Table 6A.)	Excision usually curative (BII); azithromycin PO OR clarithromycin PO for 6–12 wk (with or without rifampin) if susceptible (BII)	Antibiotic susceptibility patterns are quite variable; cultures should guide therapy; medical therapy 60%–70% effective. Newer data suggest toxicity of antimicrobials may not be worth the small clinical benefit.
– Pneumonia or disseminated infection in compromised hosts (HIV or gamma-interferon receptor deficiency)	Usually treated with 3 or 4 active drugs (eg, clarithromycin OR azithromycin, AND amikacin, cefoxitin, meropenem). Also test for ciprofloxacin, TMP/SMX, ethambutol, rifampin, linezolid, clofazimine, and doxycycline (BII).	See Chapter 11 for dosages; cultures are essential, as the susceptibility patterns of nontuberculous mycobacteria are varied.
Nocardiosis (*Nocardia asteroides* and *Nocardia brasiliensis*)[312,313]	TMP/SMX 8 mg/kg/day TMP div bid or sulfisoxazole 120–150 mg/kg/day PO div qid for 6–12 wk or longer. For severe infection, particularly in immunocompromised hosts, use ceftriaxone or imipenem AND amikacin 15–20 mg/kg/day IM, IV div q8h (AIII).	Wide spectrum of disease from skin lesions to brain abscess Surgery when indicated Alternatives: doxycycline (for children >7 y of age), amox/clav, or linezolid
Plague (*Yersinia pestis*)[314–316]	Gentamicin 7.5 mg/kg/day IV div q8h (AII)	Doxycycline 4 mg/kg/day (max 200 mg/day) PO div bid or ciprofloxacin 30 mg/kg/day PO div bid
Q fever (*Coxiella burnetii*)[317,318]	Acute stage: doxycycline 4.4 mg/kg/day (max 200 mg/day) PO div bid for 14 days (AII) for children of any age. Endocarditis and chronic disease (ongoing symptoms for 6–12 mo): doxycycline for children >7 y AND hydroxychloroquine for 18–36 mo (AIII). Seek advice from pediatric infectious disease specialist for children ≤7 y: may require TMP-SMX, 8–10 mg TMP/kg/day div q12h with doxycycline; or levofloxacin with rifampin for 18 mo.	Follow doxycycline and hydroxychloroquine serum concentrations during endocarditis/chronic disease therapy. CNS: Use fluoroquinolone (no prospective data) (BIII). Clarithromycin may be an alternative based on limited data (CIII).

Rocky Mountain spotted fever (fever, petechial rash with centripetal spread; *Rickettsia rickettsii*)[319,320]	Doxycycline 4.4 mg/kg/day (max 200 mg/day) PO div bid for 7–10 days (AI) for children of any age	Start empiric therapy early.
Tetanus (*Clostridium tetani*)[321,322]	Metronidazole 30 mg/kg/day IV, PO div q8h or penicillin G 100,000 U/kg/day IV div q6h for 10–14 days AND TIG 3,000–6,000 U IM (AII)	Wound debridement essential; IVIG may provide antibody to toxin if TIG not available. Immunize with Td or Tdap. See Chapter 14 for prophylaxis recommendations.
Toxic shock syndrome (toxin-producing strains of *S aureus* [including MRSA] or group A streptococcus)[6,7,323,324]	Empiric: vancomycin 45 mg/kg/day IV div q8h AND oxacillin/nafcillin 150 mg/kg/day IV div q6h, AND clindamycin 30–40 mg/kg/day div q8h ± gentamicin for 7–10 days (AIII)	Clindamycin added for the initial 48–72 h of therapy to decrease toxin production; IVIG has a theoretical benefit and may bind circulating toxin (CIII). For MSSA: oxacillin/nafcillin AND clindamycin ± gentamicin. For CA-MRSA: vancomycin AND clindamycin ± gentamicin. For group A streptococcus: penicillin G AND clindamycin.
Tularemia (*Francisella tularensis*)[152,325]	Gentamicin 6–7.5 mg/kg/day IM, IV div q8h; for 10–14 days (AII)	Alternatives: doxycycline (for 14–21 days) or ciprofloxacin (for 10 days)

7. Preferred Therapy for Specific Bacterial and Mycobacterial Pathogens

NOTES

- For fungal, viral, and parasitic infections, see chapters 8, 9, and 10, respectively.
- Limitations of space do not permit listing of all possible alternative antimicrobials.
- **Abbreviations:** amox/clav, amoxicillin/clavulanate (Augmentin); amp/sul, ampicillin/sulbactam (Unasyn); CA-MRSA, community-associated methicillin-resistant *Staphylococcus aureus;* CDC, Centers for Disease Control and Prevention; CNS, central nervous system; CRE, carbapenem-resistant *Enterobacteriaceae;* ESBL, extended spectrum beta-lactamase; FDA, US Food and Drug Administration; HRSA, Health Resources and Services Administration; IM, intramuscular; IV, intravenous; KPC, *Klebsiella pneumoniae* carbapenemase; MDR, multidrug resistant; MIC, minimal inhibitory concentration; MRSA, methicillin-resistant *S aureus;* MSSA, methicillin-susceptible *S aureus;* NARMS, National Antimicrobial Resistance Monitoring System for Enteric Bacteria; pen-S, penicillin-susceptible; pip/tazo, piperacillin/tazobactam (Zosyn); PO, oral; PZA, pyrazinamide; spp, species; ticar/clav, ticarcillin/clavulanate (Timentin); TMP/SMX, trimethoprim/sulfamethoxazole; UTI, urinary tract infection.

A. COMMON BACTERIAL PATHOGENS AND USUAL PATTERN OF SUSCEPTIBILITY TO ANTIBIOTICS (GRAM POSITIVE)

	Commonly Used Antibiotics (One Agent per Class Listed)			
	Penicillin	Ampicillin/ Amoxicillin	Amoxicillin/ Clavulanate	Methicillin/ Oxacillin
Enterococcus faecalis[a]	++	++	++	⦸
Enterococcus faecium[a]	++	++	++	⦸
Staphylococcus, coagulase negative	⦸	⦸	⦸	+
Staphylococcus aureus, methicillin-resistant	⦸	⦸	⦸	⦸
Staphylococcus aureus, methicillin-susceptible	⦸	⦸	⦸	+++
Streptococcus pneumoniae	+++	+++	+++	++
Streptococcus pyogenes	+++	+++	+++	+++

NOTE: +++ = very active (>90% of isolates are susceptible in most locations); ++ = some decreased susceptibility (substantially less active in vitro or resistance in isolates between 10% and 30% in some locations); + = significant resistance (30%–80% in some locations); ⦸ = don't even think about it.

[a]Need to add gentamicin or other aminoglycoside to ampicillin/penicillin or vancomycin for in vitro bactericidal activity.

Commonly Used Antibiotics (One Agent per Class Listed)					
				Approved for Adults Some Studies in Children	
Cefazolin/ Cephalexin	Vancomycin	Clindamycin	Linezolid	Daptomycin	Ceftaroline
⊘	++	⊘	++	+++	⊘
⊘	++	⊘	++	++	⊘
+	+++	++	+++	+++	+++
⊘	+++	++	+++	+++	+++
+++	+++	++	+++	+++	+++
+++	+++	+++	+++	+++	+++
+++	+++	+++	+++	+++	+++

B. COMMON BACTERIAL PATHOGENS AND USUAL PATTERN OF SUSCEPTIBILITY TO ANTIBIOTICS (GRAM NEGATIVE)[a]

	Commonly Used Antibiotics (One Agent per Class Listed)				
	Ampicillin/ Amoxicillin	**Amoxicillin/ Clavulanate**	**Cefazolin/ Cephalexin**	**Cefuroxime**	**Ceftriaxone/ Cefotaxime**
Acinetobacter spp	⊘	⊘	⊘	⊘	++
Citrobacter spp	⊘	⊘	⊘	++	++
Enterobacter spp[b]	⊘	⊘	⊘	+	++
Escherichia coli[c]	+	++	++	+++[d]	+++[d]
Haemophilus influenzae[f]	+++	+++	+++	+++	+++
Klebsiella spp[c]	⊘	⊘	++	+++	+++
Neisseria meningitidis	+++	+++	-	+++	+++
Pseudomonas aeruginosa	⊘	⊘	⊘	⊘	⊘
Salmonella, non-typhoid spp	++	+++	–	–	+++
Serratia spp[b]	⊘	⊘	⊘	+	++
Shigella spp	++	++	–	++	+++
Stenotrophomonas maltophilia	⊘	⊘	⊘	⊘	⊘

NOTE: +++ = very active (<10% of isolates are resistant in most locations); ++ = some decreased susceptibility (substantially less active in vitro with higher MICs or resistance in isolates between 10% and 30% in some locations); + = significant resistance (30%–80% in some locations); ⊘ = don't even think about it; – = not usually tested for susceptibility for treatment of infections (resistant or has not previously been considered for routine therapy, so little data exist).

[a]CDC (NARMS) statistics and SENTRY surveillance system (JMI Laboratories) as primary references; also using current antibiograms from Children's Medical Center, Dallas, TX, and Rady Children's Hospital San Diego to assess pediatric trends. When sufficient data are available, pediatric community isolate susceptibility data are used. Nosocomial resistance patterns may be quite different, usually with increased resistance, particularly in adults; please check your local/regional hospital antibiogram for your local susceptibility patterns.

[b]AmpC will be constitutively produced in low frequency in every population of organisms and will be selected out during therapy with third-generation cephalosporins if used as single agent therapy.

[c]Rare carbapenem resistant isolates in pediatrics (KPC, KPC strains)

[d]Will be resistant to virtually all current cephalosporins if ESBL producing.

[e]Follow the MIC, not the report for susceptable (S), intermediate (I), or resistant (R), as some ESBL producers will have low MICs and can be effectively treated with higher dosages.

[f]Will be resistant to ampicillin/amoxicillin if beta-lactamase producing.

Commonly Used Antibiotics (One Agent per Class Listed)

Ceftazidime	Cefepime	Meropenem/ Imipenem	Piperacillin/ Tazobactam	TMP/SMX	Ciprofloxacin	Gentamicin
++	++	+++	++	++	++	+++
++	+++	+++	++	+++	+++	+++
++	+++	+++	++	++	+++	+++
+++[d]	+++[e]	+++	+++	++	+++	+++
+++	+++	+++	+++	+++	+++	+
+++	+++[e]	+++	+++	+++	+++	+++
++	+++	+++	+++	–	+++	–
++	+++	+++	+++	⃠	+++	++
+++	+++	+++	+++	+++	+++	–
++	+++	+++	++	+++	+++	+++
+++	+++	+++	+++	+	+++	–
++	+	+	++	+++	+++	+

C. COMMON BACTERIAL PATHOGENS AND USUAL PATTERN OF SUSCEPTIBILITY TO ANTIBIOTICS (ANAEROBES)

Common Bacterial Pathogens: Anaerobes	Commonly Used Antibiotics (One Agent per Class Listed)				
	Penicillin	Ampicillin/ Amoxicillin	Amoxicillin/ Clavulanate	Cefazolin	Cefoxitin
Anaerobic streptococci	+++	+++	+++	+++	+++
Bacteroides fragilis	+	+	+++	⃠	++
Clostridia (eg, *tetani, perfringens*)	+++	+++	+++	–	++
Clostridium difficile	⃠	⃠	⃠	–	⃠

NOTE: +++ = very active (<10% of isolates are susceptible in most locations); ++ = some decreased susceptibility (substantially less active in vitro or resistance in isolates between 10% and 30% in some locations); + = significant decreased susceptibility (with high minimum inhibitory concentrations or full resistance between 30% and 80% in some locations); ⃠ = don't even think about it; – = not usually tested for susceptibility for treatment of infections (resistant or has not previously been considered for routine therapy, so little data exist).

Commonly Used Antibiotics (One Agent per Class Listed)					
Ceftriaxone/ Cefotaxime	Meropenem/ Imipenem	Piperacillin/ Tazobactam	Metronidazole	Clindamycin	Vancomycin
+++	+++	+++	+++	+++	+++
⃠	+++	+++	+++	++	x
+	+++	+++	+++	++	+++
⃠	+++	–	+++	⃠	+++

D. PREFERRED THERAPY FOR SPECIFIC BACTERIAL AND MYCOBACTERIAL PATHOGENS

Organism	Clinical Illness	Drug of Choice (evidence grade)	Alternatives
Acinetobacter baumanii[1–4]	Sepsis, meningitis, nosocomial pneumonia	Meropenem (BIII) or other carbapenem	Use culture results to guide therapy: ceftazidime, amp/sul; pip/tazo; TMP/SMX; ciprofloxacin; tigecycline; colistin. Watch for emergence of resistance *during* therapy. Consider combination therapy for life-threatening infection to prevent emergence of resistance. Inhaled colistin for pneumonia caused by MDR strains (BIII).
Actinomyces israelii[5]	Actinomycosis (cervicofacial, thoracic, abdominal)	Penicillin G; ampicillin (CIII)	Amoxicillin; doxycycline; clindamycin; ceftriaxone; imipenem
Aeromonas hydrophila[6]	Diarrhea	Ciprofloxacin (CIII)	Azithromycin, cefepime, TMP/SMX
	Sepsis, cellulitis, necrotizing fasciitis	Ceftazidime (BIII)	Cefepime; ceftriaxone, meropenem; ciprofloxacin
Aggregatibacter (formerly *Actinobacillus*) *actinomycetemcomitans*[7]	Periodontitis, abscesses (including brain), endocarditis	Ampicillin (amoxicillin) ± gentamicin (CIII)	Doxycycline; TMP/SMX; ciprofloxacin; ceftriaxone
Anaplasma (formerly *Ehrlichia*) *phagocytophilum*[8,9]	Human granulocytic anaplasmosis	Doxycycline (all ages) (AII)	Rifampin
Arcanobacterium haemolyticum[10]	Pharyngitis, cellulitis, Lemierre syndrome	Erythromycin; penicillin (BIII)	Azithromycin, amoxicillin, clindamycin; doxycycline; vancomycin
Bacillus anthracis[11]	Anthrax (cutaneous, gastro-intestinal, inhalational, meningoencephalitis)	Ciprofloxacin (regardless of age) (AIII). For invasive, systemic infection, use combination therapy.	Doxycycline; amoxicillin, levofloxacin, clindamycin; penicillin G; vancomycin, meropenem

Bacillus cereus or *subtilis*[12,13]	Sepsis; toxin-mediated gastroenteritis	Vancomycin (BIII)	Ciprofloxacin, linezolid, daptomycin
Bacteroides fragilis[14,15]	Peritonitis, sepsis, abscesses	Metronidazole (AI)	Meropenem or imipenem (AI); ticar/clav; pip/tazo (AI); amox/clav (BII). Recent surveillance suggests resistance of up to 25% for clindamycin.
Bacteroides, other spp[14,15]	Pneumonia, sepsis, abscesses	Metronidazole (BII)	Meropenem or imipenem; penicillin G or ampicillin if beta-lactamase negative
Bartonella henselae[16,17]	Cat-scratch disease	Azithromycin for lymph node disease (BII); gentamicin in combination with TMP/SMX AND rifampin for invasive disease (BIII)	Cefotaxime; ciprofloxacin; doxycycline
Bartonella quintana[18]	Bacillary angiomatosis, peliosis hepatis	Gentamicin plus doxycycline (BIII); erythromycin; ciprofloxacin (BIII)	Azithromycin; doxycycline
Bordetella pertussis, parapertussis[19,20]	Pertussis	Azithromycin (AIII); erythromycin (BII)	Clarithromycin; TMP/SMX; ampicillin
Borrelia burgdorferi, Lyme disease[21–23]	Treatment based on stage of infection (See Lyme disease in Chapter 6.)	Doxycycline if >8 y (AII); amoxicillin or erythromycin in children ≤7 y (AIII); ceftriaxone IV for meningitis (AII)	
Borrelia hermsii, turicatae, parkeri, tick-borne relapsing fever[24,25]	Relapsing fever	Doxycycline for all ages (AIII)	Penicillin or erythromycin in children intolerant of doxycycline (BIII)
Borrelia recurrentis, louse-borne relapsing fever[24,25]	Relapsing fever	Single-dose doxycycline for all ages (AIII)	Penicillin or erythromycin in children intolerant of doxycycline (BIII)

D. PREFERRED THERAPY FOR SPECIFIC BACTERIAL AND MYCOBACTERIAL PATHOGENS (cont)

Organism	Clinical Illness	Drug of Choice (evidence grade)	Alternatives
Brucella spp[26–28]	Brucellosis (See Chapter 6.)	Doxycycline AND rifampin (BIII); OR, for children <8 y: TMP/SMX AND rifampin (BIII)	For serious infection: doxycycline AND gentamicin; or TMP/SMX AND gentamicin (AIII)
Burkholderia cepacia complex[29–31]	Pneumonia, sepsis in immunocompromised children; pneumonia in children with cystic fibrosis[32]	Meropenem (BIII); for severe disease, ADD tobramycin AND TMP/SMX (AIII)	Imipenem, doxycycline; ceftazidime; pip/tazo; ciprofloxacin. Aerosolized antibiotics may provide higher concentrations in lung.[31]
Burkholderia pseudomallei[33–35]	Melioidosis	Meropenem (AIII) or ceftazidime (BIII); followed by prolonged TMP/SMX for 12 wk (AII)	TMP/SMX, doxycycline, or amox/clav for chronic disease
Campylobacter fetus[36]	Sepsis, meningitis in the neonate	Meropenem (BIII)	Cefotaxime; gentamicin; erythromycin
Campylobacter jejuni[37–39]	Diarrhea	Azithromycin (BII); erythromycin (BII)	Doxycycline; ciprofloxacin (very high rates of ciprofloxacin-resistant strains in Thailand, Hong Kong, and Spain)
Capnocytophaga canimorsus[40,41]	Sepsis after dog bite	Pip/tazo OR meropenem; amox/clav (BIII)	Clindamycin; linezolid; penicillin G; ciprofloxacin
Capnocytophaga ochracea[42]	Sepsis, abscesses	Clindamycin (BIII); amox/clav (BIII)	Meropenem; pip/tazo
Chlamydia trachomatis[43–45]	Lymphogranuloma venereum	Doxycycline (AII)	Azithromycin; erythromycin
	Urethritis, cervicitis	Doxycycline (AII)	Azithromycin; erythromycin; ofloxacin
	Inclusion conjunctivitis of newborn	Azithromycin (AIII)	Erythromycin
	Pneumonia of infancy	Azithromycin (AIII)	Erythromycin; ampicillin
	Trachoma	Azithromycin (AI)	Doxycycline; erythromycin

Chlamydophila (formerly *Chlamydia*) *pneumoniae*[46,47]	Pneumonia	Azithromycin (AII); erythromycin (AII)	Doxycycline; ciprofloxacin
Chlamydophila (formerly *Chlamydia*) *psittaci*[48]	Psittacosis	Azithromycin (AIII); erythromycin (AIII)	Doxycycline
Chromobacterium violaceum[49,50]	Sepsis, pneumonia, abscesses	Meropenem AND ciprofloxacin (AIII)	Imipenem, TMP/SMX
Citrobacter koseri (diversus) and *freundii*[51–53]	Meningitis, sepsis	Meropenem (AIII)	Cefepime; ciprofloxacin; ceftriaxone AND gentamicin; TMP/SMX Carbapenem-resistant strains now reported
Clostridium botulinum[54–56]	Botulism: foodborne; wound; potentially bioterror related	Botulism antitoxin heptavalent (equine) types A–G is now FDA approved (www.fda.gov/downloads/BiologicsBloodVaccines/BloodBloodProducts/ApprovedProducts/LicensedProductsBLAs/FractionatedPlasma Products/UCM345147.pdf). No antibiotic treatment.	For more information, call your state health department or the CDC Emergency Operations Center, 770/488-7100 (accessed October 23, 2014).
	Infant botulism	Human botulism immune globulin for infants (BabyBIG) (AII) No antibiotic treatment	BabyBIG available nationally from the California Department of Public Health at 510/231-7600 (www.infantbotulism.org) (accessed October 10, 2014, 2014)
Clostridium difficile[57,58]	Antibiotic-associated colitis (See Chapter 6, Table 6H, Gastrointestinal Infections, *Clostridium difficile*.)	Metronidazole PO (AI)	Vancomycin PO for metronidazole failures; stop the predisposing antimicrobial therapy, if possible. No pediatric data on fidaxomicin PO. No pediatric data on fecal transplantation for recurrent disease.

D. PREFERRED THERAPY FOR SPECIFIC BACTERIAL AND MYCOBACTERIAL PATHOGENS (cont)

Organism	Clinical Illness	Drug of Choice (evidence grade)	Alternatives
Clostridium perfringens[59,60]	Gas gangrene/necrotizing fasciitis/sepsis (also caused by *C sordellii, C septicum, C novyi*) Food poisoning	Penicillin G AND clindamycin for invasive infection (BII); no antimicrobials indicated for foodborne illness	Meropenem, metronidazole, clindamycin monotherapy
Clostridium tetani[61,62]	Tetanus	Metronidazole (AIII); penicillin G (BIII)	Treatment: tetanus immune globulin 3,000 to 6,000 U IM, with part injected directly into the wound. Prophylaxis for contaminated wounds: 250 U IM for those with <3 tetanus immunizations. Start/continue immunization for tetanus. Alternative antibiotics: meropenem; doxycycline, clindamycin.
Corynebacterium diphtheriae[63]	Diphtheria	Diphtheria equine antitoxin (available through CDC under an investigational protocol [www.cdc.gov/diphtheria/dat.html]) AND erythromycin or penicillin G (AIII)	Antitoxin from the CDC Emergency Operations Center, 770/488-7100; protocol: www.cdc.gov/diphtheria/downloads/protocol.pdf (accessed October 10, 2014)
Corynebacterium jeikeium[64]	Sepsis, endocarditis	Vancomycin (AIII)	Penicillin G AND gentamicin, tigecycline, linezolid, daptomycin
Corynebacterium minutissimum[65,66]	Erythrasma; bacteremia in compromised hosts	Erythromycin PO for erythrasma (BIII); vancomycin IV for bacteremia (BIII)	Topical clindamycin for cutaneous infection
Coxiella burnetii[67,68]	Q fever (See Chapter 6, Q fever.)	Acute infection: doxycycline (all ages) (AII) Chronic infection: TMP/SMX AND doxycycline (BII); OR levofloxacin AND rifampin	Alternative for acute infection: TMP/SMX

Ehrlichia chaffeensis[8,9] *Ehrlichia muris*-like[69]	Human monocytic ehrlichiosis	Doxycycline (all ages) (AII)	Rifampin
Ehrlichia ewingii[8,9]	*E ewingii* ehrlichiosis	Doxycycline (all ages) (AII)	Rifampin
Eikenella corrodens[70]	Human bite wounds; abscesses, meningitis, endocarditis	Ampicillin; penicillin G (BIII)	Amox/clav; ticar/clav; pip/tazo; amp/sul; ceftriaxone; ciprofloxacin; imipenem Resistant to clindamycin, cephalexin, erythromycin
Elizabethkingia (formerly *Chryseobacterium*) *meningoseptica*[71,72]	Sepsis, meningitis	Levofloxacin; TMP/SMX (BIII)	Add rifampin to another active drug; pip/tazo.
Enterobacter spp[53,73,74]	Sepsis, pneumonia, wound infection, UTI	Cefepime; meropenem (BII)	Ertapenem; imipenem; cefotaxime or ceftriaxone AND gentamicin; TMP/SMX; ciprofloxacin Newly emerging carbapenem-resistant strains worldwide[74,75]
Enterococcus spp[76–78]	Endocarditis, UTI, intra-abdominal abscess	Ampicillin AND gentamicin (AI)	Vancomycin AND gentamicin For vancomycin-resistant strains that are also amp-resistant: linezolid, daptomycin, tigecycline
Erysipelothrix rhusiopathiae[79]	Cellulitis (erysipeloid), sepsis, abscesses, endocarditis	Ampicillin (BIII); penicillin G (BIII)	Ceftriaxone; clindamycin, meropenem; ciprofloxacin, erythromycin Resistant to vancomycin, daptomycin, TMP/SMX
Escherichia coli See Chapter 6 for specific infection entities and references. *Increasing resistance to 3rd-generation cephalosporins due to ESBLs.*	UTI, not hospital acquired	A 2nd- or 3rd-generation cephalosporin PO, IM (BI)	Amoxicillin; TMP/SMX if susceptible. Ciprofloxacin if resistant to other options. For hospital-acquired UTI, review hospital antibiogram for choices.
	Traveler's diarrhea	Azithromycin (AII)	Rifaximin (for nonfebrile, non-bloody diarrhea for children >11 y); cefixime
	Sepsis, pneumonia, hospital-acquired UTI	A 2nd- or 3rd-generation cephalosporin IV (BI)	For ESBL-producing strains: meropenem (AIII) or other carbapenem. Ciprofloxacin if resistant to other antibiotics.
	Meningitis	Ceftriaxone; cefotaxime (AIII)	For ESBL-producing strains: meropenem (AIII)

D. PREFERRED THERAPY FOR SPECIFIC BACTERIAL AND MYCOBACTERIAL PATHOGENS (cont)

Organism	Clinical Illness	Drug of Choice (evidence grade)	Alternatives
Francisella tularensis[80,81]	Tularemia	Gentamicin (AII)	Doxycycline; ciprofloxacin
Fusobacterium spp[82,83]	Sepsis, soft tissue infection, Lemierre syndrome	Metronidazole (AIII); clindamycin (BIII)	Penicillin G; meropenem
Gardnerella vaginalis[84]	Bacterial vaginosis	Metronidazole (BII)	Tinidazole, clindamycin
Haemophilus (now *Aggregatibacter*) *aphrophilus*[85]	Sepsis, endocarditis, abscesses (including brain abscess)	Ceftriaxone (AII); OR ampicillin AND gentamicin (BII)	Ciprofloxacin, amox/clav (for strains resistant to ampicillin)
Haemophilus ducreyi[45]	Chancroid	Azithromycin (AIII); ceftriaxone (BIII)	Erythromycin; ciprofloxacin
Haemophilus influenzae[86]			
– Nonencapsulated strains	Upper respiratory tract infections	Beta-lactamase negative: ampicillin IV (AI); amoxicillin PO (AI) Beta-lactamase positive: ceftriaxone IV, IM (AI), or cefotaxime IV (AI); amox/clav (AI) OR 2nd- or 3rd-generation cephalosporins PO (AI)	Levofloxacin; azithromycin; TMP/SMX
– Type b strains	Meningitis, arthritis, cellulitis, epiglottitis, pneumonia	Beta-lactamase negative: ampicillin IV (AI); amoxicillin PO (AI) Beta-lactamase positive: ceftriaxone IV, IM (AI), or cefotaxime IV (AI); amox/clav (AI) OR 2nd- or 3rd-generation cephalosporins PO (AI)	Full IV course (10 days) for meningitis, but oral step-down therapy well documented after response to treatment for non-CNS infections.

Helicobacter pylori[87,88]	Gastritis, peptic ulcer	Clarithromycin AND amoxicillin AND omeprazole (AII)	Other regimens include metronidazole (especially for concerns of clarithromycin resistance)[89] and other proton pump inhibitors
Kingella kingae[90,91]	Osteomyelitis, arthritis	Ampicillin; penicillin G (AII)	Ceftriaxone; TMP/SMX; cefuroxime; ciprofloxacin
Klebsiella spp (*K pneumoniae, K oxytoca*)[92–94]	UTI	A 2nd- or 3rd-generation cephalosporin (AII)	Use most narrow spectrum agent active against pathogen: TMP/SMX; ciprofloxacin, gentamicin. ESBL producers should be treated with a carbapenem (meropenem, ertapenem, imipenem), but KPC-containing CREs may require ciprofloxacin or colistin.[94]
	Sepsis, pneumonia, meningitis	Ceftriaxone; cefotaxime, cefepime (AIII)	Carbapenem or ciprofloxacin if resistant to other routine antibiotics Meningitis caused by ESBL producer: meropenem KPC carbapenemase producers (CRE pathogens): ciprofloxacin, colistin
Klebsiella granulomatis[45]	Granuloma inguinale	Doxycycline (AII)	Azithromycin; TMP/SMX; ciprofloxacin
Legionella spp[95]	Legionnaires disease	Azithromycin (AI) OR levofloxacin (AII)	Erythromycin
Leptospira spp[96]	Leptospirosis	Penicillin G(AII); ceftriaxone(AII)	Amoxicillin; doxycycline; azithromycin
Leuconostoc[97]	Bacteremia	Penicillin G (AIII); ampicillin (BIII)	Clindamycin; erythromycin; doxycycline (resistant to vancomycin)
Listeria monocytogenes[98]	Sepsis, meningitis in compromised host; neonatal sepsis	Ampicillin (ADD gentamicin for severe infection) (AII)	TMP/SMX; vancomycin
Moraxella catarrhalis[99]	Otitis, sinusitis, bronchitis	Amox/clav (AI)	TMP/SMX; a 2nd- or 3rd-generation cephalosporin
Morganella morganii[100,101]	UTI, sepsis, wound infection	Cefepime (AIII); meropenem (AIII)	Pip/tazo; ceftriaxone AND gentamicin; ciprofloxacin

D. PREFERRED THERAPY FOR SPECIFIC BACTERIAL AND MYCOBACTERIAL PATHOGENS (cont)

Organism	Clinical Illness	Drug of Choice (evidence grade)	Alternatives
Mycobacterium abscessus[102,103]	Skin and soft tissue infections; pneumonia in cystic fibrosis	Clarithromycin or azithromycin (AIII); ADD amikacin ± cefoxitin for invasive disease (AIII).	Also test for susceptibility to meropenem, tigecycline, linezolid.
Mycobacterium avium complex[102,104]	Cervical adenitis, pneumonia[104]	Clarithromycin (AII); azithromycin (AII)	Surgical excision is more likely to lead to cure than sole medical therapy. May increase cure rate with addition of rifampin ± ethambutol.
	Disseminated disease in competent host, or disease in immunocompromised host	Clarithromycin or azithromycin AND ethambutol AND rifampin (AIII)	Depending on susceptibilities and the severity of illness, ADD amikacin ± ciprofloxacin.
Mycobacterium bovis[105,106]	Tuberculosis (adenitis; abdominal tuberculosis; meningitis)	Isoniazid AND rifampin (AII); add ethambutol for suspected resistance (AIII).	Add streptomycin for severe infection. *M bovis* is always resistant to PZA.
Mycobacterium chelonae[102,104,107,108]	Abscesses; catheter infection	Clarithromycin or azithromycin (AIII); ADD amikacin ± cefoxitin for invasive disease (AIII).	Also test for susceptibility to cefoxitin; TMP/SMX; doxycycline; tobramycin, imipenem; moxifloxacin, linezolid.
Mycobacterium fortuitum complex[102,108]	Skin and soft tissue infections; catheter infection	Amikacin AND meropenem (AIII) ± ciprofloxacin (AIII)	Also test for susceptibility to clarithromycin, cefoxitin; sulfonamides; doxycycline; linezolid.
Mycobacterium leprae[109]	Leprosy	Dapsone AND rifampin (for paucibacillary (1–5 patches) (AII). ADD clarithromycin (or clofazimine) for lepromatous, multibacillary (>5 patches) disease (AII).	Consult HRSA (National Hansen's Disease [Leprosy] Program) at www.hrsa.gov/hansensdisease for advice about treatment and free antibiotics: 800/642-2477 (accessed October 10, 2014).
Mycobacterium marinum/balnei[102,110]	Papules, pustules, abscesses (swimmer's granuloma)	Clarithromycin ± rifampin (AIII)	TMP/SMX AND rifampin; doxycycline

Mycobacterium tuberculosis[105,111] See Tuberculosis in Chapter 6, Table 6F, Lower Respiratory Tract Infections, for detailed recommendations for active infection, latent infection, and exposures in high-risk children.	Tuberculosis (pneumonia; meningitis; cervical adenitis; mesenteric adenitis; osteomyelitis)	For active infection: isoniazid AND rifampin AND PZA (AI) For latent infection: isoniazid daily, biweekly, or in combination with rifapentine once weekly (AII)	Add ethambutol for suspect resistance; add streptomycin for severe infection. For MDR tuberculosis, bedaquiline is now FDA approved for adults and available for children. Corticosteroids should be added to regimens for meningitis, mesenteric adenitis, and endobronchial infection (AIII).
Mycoplasma hominis[45,112,113]	Nongonococcal urethritis; neonatal infection including meningitis	Clindamycin (AIII)	Fluoroquinolones; doxycycline Usually erythromycin-resistant
Mycoplasma pneumoniae[114]	Pneumonia	Azithromycin (AI); erythromycin (BI); macrolide resistance emerging worldwide[115]	Doxycycline and fluoroquinolones are active against macrolide-susceptible and macrolide-resistant strains.
Neisseria gonorrhoeae[45]	Gonorrhea; arthritis	Ceftriaxone AND azithromycin or doxycycline (AIII)	Oral cefixime as single drug therapy no longer recommended due to increasing resistance.[116] Spectinomycin IM.
Neisseria meningitidis[117]	Sepsis, meningitis	Ceftriaxone (AI); cefotaxime (AI)	Penicillin G or ampicillin if susceptible[118] For prophylaxis following exposure: rifampin or ciprofloxacin (Ciprofloxacin-resistant strains have now been reported.)
Nocardia asteroides or *brasiliensis*[119,120]	Nocardiosis	TMP/SMX (AII); sulfisoxazole (BII); imipenem AND amikacin for severe infection (AII)	Ceftriaxone; minocycline; linezolid, levofloxacin, tigecycline
Oerskovia (now known as *Cellulosimicrobium cellulans)*[121]	Wound infection; catheter infection	Vancomycin ± rifampin (AIII)	Linezolid; resistant to beta-lactams, macrolides, clindamycin, aminoglycosides

D. PREFERRED THERAPY FOR SPECIFIC BACTERIAL AND MYCOBACTERIAL PATHOGENS (cont)

Organism	Clinical Illness	Drug of Choice (evidence grade)	Alternatives
Pasteurella multocida[122]	Sepsis, abscesses, animal bite wound	Penicillin G (AIII); ampicillin (AIII); amoxicillin (AIII)	Amox/clav; ticar/clav; pip/tazo; doxycycline; ceftriaxone; cefpodoxime; TMP/SMX Not usually susceptible to clindamycin
Peptostreptococcus[123]	Sepsis, deep head/neck space and intra-abdominal infection	Penicillin G (AII); ampicillin (AII)	Clindamycin; vancomycin; meropenem, imipenem, metronidazole
Plesiomonas shigelloides[124,125]	Diarrhea, neonatal sepsis, meningitis	Antibiotics may not be necessary to treat diarrhea: 2nd- and 3rd-generation cephalosporins (AIII); azithromycin (BIII); ciprofloxacin (CIII). For meningitis/sepsis: ceftriaxone.	Meropenem; pip/tazo
Prevotella (*Bacteroides*) spp,[126] *melaninogenica*	Deep head/neck space abscess; dental abscess	Metronidazole (AII); meropenem or imipenem (AII)	Pip/tazo; clindamycin
Propionibacterium acnes[127,128]	In addition to acne, invasive infection: sepsis, post-op wound infection	Penicillin (AIII); vancomycin (AIII) wound infection	Cefotaxime; doxycycline; clindamycin; linezolid
Proteus mirabilis[129]	UTI, sepsis, meningitis	Ceftriaxone (AII); cefotaxime (AII)	Aminoglycosides. Increasing resistance to ampicillin, TMP/SMX, and fluoroquinolones, particularly in nosocomial isolates. Colistin resistant.
Proteus vulgaris, other spp (indole-positive strains)[53]	UTI, sepsis, meningitis	Cefepime; ciprofloxacin, gentamicin (BIII)	Meropenem or other carbapenem; pip/tazo; TMP/SMX. Colistin resistant.
Providencia spp[53,74,130]	Sepsis	Cefepime; ciprofloxacin, gentamicin (BIII)	Meropenem or other carbapenem; pip/tazo; TMP/SMX. Colistin resistant.

Pseudomonas aeruginosa[74,131–135]	UTI	Cefepime (AII); other antipseudomonal beta-lactams	Tobramycin; amikacin; ciprofloxacin
	Nosocomial sepsis, pneumonia	Cefepime (AI) or meropenem (AI); OR pip/tazo AND tobramycin (BI); ceftazidime AND tobramycin (BI)	Ceftazidime AND tobramycin (BII); ciprofloxacin AND tobramycin. Controversy regarding clinical benefit in outcomes using beta-lactam AND aminoglycoside combinations. May decrease emergence of resistance.
	Pneumonia in cystic fibrosis[136–138] See Cystic Fibrosis in Chapter 6, Table 6F, Lower Respiratory Tract Infections.	Cefepime (AII) or meropenem (AI); OR ceftazidime AND tobramycin (BII); ADD aerosol tobramycin (AI). Azithromycin provides benefit in prolonging interval between exacerbations.	Inhalational antibiotics for prevention of acute exacerbations: tobramycin, aztreonam, colistin. Many organisms are multidrug resistant; consider ciprofloxacin or colistin parenterally; in vitro synergy testing may suggest effective combinations.[138] For multidrug-resistant organisms, colistin aerosol (AIII).
Pseudomonas cepacia, mallei, or *pseudomallei* (See Burkholderia.)			
Rhodococcus equi[139]	Necrotizing pneumonia	Imipenem AND vancomycin (AIII)	Dual drug combination therapy with ciprofloxacin AND azithromycin or rifampin
Rickettsia[68,140,141]	Rocky Mountain spotted fever, Q fever, typhus, rickettsial pox	Doxycycline (all ages) (AII)	Chloramphenicol is less effective than doxycycline.
Salmonella, non-*typhi*[142–144]	Gastroenteritis; focal infections; bacteremia	Ceftriaxone (AII); cefixime (AII); azithromycin (AII)	For susceptible strains: ciprofloxacin; TMP/SMX; ampicillin; resistance to fluoroquinolones detected by nalidixic acid testing
Salmonella typhi[145]	Typhoid fever	Azithromycin (AII); ceftriaxone (AII); ciprofloxacin (AII)	For susceptible strains: TMP/SMX; ampicillin
Serratia marcescens[53,74,130]	Nosocomial sepsis, pneumonia	Cefepime (AII); a carbapenem (AII)	Ceftriaxone or cefotaxime AND gentamicin; or ciprofloxacin

D. PREFERRED THERAPY FOR SPECIFIC BACTERIAL AND MYCOBACTERIAL PATHOGENS (cont)

Organism	Clinical Illness	Drug of Choice (evidence grade)	Alternatives
Shewanella spp[146]	Wound infection, nosocomial pneumonia, peritoneal-dialysis peritonitis, ventricular shunt infection, neonatal sepsis	Ceftazidime (AIII); gentamicin (AIII)	Ampicillin, meropenem, pip/tazo, ciprofloxacin
Shigella spp[147,148]	Enteritis, UTI, prepubertal vaginitis	Ceftriaxone (AII); azithromycin[149] (AII); cefixime (AII); ciprofloxacin[150] (AII)	Resistance to azithromycin now reported. Use most narrow spectrum agent active against pathogen: ampicillin (not amoxicillin for enteritis); TMP/SMX.
Spirillum minus[151,152]	Rat-bite fever (sodoku)	Penicillin G IV (AII); for endocarditis, ADD gentamicin or streptomycin (AIII).	Ampicillin; doxycycline; cefotaxime, vancomycin, streptomycin
Staphylococcus aureus (See chapters 4 and 6 for specific infections.)[153,154]			
– Mild-moderate infections	Skin infections, mild–moderate	MSSA: a 1st-generation cephalosporin (cefazolin IV, cephalexin PO) (AI); oxacillin/nafcillin IV (AI), dicloxacillin PO (AI) MRSA: vancomycin IV, or clindamycin IV or PO, or TMP/SMX PO (AII)	For MSSA: amox/clav For CA-MRSA: linezolid IV, PO; daptomycin IV
– Moderate-severe infections, treat empirically for CA-MRSA	Pneumonia, sepsis, myositis, osteomyelitis, etc	MSSA: oxacillin/nafcillin IV (AI); a 1st-generation cephalosporin (cefazolin IV) (AI) ± gentamicin (AIII) MRSA: vancomycin (AII) or clindamycin (AII); ± gentamicin ± rifampin (AIII)	For CA-MRSA: linezolid (AII); OR daptomycin for non-pulmonary infection (AII) (studies underway in children); ceftaroline IV (studies underway in children)
Staphylococcus, coagulase negative[155,156]	Nosocomial bacteremia (neonatal bacteremia), infected intravascular catheters, CNS shunts, UTI	Vancomycin (AII)	If susceptible: nafcillin (or other anti-staph beta-lactam); rifampin (in combination); clindamycin, linezolid; ceftaroline IV (studies underway in children)

Stenotrophomonas maltophilia[157,158]	Sepsis	TMP/SMX (AII)	Ceftazidime; ticar/clav; doxycycline; levofloxacin
Streptobacillus moniliformis[151,152]	Rat-bite fever (Haverhill fever)	Penicillin G (AIII); ampicillin (AIII); for endocarditis, ADD gentamicin or streptomycin (AIII).	Doxycycline; ceftriaxone; carbapenems; clindamycin; vancomycin
Streptococcus, group A[159]	Pharyngitis, impetigo, adenitis, cellulitis, necrotizing fasciitis	Penicillin (AI); amoxicillin (AI)	A 1st-generation cephalosporin (cefazolin or cephalexin) (AI); clindamycin (AI); a macrolide (AI), vancomycin (AIII) For relapsing streptococcal pharyngitis, clindamycin or amox/clav (AIII)
Streptococcus, group B[160]	Neonatal sepsis, pneumonia, meningitis	Penicillin (AII) or ampicillin (AII) ± gentamicin (AIII)	Vancomycin (AIII)
Streptococcus, milleri/anginosus group (*S intermedius, anginosus,* and *constellatus;* includes some beta-hemolytic group C and group G streptococci)[161–163]	Pneumonia, sepsis, skin and soft tissue infection, sinusitis,[164] arthritis, brain abscess, meningitis	Penicillin G (AIII); ampicillin (AIII); ADD gentamicin for serious infection (AIII). Many strains show decreased susceptibility to penicillin, requiring higher dosages.	Clindamycin; a 1st-generation cephalosporin; vancomycin
Streptococcus pneumoniae[165–168] With widespread use of conjugate pneumococcal vaccines, antibiotic resistance in pneumococci has decreased substantially.[168]	Sinusitis, otitis[165]	Amoxicillin, high-dose (90 mg/kg/day) (AII)	Amox/clav; cefdinir; cefpodoxime; cefuroxime; clindamycin; OR ceftriaxone IM
	Meningitis	Ceftriaxone (AI) or cefotaxime (AI); AND vancomycin for possible ceftriaxone-resistant strains (AIII)	Penicillin G alone for pen-S strains; ceftriaxone alone for ceftriaxone-susceptible strains
	Pneumonia,[114] osteomyelitis/arthritis, sepsis	Ampicillin (AII); ceftriaxone (AI); cefotaxime (AI)	Penicillin G for pen-S strains (AI)
Streptococcus, viridans group (alpha-hemolytic streptococci, most commonly *S sanguis, S oralis* [*mitis*], *S salivarius, S mutans, S morbillorum*)[169]	Endocarditis	Penicillin G ± gentamicin (AII) OR ceftriaxone ± gentamicin (AII)	Vancomycin

D. PREFERRED THERAPY FOR SPECIFIC BACTERIAL AND MYCOBACTERIAL PATHOGENS (cont)

Organism	Clinical Illness	Drug of Choice (evidence grade)	Alternatives
Treponema pallidum[45,170]	Syphilis	Penicillin G (AII)	Desensitize to penicillin preferred to alternate therapies. Doxycycline; ceftriaxone.
Ureaplasma urealyticum[45,171]	Genitourinary infections Neonatal pneumonia (Therapy may not be effective.)	Azithromycin (AII) Azithromycin (AIII)	Erythromycin; doxycycline, ofloxacin (for adolescent genital infections)
Vibrio cholerae[172,173]	Cholera	Doxycycline (AI) or azithromycin (AII)	If susceptible: ciprofloxacin; TMP/SMX
Vibrio vulnificus[174,175]	Sepsis, necrotizing fasciitis	Doxycycline AND ceftazidime (AII)	Ciprofloxacin AND cefotaxime
Yersinia enterocolitica[176,177]	Diarrhea, mesenteric enteritis, reactive arthritis, sepsis	TMP/SMX for enteritis (AIII); ciprofloxacin or ceftriaxone for invasive infection (AIII)	Gentamicin, doxycycline
Yersinia pestis[178,179]	Plague	Gentamicin (AIII)	Doxycycline; TMP/SMX, ciprofloxacin
Yersinia pseudotuberculosis[177,180]	Mesenteric adenitis; Far East scarlet fever; reactive arthritis	TMP/SMX (AIII) or ciprofloxacin (AIII)	Ceftriaxone; gentamicin, doxycycline

8. Preferred Therapy for Specific Fungal Pathogens

NOTES

- See Chapter 2 for discussion of the differences between polyenes, azoles, and echinocandins.
- **Abbreviations:** AmB, amphotericin B; AmB-D, amphotericin B deoxycholate, the conventional standard AmB (original trade name Fungizone); ABLC, amphotericin B lipid complex (Abelcet); bid, twice daily; CNS, central nervous system; CSF, cerebrospinal fluid; div, divided; ECMO, extracorporeal membrane oxygenation; HIV, human immunodeficiency virus; L-AmB, liposomal amphotericin B (AmBisome); IV, intravenous; PO, orally; qd, once daily; qid, 4 times daily; spp, species; TMP/SMX, trimethoprim/sulfamethoxazole.

A. OVERVIEW OF FUNGAL PATHOGENS AND USUAL PATTERN OF SUSCEPTIBILITY TO ANTIFUNGALS

Fungal Species	Amphotericin B Formulations	Fluconazole	Itraconazole	Voriconazole	Posaconazole	Flucytosine	Caspofungin, Micafungin, or Anidulafungin
Aspergillus calidoustus	++	–	+	–	–	–	++
Aspergillus fumigatus	+	–	+	++	+	–	+
Aspergillus terreus	–	–	+	++	+	–	+
Blastomyces dermatitidis	++	+	++	+	+	–	–
Candida albicans	+	++	+	+	+	+	++
Candida glabrata	+	–	–	+/–	+/–	+	+/-
Candida guilliermondii	+	+	+	+	+	+	+/–
Candida krusei	+	–	–	+	+	+	++
Candida lusitaniae	–	++	+	+	+	+	+
Candida parapsilosis	++	++	+	+	+	+	+/–
Candida tropicalis	+	++	+	+	+	+	++
Coccidioides immitis	++	+	++	+	+	–	–
Cryptococcus spp	++	+	+	+	+	++	–
Fusarium spp	+/-	–	–	++	+	–	–

Histoplasma capsulatum	++	+	++	+	+	–	–
Mucor spp	++	–	+/–	–	+	–	–
Paracoccidioides spp	+	+	++	+	+	–	–
Penicillium spp	+/–	–	++	+	+	–	–
Rhizopus spp	++	–	–	–	+	–	–
Scedosporium apiospermum	–	–	+	++	+	–	–
Scedosporium prolificans	–	–	+/–	+/–	+/–	–	–
Sporothrix spp	+	+	++	+	+	–	–
Trichosporon spp	–	+	+	++	+	–	–

NOTE: ++ = preferred therapy(ies); + = usually active; +/– =variably active; – = usually not active.

B. SYSTEMIC INFECTIONS

Infection	Therapy (evidence grade)	Comments
Prophylaxis		
Prophylaxis of invasive fungal infection in patients with hematologic malignancies[1–4]	Fluconazole 6 mg/kg/day for prevention of infection (AII)	Fluconazole is not effective against molds and some strains of *Candida*. Posaconazole PO, voriconazole PO, and micafungin IV are effective in adults in preventing yeast and mold infections but are not well studied in children for this indication.[5]
Prophylaxis of invasive fungal infection in patients with solid organ transplants[6–8]	Fluconazole 6 mg/kg/day for prevention of infection (AII)	AmB, caspofungin, micafungin, voriconazole, or posaconazole may be effective in preventing infection.
Treatment		
Aspergillosis[9–11]	Voriconazole 18 mg/kg/day IV div q12h for a loading dose on the first day, then 16 mg/kg/day IV div q12h as a maintenance dose for children 2–12 y. In children >12 y, use adult dosing (load 12 mg/kg/day IV div q12h on first day, then 8 mg/kg/day div q12h as a maintenance dose) (AII). When stable, may switch from voriconazole IV to voriconazole PO at a dose of 18 mg/kg/day div bid for children 2–12 y and 400 mg/day div bid for children >12 y (AIII). These are only initial dosing recommendations; continued dosing is guided by trough serum concentrations. Alternatives: caspofungin 70 mg/m^2 IV loading dose on day 1 (max dose 70 mg), followed by 50 mg/m^2 IV (max dose 70 mg) on subsequent days (BII) OR L-AmB 5 mg/kg/day as 3–4 h infusions (in adults, higher dosages have not produced improved outcome)[12] (AII).	Voriconazole is the preferred primary antifungal therapy for all clinical forms of infection. Optimal voriconazole trough serum concentrations (generally thought to be >1–2 µg/mL) are important for success, but it is critical to monitor trough concentrations to guide therapy due to high inter-patient variability.[13] Low voriconazole concentrations are a leading cause of clinical failure. Micafungin likely has equal efficacy to caspofungin against aspergillosis.[14] Total treatment course is at least 6 wk or until disease controlled. Salvage therapy options include a change of antifungal class (using L-AmB or an echinocandin), switching to posaconazole (trough concentrations >0.7 µg/mL), or using combination antifungal therapy.

		The addition of anidulafungin to voriconazole as combination therapy found no clear statistical benefit to the combination over voriconazole monotherapy.[15] In vitro data suggest some synergy with 2 (but not 3) drug combinations: an azole plus an echinocandin is the most well studied. If employed, this is likely best initially when voriconazole trough concentrations may not be appropriate yet. Azole-resistant *Aspergillus fumigatus* is increasing, confirm antifungal susceptibility in evaluating causes of clinical failure. Voriconazole and AmB are fungicidal, while the echinocandins are fungistatic against most *Aspergillus* spp. Return of immune function is paramount to treatment success; for children receiving corticosteroids, decreasing the corticosteroid dosage or changing to steroid-sparing protocols are also important.
Blastomycosis (North American)[16–18]	For moderate to severe disease: ABLC or L-AmB 5 mg/kg IV daily as 3–4 h infusion for 1–2 wk or until improvement noted, followed by oral solution itraconazole 10 mg/kg/day div bid (max 400 mg/day) PO for a total of 12 mo (AIII) For mild-moderate disease: oral solution itraconazole 10 mg/kg/day div bid (max 400 mg/day) PO for a total of 6–12 mo (AIII)	Itraconazole oral solution provides greater and more reliable absorption than capsules; serum concentrations of itraconazole should be determined 2 wk after start of therapy to ensure adequate drug exposure (maintain trough concentrations >0.5 µg/mL). Alternative to itraconazole: 12 mg/kg/day fluconazole (BIII). Patients with extrapulmonary blastomycosis should receive at least 12 mo of total therapy. CNS blastomycosis should begin with ABLC/L-AmB for 4–6 wk, followed by an azole (fluconazole preferred, at 12 mg/kg/day) for a total therapy of at least 12 mo and until resolution of CSF abnormalities. Lifelong itraconazole if immunosuppression cannot be reversed.

B. SYSTEMIC INFECTIONS (cont)

Infection	Therapy (evidence grade)	Comments
Candidiasis[19] (See Chapter 2.)		
– Disseminated infection	For neutropenic patients An echinocandin is recommended. Caspofungin 70 mg/m^2 IV loading dose on day 1 (max dose 70 mg), followed by 50 mg/m^2 IV (max dose 70 mg) on subsequent days (AII); OR micafungin 2–4 mg/kg/day q24h (max dose 150 mg) (BIII)[20]; preterm neonates require 10 mg/kg/day to achieve adequate drug exposure (BIII)[19] OR ABLC or L-AmB 5 mg/kg/day IV q24h (BII). For neutropenic but less critically ill patients with no recent azole exposure, fluconazole (12 mg/kg/day q24h) is an alternative. For non-neutropenic patients Fluconazole (12 mg/kg/day) is recommended in those patients who are less critically ill and with no recent azole exposure. An echinocandin is recommended in those non-neutropenic patients who are more critically ill, patients who have had recent azole exposure, or patients at risk for *Candida glabrata* or *Candida krusei*. L-AmB or ABLC (5 mg/kg/day) are alternatives, and voriconazole could be used for step-down oral therapy for voriconazole-susceptible *Candida krusei* or *Candida glabrata*, but otherwise offers little advantage over fluconazole. For CNS infections AmB-D 1 mg/kg/day or L-AmB/ABLC (5 mg/kg/day) AND flucytosine 100 mg/kg/day PO div q6h (AII) until initial clinical response, followed by step-down therapy with fluconazole (12 mg/kg/day); echinocandins do not achieve therapeutic concentrations in CSF.	Prompt removal of infected IV catheter or any infected devices is critical to success. For infections with *C krusei* or *C glabrata*, an echinocandin is preferred; however, there are increasing reports of some *C glabrata* resistance to echinocandins. Transition to an azole as step-down therapy only after confirmation of isolate susceptibility. Patients already receiving an empiric azole who are clinically improving can remain on the azole. For infections with *Candida parapsilosis*, fluconazole or ABLC/L-AmB is preferred. Patients already receiving an empiric echinocandin who are clinically improving can remain on the echinocandin. Therapy is for 2 wk after negative cultures in pediatric patients but 3 wk in neonates due to higher rate of meningitis and dissemination. Load with fluconazole at 25 mg/kg on day 1, followed by 12 mg/kg/day q24h to achieve steady state more rapidly. For children on ECMO, 35 mg/kg load followed by 12 mg/kg/day is also likely to be beneficial.

– Oropharyngeal, esophageal[19,20]	Oropharyngeal: mild disease; clotrimazole 10 mg troches PO 5 times daily OR nystatin 100,000 U/mL, 4–6 mL 4 times daily for 7–14 days. Moderate-severe disease: fluconazole 3–6 mg/kg qd PO for 7–14 days (AII). Esophageal: oral fluconazole (6–12 mg/kg/day) for 14–21 days. If cannot tolerate oral therapy, use fluconazole IV OR ABLC/L-AmB/AmB-D OR an echinocandin.	For fluconazole-refractory disease: itraconazole OR posaconazole OR AmB IV OR an echinocandin for 14–28 days. Esophageal disease always requires systemic antifungal therapy. Suppressive therapy (3 times weekly) with fluconazole is recommended for recurrent infections.
– Neonatal candidiasis[21]	L-AmB/ABLC (5 mg/kg/day) or AmB-D (1 mg/kg/day). Some would not recommend lipid AmB formulations if urinary tract involvement is possible. Theoretical risk of less urinary tract penetration by lipid AmB compared to AmB-D. Fluconazole (12 mg/kg/day, after loading dose of 25 mg/kg) is an alternative (BIII). Therapy is for 3 wk (not 2 wk as in pediatric patients). For treatment of neonates and young infants (<120 days) on ECMO, fluconazole load with 35 mg/kg on day 1, followed by 12 mg/kg/day q24h (BII).	Nurseries with high rates of candidiasis (generally thought to be >10%) should consider fluconazole prophylaxis (AI) (6 mg/kg twice weekly) in high-risk neonates (birth weight <1,000 g). Lumbar puncture and thorough retinal examination recommended (BIII). Imaging of genitourinary tract, liver, and spleen recommended if persistently positive cultures (BIII). Assume meningoencephalitis in the neonate due to the high incidence of this complication. Role of flucytosine in neonates with meningitis is questionable and not routinely recommended due to toxicity concerns. Echinocandins are generally used in cases of antifungal resistance.
– Peritonitis (secondary to peritoneal dialysis)[22]	Fluconazole 200 mg intraperitoneal q24h (AII)	Remove peritoneal dialysis catheter; replace after 4–6 wk of treatment, if possible. High-dosage oral fluconazole may also be used. AmB should not be instilled into the peritoneal cavity.

B. SYSTEMIC INFECTIONS (cont)

Infection	Therapy (evidence grade)	Comments
– Urinary tract infection	Cystitis: fluconazole 6 mg/kg qd IV or PO for 2 wk (AIII) Pyelonephritis: fluconazole 6–12 mg/kg qd IV or PO for 2 wk (AII)	Removing Foley catheter, if present, may lead to a spontaneous cure in the normal host; check for additional upper urinary tract disease. For fluconazole-resistant organisms, AmB-D is an alternative. AmB-D bladder irrigation is not generally recommended due to high relapse rate (an exception may be in fluconazole-resistant *Candida*). For renal collecting system fungus balls, surgical debridement may be required in non-neonates (BIII). Echinocandins have poor urinary concentrations.
– Vulvovaginal[23]	Topical vaginal cream/tablets/suppositories (alphabetic order): butoconazole, clotrimazole, econazole, fenticonazole, miconazole, sertaconazole, terconazole, or tioconazole for 3–7 days OR fluconazole 10 mg/kg (max 150 mg) as a single dose (AII)	No topical agent is clearly superior. Avoid azoles during pregnancy. For recurring disease, consider 10–14 days of induction with topical or systemic azole followed by fluconazole once weekly for 6 mo.
– Cutaneous candidiasis	Topical therapy (alphabetic order): ciclopirox, clotrimazole, econazole, haloprogin, ketoconazole, miconazole, oxiconazole, sertaconazole, sulconazole	Fluconazole 3–6 mg/kg/day PO qd for 5–7 days
– Chronic mucocutaneous[19]	Fluconazole 3–6 mg/kg daily PO until lesions clear (AII)	Alternative: itraconazole 5 mg/kg PO solution q24h Relapse common
Chromoblastomycosis[24,25]	Itraconazole oral solution 10 mg/kg/day div bid PO for 12–18 mo, in combination with surgical excision or repeated cryotherapy (AIII)	Alternative: terbinafine or an AmB

Coccidioidomycosis[26–30]	For moderate infections: fluconazole 12 mg/kg IV, PO q24h (AII). For severe pulmonary disease: AmB-D 1 mg/kg/day IV q24h; OR ABLC/ L-AmB 5 mg/kg/day IV q24h (AIII) as initial therapy until clear improvement, followed by an oral azole for total therapy of up to 12 mo, depending on genetic or immunocompromised risk factors. For meningitis: fluconazole 12 mg/kg/day IV q24h (AII); for failures, intrathecal AmB-D (0.1–1.5 mg/dose) OR voriconazole IV (AIII). Lifelong azole suppressive therapy may be required. For extrapulmonary (non-meningeal), particularly for osteomyelitis: itraconazole solution 10 mg/kg/day div bid for 12 mo appears more effective than fluconazole (AIII), and AmB as an alternative if worsening.	Mild pulmonary disease does not require therapy in the normal host and only requires periodic reassessment. Posaconazole also active, but little experience in children. Treat until serum cocci complement fixation titers drop to 1:8 or 1:4, about 3–6 mo. Disease in immunocompromised hosts may need to be treated longer, including potentially lifelong azole secondary prophylaxis. Watch for relapse up to 1–2 y after therapy.
Cryptococcosis[31–34]	For mild-moderate pulmonary disease: fluconazole 12 mg/kg/day IV, PO q24h for 6–12 mo (AII). For meningitis or severe pulmonary disease: induction therapy with AmB-D 1-1.5 mg/kg/day IV q24h OR ABLC/L-AmB 5 mg/kg/day q24h; AND flucytosine 100 mg/kg/day PO div q6h for a minimum of 2 wk until CSF cleared, FOLLOWED BY consolidation therapy with fluconazole (12 mg/kg/day) for a minimum of 8 more wk (AI).	Monitor flucytosine serum trough concentrations to keep peaks <80–100 µg/mL (and ideally 60–80 µg/mL) to prevent neutropenia. For HIV-positive patients, continue maintenance therapy with fluconazole (6 mg/kg/day) indefinitely. In organ transplant recipients, continue maintenance fluconazole (6 mg/kg/day) for 6–12 mo after consolidation therapy. For cryptococcal relapse, restart induction therapy and determine antifungal susceptibility of relapse isolate.

B. SYSTEMIC INFECTIONS (cont)

Infection	Therapy (evidence grade)	Comments
Fusarium, Scedosporium prolificans, and ***Pseudallescheria boydii*** (and its asexual form, ***Scedosporium apiospermum***)[35,36]	Voriconazole 18 mg/kg/day IV div q12h for a loading dose on the first day, then 16 mg/kg/day IV div q12h as a maintenance dose for children 2–12 y. In children >12 y, use adult dosing (load 12 mg/kg/day IV div q12h on first day, then 8 mg/kg/day div q12h as a maintenance dose) (AII). When stable, may switch from voriconazole IV to voriconazole PO at a dose of 18 mg/kg/day div bid for children 2–12 y and 400 mg/day div bid for children >12 y (AIII).	Optimal voriconazole trough concentrations (generally thought to be >1–2 µg/mL) are important. Resistant to AmB in vitro. Alternatives: echinocandins have been successful at salvage therapy in combination anecdotally; posaconazole (trough concentrations >0.7 µg/mL) likely helpful; while there are reports of combinations with terbinafine, terbinafine does not obtain good tissue concentrations for these disseminated infections. These can be very resistant infections, so highly recommend antifungal susceptibility testing.
Histoplasmosis[37,38]	For severe pulmonary disease: AmB-D 1 mg/kg/day q24h OR ABLC/L-AmB 5 mg/kg/day q24h for 1–2 wk, FOLLOWED BY itraconazole 10 mg/kg/day div bid to complete a total of 12 wk (AIII). For mild-moderate acute pulmonary disease, itraconazole 10 mg/kg/day PO solution div bid for 6–12 wk (AIII).	Mild disease may not require therapy and, in most cases, resolves in 1 mo. For disease with respiratory distress, ADD corticosteroids in first 1–2 wk of antifungal therapy. Progressive disseminated or CNS disease requires AmB therapy for the initial 4–6 wk. Potential lifelong suppressive itraconazole if cannot reverse immunosuppression.
Paracoccidioidomycosis[39–41]	Itraconazole 10 mg/kg/day PO solution div bid for 6 mo (AIII) OR ketoconazole 5 mg/kg/day PO q24h for 6 mo (BIII)	Alternatives: voriconazole; sulfadiazine or TMP/SMX for 3–5 y. AmB is another alternative and may be combined with sulfa or azole antifungals.

Phaeohyphomycosis (dematiaceous, pigmented fungi)[35,42]	Voriconazole 18 mg/kg/day IV div q12h for a loading dose on the first day, then 16 mg/kg/day IV div q12h as a maintenance dose for children 2–12 y. In children >12 y, use adult dosing (load 12 mg/kg/day IV div q12h on first day, then 8 mg/kg/day div q12h as a maintenance dose) (AII). When stable, may switch from voriconazole IV to voriconazole PO at a dose of 18 mg/kg/day div bid for children 2–12 y and 400 mg/day div bid for children >12 y (AIII). Alternatives could include posaconazole (trough concentrations >0.7 µg/mL), combination therapy with an echinocandin and an azole or an echinocandin and AmB (AIII).	Surgery is essential; antifungal susceptibilities are variable. Optimal voriconazole trough concentrations (generally thought to be >1–2 µg/mL) are important.
***Pneumocystis jiroveci* (*carinii*) pneumonia**[43]	Severe disease: preferred regimen is TMP/SMX, 15–20 mg TMP component/kg/day IV div q8h (AI) OR, for TMP/SMX intolerant or TMP/SMX treatment failure, pentamidine isethionate 4 mg base/kg/day IV daily (BII); for 3 wk. Mild-moderate disease: start with IV therapy, then after acute pneumonitis is resolved, TMP/SMX, 20 mg TMP component/kg/day PO div qid for 3 wk total treatment course (AII).	Alternatives: TMP AND dapsone; OR primaquine AND clindamycin; OR atovaquone. Prophylaxis: preferred regimen is TMP/SMX (5 mg TMP component/kg/day) PO div bid, 3 times/wk on consecutive days; OR same dose, given qd, every day; OR atovaquone: 30 mg/kg/day for infants 1–3 mo; 45 mg/kg/day for infants/children 4–24 mo; and 30 mg/kg/day for children >24 mo; OR dapsone 2 mg/kg (max 100 mg) PO qd, OR dapsone 4 mg/kg (max 200 mg) PO once weekly. Use steroid therapy for more severe disease.

B. SYSTEMIC INFECTIONS (cont)

Infection	Therapy (evidence grade)	Comments
Sporotrichosis[44]	For cutaneous/lymphocutaneous: itraconazole 10 mg/kg/day div bid PO solution for 2–4 wk after all lesions gone (generally total of 3–6 mo) (AII). For serious pulmonary or disseminated infection or disseminated sporotrichosis: ABLC/L-AmB at 5 mg/kg/day q24h until stable, then step-down therapy with itraconazole PO for a total of 12 mo (AIII). For less severe disease, itraconazole for 12 mo.	If no response for cutaneous disease, treat with higher itraconazole dose, terbinafine, or saturated solution of potassium iodide. Fluconazole is less effective. Obtain serum concentrations of itraconazole after 2 wk of therapy, want serum trough concentration >0.5 µg/mL. For meningeal disease, initial AmB should be 4–6 wk before change to itraconazole for at least 12 mo of therapy. Surgery may be necessary in osteoarticular or pulmonary disease.
Zygomycosis (mucormycosis)[45–48]	Requires aggressive surgery with antifungal therapy: ABLC/L-AmB at 5 mg/kg/day q24h (AIII). For AmB failures, posaconazole may be effective against most strains (AIII).	Following clinical response with AmB, long-term oral step-down therapy with posaconazole (trough concentrations >0.7 µg/mL) can be attempted for 2–6 mo. Some experts recommend initial combination therapy with L-AmB + caspofungin or micafungin. Voriconazole has NO activity against *Zygomycetes*.

C. LOCALIZED MUCOCUTANEOUS INFECTIONS

Infection	Therapy (evidence grade)	Comments
Dermatophytoses		
– Scalp (tinea capitis, including kerion)[49–51]	Griseofulvin ultramicrosized 10–15 mg/kg/day or microsized 20–25 mg/kg/day qd PO for 2 mo or longer (AII) (taken with milk or fatty foods to augment absorption). For kerion, treat concurrently with prednisone (1–2 mg/kg/day for 1–2 wk) (AIII).	No need to routinely follow liver function tests in normal healthy children taking griseofulvin. 2.5% selenium sulfide shampoo, or 2% ketoconazole shampoo, 2–3 times/wk should be used concurrently to prevent recurrences. Alternatives: terbinafine PO (4 wk), itraconazole solution 5 mg/kg PO qd, or fluconazole PO; terbinafine superior for *Trichophyton tonsurans,* but griseofulvin superior for *Microsporum canis.*
– Tinea corporis (infection of trunk/limbs/face) – Tinea cruris (infection of the groin) – Tinea pedis (infection of the toes/feet)	Alphabetic order of topical agents: butenafine, ciclopirox, clotrimazole, econazole, haloprogin, ketoconazole, miconazole, naftifine, oxiconazole, sertaconazole, sulconazole, terbinafine, and tolnaftate (AII); apply daily for 4 wk	For unresponsive tinea lesions, use griseofulvin PO in dosages provided above; fluconazole PO, itraconazole PO; OR terbinafine PO. For tinea pedis: Terbinafine PO or itraconazole PO are preferred over other oral agents. Keep skin as clean and dry as possible, particularly for tinea cruris and tinea pedis.
– Tinea unguium (onychomycosis)[51,52]	Topical 8% ciclopirox nail lacquer solution applied daily for 6–12 mo (AII); OR itraconazole 5 mg/kg PO solution q24h (AII)	Recurrence or partial response common Alternative: terbinafine PO 500 mg daily (adult dosage) for 1 wk per mo for 3 mo (hands) or 6–12 mo (toes) until new nail growth; requires systemic treatment (not topical)
– Tinea versicolor (also pityriasis versicolor)[51,53]	Apply topically: selenium sulfide 2.5% lotion or 1% shampoo daily, leave on 30 min, then rinse; for 7 d, then monthly for 6 mo (AIII); OR ciclopirox 1% cream for 4 wk (BII); OR terbinafine 1% solution (BII); OR ketoconazole 2% shampoo daily for 5 days (BII) For small lesions, topical clotrimazole, econazole, haloprogin, ketoconazole, miconazole, or naftifine	For lesions that fail to clear with topical therapy or for extensive lesions: fluconazole PO or itraconazole PO are equally effective. Recurrence common.

9. Preferred Therapy for Specific Viral Pathogens

NOTE

- **Abbreviations:** AIDS, acquired immunodeficiency syndrome; ART, antiretroviral therapy; ARV, antiretroviral; bid, twice daily; BSA, body surface area; CDC, Centers for Disease Control and Prevention; CMV, cytomegalovirus; CrCl, creatinine clearance; div, divided; EBV, Epstein-Barr virus; FDA, US Food and Drug Administration; G-CSF, granulocyte-colony stimulating factor; HAART, highly active antiretroviral therapy; HBV, hepatitis B virus; HCV, hepatitis C virus; HHS, US Department of Health and Human Services; HIV, human immunodeficiency virus; HSV, herpes simplex virus; IG, immune globulin; IFN, interferon; IM, intramuscular; IV, intravenous; NRTI, nucleoside analog reverse transcriptase inhibitor; PO, orally; postmenstrual age, weeks of gestation since last menstrual period PLUS weeks of chronologic age since birth; PTLD, posttransplant lymphoproliferative disorder; qd, once daily; qid, 4 times daily; RSV, respiratory syncytial virus; SQ, subcutaneous; tid, 3 times daily.

A. OVERVIEW OF NON-HIV VIRAL PATHOGENS AND USUAL PATTERN OF SUSCEPTIBILITY TO ANTIVIRALS

Virus	Acyclovir	Adefovir	Boceprevir	Cidofovir	Entecavir	Famciclovir	Foscarnet	Ganciclovir
Cytomegalovirus				+			+	++
Hepatitis B virus		+			++			
Hepatitis C virus			+					
Herpes simplex virus	++					++	+	+
Influenza A and B								
Varicella-zoster virus	++					++	+	+

Virus	Interferon alfa-2b	Lamivudine	Oseltamivir	Pegylated interferon alfa-2a	Ribavirin	Simeprevir
Cytomegalovirus						
Hepatitis B virus	+	+		++		
Hepatitis C virus				++	++	++
Herpes simplex virus						
Influenza A and B			++			
Varicella-zoster virus						

Virus	Sofosbuvir	Telaprevir	Telbivudine	Tenofovir	Valacyclovir	Valganciclovir	Zanamivir
Cytomegalovirus						++	
Hepatitis B virus			+	++			
Hepatitis C virus	++	+					
Herpes simplex virus					++	+	
Influenza A and B							+
Varicella-zoster virus					++		

NOTE: ++ = preferred therapy(ies); + = acceptable therapy.

B. PREFERRED THERAPY FOR SPECIFIC VIRAL PATHOGENS

Infection	Therapy (evidence grade)	Comments
Adenovirus (pneumonia or disseminated infection in immunocompromised hosts)[1]	Cidofovir and ribavirin are active in vitro, but no prospective clinical data exist and both have significant toxicity. Two cidofovir dosing schedules have been employed in clinical settings: (1) 5 mg/kg/dose IV once weekly or (2) 1–1.5 mg/kg/dose IV 3 times/wk. If parenteral cidofovir is utilized, IV hydration and oral probenecid should be used to reduce renal toxicity.	The orally bioavailable lipophilic derivative of cidofovir, CMX001 (brincidofovir), is under investigation for the treatment of adenovirus in immunocompromised hosts. It is not yet commercially available.
Cytomegalovirus		
– Neonatal[2]	See Chapter 5.	
– Immunocompromised (HIV, chemotherapy, transplant-related)[3–15]	For induction: ganciclovir 10 mg/kg/day IV div q12h for 14–21 days (AII) (may be increased to 15 mg/kg/day IV div q12h). For maintenance: 5 mg/kg IV q24h for 5–7 days per week. Duration dependent on degree of immunosuppression (AII). CMV hyperimmune globulin may decrease morbidity in bone marrow transplant patients with CMV pneumonia (AII).	Use foscarnet or cidofovir for ganciclovir-resistant strains; for HIV-positive children on HAART, CMV may resolve without therapy. Also used for prevention of CMV disease posttransplant for 100–120 days. Data on valganciclovir dosing in young children for treatment of retinitis are unavailable, but consideration can be given to transitioning from IV ganciclovir to oral valganciclovir after improvement of retinitis is noted. Limited data on oral valganciclovir in neonates[16,17] (32 mg/kg/day PO div bid) and children dosing by BSA (dose [mg] = 7 × BSA × CrCl).[5]
– Prophylaxis of infection in immunocompromised hosts[4,18]	Ganciclovir 5 mg/kg IV daily (or 3 times/wk) (started at engraftment for stem cell transplant patients) (BII) Valganciclovir oral solution (50 mg/mL) at total dose in milligrams = 7 x BSA x CrCl (use maximum CrCl 150 mL/min/1.73 m^2) orally once daily with food for children 4 mo–16 y (max dose 900 mg/day) for primary prophylaxis in HIV patients[19] who are CMV antibody positive and have severe immunosuppression (CD4 count <50 cells/mm^3 in children ≥6 y; CD4 percentage <5% in children <6 y) (CIII)	Neutropenia is a complication with ganciclovir prophylaxis and may be addressed with G-CSF. Prophylaxis and preemptive strategies are effective; neither has been shown clearly superior to the other.[9]

B. PREFERRED THERAPY FOR SPECIFIC VIRAL PATHOGENS (cont)

Infection	Therapy (evidence grade)	Comments
Epstein-Barr virus		
– Mononucleosis, encephalitis[20–22]	Limited data suggest small clinical benefit of valacyclovir in adolescents for mononucleosis (3 g/day div tid for 14 days) (CIII). For EBV encephalitis: ganciclovir IV OR acyclovir IV (AIII).	No prospective data on benefits of acyclovir IV or ganciclovir IV in EBV clinical infections of normal hosts. Patients suspected to have infectious mononucleosis should not be given ampicillin or amoxicillin, which cause nonallergic morbilliform rashes in a high proportion of patients with active EBV infection (AII). Therapy with short-course corticosteroids (prednisone 1 mg/kg per day, orally [maximum 20 mg/day], for 7 days with subsequent tapering) may have a beneficial effect on acute symptoms in patients with marked tonsillar inflammation with impending airway obstruction, massive splenomegaly, myocarditis, hemolytic anemia, or hemophagocytic lymphohistiocytosis (BIII).
– Posttransplant lymphoproliferative disorder[23,24]	Ganciclovir (AIII)	Decrease immune suppression if possible, as this has the most impact on control of EBV; rituximab, methotrexate have been used but without controlled data. Preemptive treatment with ganciclovir may decrease PTLD in solid organ transplants.

Hepatitis B virus (chronic)[25–38]	IFN-alpha 3 million U/m^2 BSA SQ 3 times/wk for 1 wk, followed by dose escalation to 6 million U/m^2 BSA (max 10 million U/dose), to complete a 24-wk course for children 1–18 y; OR lamivudine 3 mg/kg/day (max 100 mg) PO q24h for 52 wk for children ≥2 y (children coinfected with HIV and HBV should use the approved dose for HIV) (AII); OR adefovir for children ≥12 y (10 mg PO q24h for a minimum of 12 mo; optimum duration of therapy unknown) (BII); OR entecavir for children ≥16 y (0.5 mg qd in patients who have not received prior nucleoside therapy; 1 mg qd in patients who are previously treated [not first choice in this setting]); optimum duration of therapy unknown (BII)	Indications for treatment of chronic HBV infection, with or without HIV coinfection, are: (1) evidence of ongoing HBV viral replication, as indicated by serum HBV DNA (>20,000 without HBeAg positivity or >2,000 IU/mL with HBeAg positivity) for >6 mo and persistent elevation of serum transaminase levels for >6 mo, or (2) evidence of chronic hepatitis on liver biopsy (BII). Antiviral therapy is not warranted in children without necroinflammatory liver disease (BIII). Treatment is not recommended for children with immunotolerant chronic HBV infection (ie, normal serum transaminase levels despite detectable HBV DNA) (BII). Standard IFN-alfa (IFN-2a or -2b) is recommended for treating chronic HBV infection with compensated liver disease in HIV-uninfected children aged ≥2 y who warrant treatment (AI). IFN-alfa therapy in combination with oral antiviral therapy cannot be recommended for pediatric HBV infection in HIV-uninfected children until more data are available (BII). In HIV/HBV-coinfected children who do not require ART for their HIV infection, IFN-alpha therapy is the preferred agent to treat chronic HBV (BIII), whereas adefovir can be considered in children ≥12 y (BIII). Treatment options for HIV/HBV-coinfected children who meet criteria for HBV therapy and who are already receiving lamivudine- or emtricitabine-containing HIV-suppressive ART, include the standard IFN-alpha therapy to the ARV regimen (BIII), or adefovir if the child can receive adult dosing (BIII), or use of tenofovir disoproxil fumarate in lamivudine (or emtricitabine)-containing ARV regimen in children ≥2 y (BIII). HIV/HBV-coinfected children should not be given lamivudine (or emtricitabine) without additional anti-HIV drugs for treatment of chronic HBV (CIII).[19]
		Alternatives Tenofovir (adult and adolescent dose [≥12 y] 300 mg qd). Telbivudine (adult dose 600 mg qd). There are not sufficient clinical data to identify the appropriate dose for use in children. Lamivudine approved for children ≥2 y, but antiviral resistance develops on therapy in 30%. Entecavir is superior to lamivudine in the treatment of chronic HBV infection and is the most potent anti-HBV agent available.

B. PREFERRED THERAPY FOR SPECIFIC VIRAL PATHOGENS (cont)

Infection	Therapy (evidence grade)	Comments
Hepatitis C virus (chronic)[39–45]	Pegylated IFN-alpha: 2a 180 µg/1.73 m^2 BSA SQ once per wk (maximum dose 180 µg) OR 2b 60 µg/m^2 BSA once per wk PLUS Ribavirin (oral) 7.5 mg/kg body weight twice daily (fixed dose by weight recommended) 25–36 kg: 200 mg am and pm >36–49 kg: 200 mg in am and 400 mg in pm >49–61 kg: 400 mg in am and pm >61–75 kg: 400 mg in am and 600 mg in pm >75 kg: 600 mg in am and pm Treatment duration: 24–48 wk (AII)	Treatment of children aged <3 y who have HCV infection usually is not recommended (BIII). HCV-infected, HIV-uninfected children ≥3 y should be individualized because HCV usually causes mild disease in this population and few data exist to identify risk factors differentiating those at greater risk for progression of liver disease. Those who are chosen for treatment should receive combination therapy with IFN-alpha and ribavirin for 48 wk for genotype 1 and 24 wk for genotypes 2 or 3 (AI). Treatment should be considered for all HIV/HCV-coinfected children aged >3 y who have no contraindications to treatment (BIII). A liver biopsy to stage disease is recommended before deciding whether to initiate therapy for chronic HCV genotype 1 infection (BIII). However, some specialists would treat children infected with HCV genotypes 2 or 3 without first obtaining a liver biopsy (BIII). Treatment of HCV-infected children, regardless of HIV status, should include IFN-alpha plus ribavirin combination therapy (AI). Duration of treatment for HIV/HCV-coinfected children should be 48 wk, regardless of HCV genotype (BIII). IFN-alpha therapy is contraindicated for children with decompensated liver disease, substantial cytopenias, renal failure, severe cardiac or neuropsychiatric disorders, and non–HCV-related autoimmune disease (AII).[19] Several new direct-acting antiviral agents have recently been approved for use in adults, with several more in clinical trials. These drugs include protease inhibitors (the 1st-generation agents telaprevir and boceprevir and 2nd-generation agents simeprevir and faldaprevir [FDA approval pending]), NS5B polymerase inhibitors (sofosbuvir), and inhibitors of the nonstructural NS5A enzyme replication complex of HCV (daclatasvir). Clinical trials in adults of these agents, with or without IFN and ribavirin co-therapies, have yielded cure rates of >90% for certain genotypes. These agents may be tested and approved for use in children in the near future. No recommendations for use of these agents in children can be made at this time.

Herpes simplex virus		
– Third trimester maternal suppressive therapy[46,47]	Acyclovir or valacyclovir maternal suppressive therapy in pregnant women reduces HSV recurrences and viral shedding at the time of delivery but does not fully prevent neonatal HSV[48] (BIII).	
– Neonatal	See Chapter 5.	
– Mucocutaneous (normal host)	Acyclovir 80 mg/kg/day PO div qid (max dose: 800 mg) for 5–7 days, or 15 mg/kg/day IV as 1–2 h infusion div q8h (AII) Suppressive therapy for frequent recurrence (no pediatric data): 20 mg/kg/dose given bid or tid (max dose: 400 mg) for 6–12 mo; then reevaluate need (AIII) Valacyclovir 20 mg/kg/dose (max dose: 1 g) PO bid[49] for 5–7 days (BII)	Foscarnet for acyclovir-resistant strains. Immunocompromised hosts may require 10–14 days of therapy. Topical acyclovir not efficacious and therefore is not recommended.
– Genital	Adult doses: acyclovir 400 mg PO tid, for 7–10 days; OR valacyclovir 1 g PO bid for 10 days; OR famciclovir 250 mg PO tid for 7–10 days (AI)	All 3 drugs have been used as prophylaxis to prevent recurrence. Topical acyclovir not efficacious and therefore is not recommended.
– Encephalitis	Acyclovir 60 mg/kg/day IV as 1–2 h infusion div q8h; for 21 days for infants ≤4 mo. For older infants and children, 45–60 mg/kg/day IV (AIII).	Safety of high-dose acyclovir (60 mg/kg/day) not well defined beyond the neonatal period; can be used but monitor for neurotoxicity and nephrotoxicity.
– Keratoconjunctivitis	1% trifluridine, 0.1% idoxuridine, or 0.15% ganciclovir ophthalmic gel (AII)	Treat in consultation with an ophthalmologist. Topical steroids may be helpful when used together with antiviral agents.
Human herpesvirus 6		
– Immunocompromised children[50]	No prospective comparative data; ganciclovir 10–20 mg/kg/day IV div q12h used in case report (AIII)	May require high dose to control infection; safety and efficacy not defined at high doses.

B. PREFERRED THERAPY FOR SPECIFIC VIRAL PATHOGENS (cont)

Infection	Therapy (evidence grade)	Comments
Human immunodeficiency virus		
Current information on HIV treatment and opportunistic infections for children[51] is posted at http://aidsinfo.nih.gov/ContentFiles/PediatricGuidelines.pdf (accessed October 13, 2014); other information on HIV programs is available at www.cdc.gov/hiv/policies/index.html (accessed October 13, 2014). Consult with an HIV expert, if possible, for current recommendations.		
– **Therapy of HIV infection** State-of-the-art therapy is rapidly evolving with introduction of new agents and combinations; currently there are 23 individual ARV agents approved for use by the FDA that have pediatric indications, as well as multiple combinations; guidelines for children and adolescents are continually updated on the AIDSINFO and CDC Web sites given previously.	Effective therapy (HAART) consists of ≥3 agents, including 2 nucleoside reverse transcriptase inhibitors, plus a protease inhibitor or non-nucleoside reverse transcriptase inhibitor (integrase inhibitors are currently available for 2nd-line therapy options); many different combination regimens give similar treatment outcomes; choice of agents depends on the age of the child, viral load, consideration of potential viral resistance, and extent of immune depletion, in addition to judging the child's ability to adhere to the regimen.	Assess drug toxicity (based on the agents used) and virologic/immunologic response to therapy (quantitative plasma HIV and CD4 count) initially monthly and then every 3–6 mo during the maintenance phase.
– Children of any age	Any child with AIDS or significant HIV-related symptoms (clinical category C and most B conditions) should be treated (AI).	Adherence counseling and appropriate ARV formulations are critical for successful implementation.
– First year of life	HAART with ≥3 drugs is now recommended for all infants ≤12 mo, regardless of clinical status or laboratory values (AI for <12 wk; AII for 12–52 wk).	Preferred therapy in the first year of life is zidovudine plus lamivudine plus lopinavir/ritonavir (toxicity concerns preclude its use until a postmenstrual age of 42 wk and a postnatal age of at least 14 days is reached).

– HIV-infected children ≥1 y who are asymptomatic or have mild symptoms	Treat with the following CD4 values: Age 1–<3 y with CD4 <1,000 or <25% (AII) Age 3–<5 y with CD4 <750 <25% (AII) Age ≥5 y with CD4 <350 (AI) or CD4 350–500 (BII)	Preferred regimens comprise zidovudine plus lamivudine (at any age) OR abacavir plus lamivudine (>3 mo) OR tenofovir plus emtricitabine aka Truvada (adolescents/Tanner stage 4 or 5) PLUS lopinavir/ritonavir (any age >2 wk) OR efavirenz (≥3 y) OR atazanavir/ritonavir (≥6 y).
– HIV-infected children ≥1 y who are asymptomatic or have mild symptoms	Consider treatment with the following CD4 values: Age 1–<3 y with CD4 ≥1,000 or ≥25% (BIII) Age 3–<5 y with CD4 ≥750 or ≥25% (BIII) Age ≥5 y with CD4 >500 (BIII)	Expert opinion has migrated toward treatment consideration even in mild clinical situations. Treatment deferral and monitoring of clinical course, CD4 count, and plasma HIV RNA on a 3- to 4-mo basis is an option.
– Any child ≥1 y	Treat when viral load ≥100,000 copies/mL (AII).	Most experts now recommend treatment in settings of high viral load.
– Antiretroviral-experienced child	Consult with HIV specialist.	Consider treatment history and drug resistance testing and assess adherence.
– **HIV exposures, nonoccupational**	Therapy recommendations for exposures available on the CDC Web site at www.cdc.gov/hiv/guidelines/preventing.html (accessed October 13, 2014), based on assessment of risk of HIV exposure.	Prophylaxis remains unproven; consider individually regarding risk, time from exposure, and likelihood of adherence; prophylactic regimens administered for 4 wk.
– Negligible exposure risk (urine, nasal secretions, saliva, sweat, or tears—no visible blood in secretions) OR >72 h since exposure	Prophylaxis not recommended (BIII)	
– Significant exposure risk (blood, semen, vaginal, or rectal secretions from a known HIV-infected individual) AND <72 h since exposure	Prophylaxis recommended (BIII): Combivir (zidovudine/lamivudine) or Truvada (tenofovir/emtricitabine) PLUS efavirenz or Kaletra (lopinavir/ritonavir). Since the last HHS/CDC guidelines in 2005, raltegravir or darunavir/ritonavir in place of efavirenz or lopinavir/ritonavir has gained some favor among experts.	Preferred prophylactic regimens – Based on treatment regimens for infected individuals – 28-day regimen In the event of poor adherence or toxicity, some experts consider 2 NRTI regimens, such as Combivir (zidovudine/lamivudine) or Truvada (tenofovir/emtricitabine) (BIII).
– HIV exposure, occupational[52]	See guidelines on CDC Web site at www.cdc.gov/hiv/guidelines/preventing.html (accessed October 13, 2014).	

B. PREFERRED THERAPY FOR SPECIFIC VIRAL PATHOGENS (cont)

Infection	Therapy (evidence grade)	Comments
Influenza virus Recommendations for the treatment of influenza can vary from season to season; access the American Academy of Pediatrics Web site (www.aap.org) and the CDC Web site (www.cdc.gov/flu/professionals/antivirals/antiviral-agents-flu.htm, accessed October 13, 2014) for the most current, accurate information.		
Influenza A and B		
– Treatment[53–55]	Oseltamivir Preterm, <38 wk postmenstrual age: 1 mg/kg/dose PO bid Preterm, 38–40 wk postmenstrual age: 1.5 mg/kg/dose PO bid Preterm, >40 wk postmenstrual age: 3.0 mg/kg/dose PO bid[53] Term, birth–8 mo: 3.0 mg/kg/dose PO bid 9–11 mo: 3.5 mg/kg/dose PO bid[54] 12–23 mo: 30 mg/dose PO bid 2–12 y: ≤15 kg: 30 mg, bid; 16–23 kg: 45 mg, bid; 24–40 kg: 60 mg, bid; >40 kg: 75 mg, bid ≥13 y: 75 mg, bid, OR Zanamivir ≥7 y: 10 mg by inhalation, bid for 5 days	Oseltamivir currently is drug of choice for treatment of influenza infections. For patients 12–23 mo, the original FDA-approved unit dose of 30 mg/dose may provide inadequate drug exposure; 3.5 mg/kg/dose PO bid has been studied,[54] but study population sizes were small. The adamantanes, amantadine and rimantadine, currently are not effective for treatment due to near-universal resistance of influenza A.
– Chemoprophylaxis	Oseltamivir 3 mo–12 y: The prophylaxis does is *one half* of the treatment does for all ages; the same mg dose that is given twice daily for treatment is given once daily for prophylaxis. Zanamivir ≥5 y: 10 mg by inhalation, qd for as long as 28 days (community outbreaks) or 10 days (household setting)	Oseltamivir currently is drug of choice for chemoprophylaxis of influenza infection. Unless the situation is judged critical, oseltamivir chemoprophylaxis not recommended for patients <3 mo because of limited safety and efficacy data in this age group. The adamantanes, amantadine and rimantadine, currently are not effective for chemoprophylaxis due to near-universal resistance of influenza A.

Measles[56]	No prospective data on antiviral therapy. Ribavirin is active against measles virus in vitro. Vitamin A is beneficial in children with measles and is recommended by the World Health Organization for all children with measles regardless of their country of residence (qd dosing for 2 days): for children ≥1 y: 200,000 IU; for infants 6–12 mo: 100,000 IU; for infants <6 mo: 50,000 IU (BII).	IG prophylaxis for exposed, susceptible children: 0.5 mL/kg (max 15 mL) IM
Respiratory syncytial virus[57]		
– Therapy (severe disease in compromised host)	Ribavirin (6-g vial to make 20 mg/mL solution in sterile water), aerosolized over 18–20 h daily for 3–5 days (BII)	Aerosol ribavirin provides a small benefit and should only be used for life-threatening infection with RSV. Airway reactivity with inhalation precludes routine use.
– Prophylaxis (palivizumab, Synagis for high-risk infants) (BI)[57]	Prophylaxis: palivizumab (a monoclonal antibody) 15 mg/kg IM monthly for the following high-risk infants (AI): In the first year of life, palivizumab prophylaxis is recommended for infants born before 29 wk 0 days' gestation. Palivizumab prophylaxis is not recommended for otherwise healthy infants born at or after 29 wk 0 days' gestation. In the first year of life, palivizumab prophylaxis is recommended for preterm infants with chronic lung disease of prematurity, defined as birth at <32 wk 0 days' gestation and a requirement for >21% oxygen for at least 28 days after birth. Clinicians may administer palivizumab prophylaxis in the first year of life to certain infants with hemodynamically significant heart disease.	Palivizumab does not provide benefit in the treatment of an active RSV infection In Florida, the RSV season lasts 5 mo but starts earlier than in the rest of the United States.[27] Palivizumab prophylaxis is not recommended in the second year of life except for children who required at least 28 days of supplemental oxygen after birth and who continue to require medical intervention (supplemental oxygen, chronic corticosteroid, or diuretic therapy). Monthly prophylaxis should be discontinued in any child who experiences a breakthrough RSV hospitalization. Children with pulmonary abnormality or neuromuscular disease that impairs the ability to clear secretions from the upper airways may be considered for prophylaxis in the first year of life. Children <24 mo who will be profoundly immunocompromised during the RSV season may be considered for prophylaxis.

B. PREFERRED THERAPY FOR SPECIFIC VIRAL PATHOGENS (cont)

Infection	Therapy (evidence grade)	Comments
Respiratory syncytial virus[57] (cont)		
	Clinicians may administer up to a maximum of 5 monthly doses of palivizumab (15 mg/kg per dose) during the RSV season to infants who qualify for prophylaxis in the first year of life. Qualifying infants born during the RSV season may require fewer doses; for example, infants born in January would receive their last dose in March.	Insufficient data are available to recommend palivizumab prophylaxis for children with cystic fibrosis or Down syndrome. The burden of RSV disease and costs associated with transport from remote locations may result in a broader use of palivizumab for RSV prevention in Alaska Native populations and possibly in selected other American Indian populations. Palivizumab prophylaxis is not recommended for prevention of health care–associated RSV disease.
Varicella-zoster virus[58]		
– Infection in a normal host	Acyclovir 80 mg/kg/day (max single dose 800 mg) PO div qid for 5 days (AI)	The sooner antiviral therapy can be started, the greater the clinical benefit.
– Severe primary chickenpox, disseminated infection (cutaneous, pneumonia, encephalitis, hepatitis); immunocompromised host with primary chickenpox or disseminated zoster	Acyclovir 30 mg/kg/day IV as 1–2 h infusion div q8h; for 10 days (acyclovir doses of 45–60 mg/kg/day in 3 div doses IV should be used for disseminated or central nervous system infection). Dosing can also be provided as 1,500 mg/m^2/day IV div q8h. Duration in immunocompromised children: 7–14 days, based on clinical response (AI)°.	Oral valacyclovir, famciclovir, foscarnet also active

10. Preferred Therapy for Specific Parasitic Pathogens

NOTES

- For some parasitic diseases, therapy may be available only from the Centers for Disease Control and Prevention (CDC), as noted. Consultation is available from the CDC for parasitic disease diagnostic services (http://dpd.cdc.gov/dpdx/Default.htm, accessed October 13, 2014), parasitic disease testing, and experimental therapy at 404/639-3670; for malaria, 770/488-7788 (please refer to MALARIA). Antiparasitic drugs available from the CDC can be reviewed and requested at www.cdc.gov/laboratory/drugservice/formulary.html (accessed October 13, 2014).
- **Abbreviations:** AFB, acid-fast bacteria; AmB, amphotericin B; A-P, atovaquone/proguanil; bid, twice daily; BP, blood pressure; CDC, Centers for Disease Control and Prevention; CNS, central nervous system; CrCl, creatinine clearance; CSF, cerebrospinal fluid; DEC, diethylcarbamazine; div, divided; ECG, electrocardiogram; FDA, US Food and Drug Administration; G6PD, glucose-6-phosphate dehydrogenase; GI, gastrointestinal; HAART, highly active antiretroviral therapy; HIV, human immunodeficiency virus; IM, intramuscular; IV, intravenous; PO, orally; qd, once daily; qid, 4 times daily; qod, every other day; spp, species; tab, tablet; tid, 3 times daily; TMP/SMX, trimethoprim/sulfamethoxazole; UV, ultraviolet.

Disease/Organism	Treatment	Comments
AMEBIASIS[1–5]		
ENTERITIS/LIVER ABSCESS		
Entamoeba histolytica		
– Asymptomatic carrier	Paromomycin 30 mg/kg/day PO div tid for 7 days; OR iodoquinol 30–40 mg/kg/day (max 2 g) PO div tid for 20 days; OR diloxanide furoate (not commercially available in the US) 20 mg/kg/day PO div tid for 10 days (CII)	Follow-up stool examination to ensure eradication of carriage; screen/treat positive close contacts.
– Mild to moderate colitis	Metronidazole 30–40 mg/kg/day PO div tid for 10 days; OR tinidazole 50 mg/kg/day PO (max 2 g) qd for 3 days FOLLOWED by paromomycin or iodoquinol as above to eliminate cysts (BII)	Avoid anti-motility drugs, steroids. Take tinidazole with food to decrease GI side effects; if unable to take tabs, pharmacists can crush tabs and mix with syrup. Nitazoxanide (see GIARDIASIS) may also be effective.
– Severe colitis, liver abscess	Metronidazole 35–40 mg/kg/day IV q8h, switch to PO when tolerated, for 10 days; OR tinidazole (age ≥3 y) 50 mg/kg/day PO (max 2 g) qd for 5 days FOLLOWED by paromomycin or iodoquinol as above to eliminate cysts (BII)	Serologic assays >95% positive in extraintestinal amebiasis. Percutaneous or surgical drainage may be indicated for large liver abscesses or inadequate response to medical therapy. Chloroquine plus metronidazole or tinidazole followed by luminal agent considered alternative for liver abscess.
MENINGOENCEPHALITIS[6–12]		
Naegleria, Acanthamoeba, Balamuthia, Hartmannella spp	AmB 1.5 mg/kg/day IV in 2 doses for 3 days, then 1 mg/kg/day for 6 days plus 1.5 mg/day intrathecally for 2 days, then 1 mg/day qod for 8 days; consider alternative 1–1.5 mg/kg/day qd for 3–4 wk or longer, PLUS azithromycin 20 mg/kg IV qd, fluconazole 12 mg/kg IV qd, and rifampin 10 mg/kg (max 600 mg) IV qd for *Naegleria.*	Treatment outcomes usually unsuccessful; early therapy (even before diagnostic confirmation if indicated) may improve survival. *Acanthamoeba* may be susceptible in vitro to fluconazole or ketoconazole, flucytosine, pentamidine, and sulfadiazine; voriconazole and miltefosine active against *Acanthamoeba* (alone or in combination with pentamidine).

		Acanthamoeba keratitis should be evaluated by an ophthalmologist; topical therapies for keratitis include 0.02% chlorhexidine or polyhexamethylene biguanide (0.02%), alone or combined with propamidine isethionate or hexamidine (topical therapies not approved in US but available at compounding pharmacies). Oral voriconazole may be beneficial for keratitis in addition to topical therapy. Prolonged therapy (>3–6 mo) often needed. *Balamuthia* may be susceptible in vitro to pentamidine, azithromycin/clarithromycin, fluconazole, sulfadiazine, flucytosine, and miltefosine (CIII). Surgical resection of CNS lesions may be beneficial. Miltefosine is available from CDC for treatment of free-living amebae and may improve.
Ancylostoma caninum	See EOSINOPHILIC COLITIS.	
Ancylostoma duodenale	See HOOKWORM.	
ANGIOSTRONGYLIASIS[13–18]		
Angiostrongylus cantonensis	Albendazole 20 mg/kg/day PO div bid for 14 days (CIII)	Most patients recover without antiparasitic therapy; treatment may provoke severe neurologic symptoms but may shorten duration of headache. Corticosteroids, analgesics, and repeat lumbar puncture may be of benefit.
Angiostrongylus costaricensis	Thiabendazole 50–75 mg/kg/day (max 3 g) PO div tid for 3 days (CIII)	Surgery sometimes needed to remove severely inflamed intestine. No well-proven treatment for either *Angiostrongylus* spp. Note: Thiabendazole has been discontinued in the United States but may be available elsewhere.

Disease/Organism	Treatment	Comments
ASCARIASIS (*Ascaris lumbricoides*)[19]	Albendazole 400 mg PO once (BII); OR ivermectin 150–200 µg/kg PO once (CII)	Follow-up stool ova and parasite examination after therapy not essential. Take albendazole with food. Nitazoxanide also effective against intestinal helminths. Albendazole has theoretical risk of causing seizures in patients coinfected with cysticercosis.
BABESIOSIS (*Babesia* spp)[20–22]	Clindamycin 30 mg/kg/day PO div tid, PLUS quinine 25 mg/kg/day PO div tid for 7 days (BII); OR atovaquone 40 mg/kg/day div bid, PLUS azithromycin 12 mg/kg/day for 7 days (CII)	Clindamycin (IV) and quinine preferred for severe disease; prolonged therapy, daily monitoring of hematocrit and percentage of parasitized red blood cells, and exchange blood transfusion may be of benefit for severe disease.
Balantidium coli[23]	Tetracycline (patient >7 y) 40 mg/kg/day PO div qid for 10 days (max 2 g/day) (BII); OR metronidazole 35–50 mg/kg/day PO div tid for 5 days; OR iodoquinol 40 mg/kg/day (max 2 g/day) PO div tid for 20 days (CII)	Repeated stool examination may be needed for diagnosis; prompt stool examination may increase detection of rapidly degenerating trophozoites. Nitazoxanide may also be effective.
Baylisascaris procyonis (raccoon roundworm)[24,25]	For CNS infection: albendazole 50 mg/kg/day PO div q12h AND high-dose corticosteroid therapy (CIII)	Therapy generally unsuccessful to prevent fatal outcome or severe neurologic sequelae once CNS disease present. Steroids may be of value in decreasing inflammation with therapy of CNS or ocular infection. Retinal worms may be killed by direct photocoagulation. Consider prophylactic albendazole (25–50 mg/kg PO daily for 10–20 days) for children who may have ingested soil contaminated with raccoon feces. If albendazole not immediately available, ivermectin may be useful in the interim.
Blastocystis hominis[26,27]	Metronidazole 30 mg/kg/day PO div tid for 10 days; OR iodoquinol 40 mg/kg/day (max 2 g) PO div tid for 20 days; OR nitazoxanide (as for *Cryptosporidium*) (CII)	Normal hosts may not need therapy; reexamination of stool for other parasites (eg, *Giardia*) may be of value. Metronidazole resistance may occur.

Pathogen	Therapy	Comments
CHAGAS DISEASE (*Trypanosoma cruzi*)[28,29]	See TRYPANOSOMIASIS.	
Clonorchis sinensis	See FLUKES.	
CRYPTOSPORIDIOSIS (*Cryptosporidium parvum*)[30–34]	Nitazoxanide, age 12–47 mo, 5 mL (100 mg) bid for 3 days; age 4–11 y, 10 mL (200 mg) bid for 3 days; age ≥12 y, 500 mg (tab or suspension) PO bid for 3 days (BII); OR paromomycin 30 mg/kg/day div bid–qid (CII); OR azithromycin 10 mg/kg/day for 5 days (CII); repeated treatment courses may be needed.	Disease may be self-limited in immunocompetent hosts. In HIV-infected patients not receiving HAART, medical therapy may have limited efficacy.
CUTANEOUS LARVA MIGRANS or CREEPING ERUPTION[35,36] (dog and cat hookworm) (*Ancylostoma caninum, Ancylostoma braziliense, Uncinaria stenocephala*)	Albendazole 15 mg/kg/day PO qd for 3 days (BII); OR ivermectin 200 µg/kg PO once (BII)	Albendazole bioavailability increased with food, especially fatty meals
Cyclospora spp[37,38] (cyanobacterium-like agent)	TMP/SMX 10 mg TMP/kg/day PO div bid for 5–10 days (BIII); OR ciprofloxacin 30 mg/kg/day div bid for 7 days	HIV-infected patients may require higher doses/longer therapy. Nitazoxanide may also be effective.
CYSTICERCOSIS[39–41] (*Cysticercus cellulosae*)	Albendazole 15 mg/kg/day PO div bid (max 800 mg/day) for 8–30 days (CII); OR praziquantel 50–100 mg/kg/day PO div tid for 15–30 days (Phenytoin decreases praziquantel concentration.) (CII)	For CNS disease with multiple lesions, give steroids and anticonvulsants before first dose; for CNS disease with few lesions, steroid pretreatment not required.[30,31] Contraindicated for eye or spinal cord lesions (pretreatment ophthalmologic examination recommended and surgery as indicated). Treatment controversial, especially for single lesion disease.
DIENTAMEBIASIS[42,43] (*Dientamoeba fragilis*)	Paromomycin 25 mg/kg/day PO div tid for 7 days; OR iodoquinol 40 mg/kg/day (max 2 g) PO div tid for 20 days; OR metronidazole 30 mg/kg/day PO div tid for 10 days (BII)	Asymptomatic colonization more common in adults than children. Take paromomycin with meals and iodoquinol after meals.
Diphyllobothrium latum	See TAPEWORMS.	

Disease/Organism	Treatment	Comments
ECHINOCOCCOSIS		
Echinococcus granulosus, Echinococcus multilocularis[44,45]	Albendazole 15 mg/kg/day PO div bid (max 800 mg/day) for 1–6 mo alone (CIII) or combined with praziquantel 50–75 mg/kg/day daily (BII) for 15 days ± once weekly dose for additional 3–6 mo	Surgical excision may be the only reliable therapy; ultrasound-guided percutaneous aspiration–injection–re-aspiration plus albendazole may be effective for hepatic hydatid cysts.
Entamoeba histolytica	See AMEBIASIS.	
Enterobius vermicularis	See PINWORMS.	
Fasciola hepatica	See FLUKES.	
EOSINOPHILIC COLITIS (*Ancylostoma caninum*)[46]	Albendazole 400 mg PO once (BIII)	Endoscopic removal may be considered if medical treatment not successful.
EOSINOPHILIC MENINGITIS	See ANGIOSTRONGYLIASIS.	
FILARIASIS[47]		Ivermectin may be effective for killing *Wuchereria, Brugia,* and *Loa loa* microfilariae; in heavy infections or when coinfection with *Onchocerca volvulus* possible, consider ivermectin initially to reduce microfilaremia before giving DEC (decreased risk of encephalopathy or severe allergic or febrile reaction).
– River blindness (*Onchocerca volvulus*)	Ivermectin 150 µg/kg PO once (AII); repeat q6–12mo until asymptomatic and no ongoing exposure	Antihistamines or corticosteroids are of benefit for allergic reactions.
– *Wuchereria bancrofti, Brugia malayi, Mansonella streptocerca*	*W bancrofti, B malayi, Brugia timori, M streptocerca:* DEC (from CDC) 1 mg/kg PO after food on day 1; then 3 mg/kg/day div tid on day 2; then 3–6 mg/kg/day div tid on day 3; then 6 mg/kg/day div tid on days 4–14 (AII)	Avoid DEC with *Onchocerca* coinfection.
Mansonella ozzardi	Ivermectin 150 µg/kg PO once may be effective.	DEC not effective
Mansonella perstans	Albendazole 400 mg PO bid for 10 days	DEC and ivermectin not effective; doxycycline beneficial for infection acquired in West Africa

Loa loa	DEC (from CDC) as above, then 9 mg/kg/day div tid on days 14–21 (AII)	
Tropical pulmonary eosinophilia[48]	DEC (from CDC) 6 mg/kg/day PO div tid for 14 days; antihistamines/corticosteroids for allergic reactions (CII)	
FLUKES		
Chinese liver fluke[49] (*Clonorchis sinensis*) and others (*Fasciolopsis, Heterophyes, Metagonimus, Metorchis, Nanophyetus, Opisthorchis*)	Praziquantel 75 mg/kg PO div tid for 2 days (BII); OR albendazole 10 mg/kg/day PO for 7 days (CIII)	Take praziquantel with liquids and food.
Lung fluke[50,51] (*Paragonimus westermani* and other *Paragonimus* lung flukes)	Praziquantel 75 mg/kg PO div tid for 2 days (BII)	Triclabendazole (5 mg/kg qd for 3 days or 10 mg/kg bid for 1 day) may also be effective; triclabendazole should be taken with food to facilitate absorption.
Sheep liver fluke[52] (*Fasciola hepatica*)	Triclabendazole (from CDC) 10 mg/kg PO once (BII) OR nitazoxanide PO (take with food), age 12–47 mo, 100 mg/dose bid for 7 days; age 4–11 y, 200 mg/dose bid for 7 days; age ≥12 y, 1 tab (500 mg)/dose bid for 7 days (CII)	Bithionol 30–50 mg/kg PO div qid on alternate days for 10–15 doses is an alternative but availability limited (no longer available from CDC).
GIARDIASIS (*Giardia lamblia*)[53–55]	Metronidazole 30–40 mg/kg/day PO div tid for 7–10 days (BII); OR nitazoxanide PO (take with food), age 12–47 mo, 100 mg/dose bid for 7 days; age 4–11 y, 200 mg/dose bid for 7 days; age ≥12 y, 1 tab (500 mg)/dose bid for 7 days (BII); OR tinidazole 50 mg/kg/day (max 2 g) for 1 day (BII)	If therapy inadequate, another course of the same agent usually curative. Alternatives: furazolidone 6 mg/kg/day in 4 doses for 7–10 days; OR paromomycin 30 mg/kg/day div tid for 5–10 days; OR albendazole 10 mg/kg/day PO for 5 days (CII). Prolonged courses may be needed for immunocompromised conditions (eg, hypogammaglobulinemia). Treatment of asymptomatic carriers not usually recommended.

Disease/Organism	Treatment	Comments
HOOKWORM[56]		
Necator americanus, Ancylostoma duodenale	Albendazole 10 mg/kg (max 400 mg) once (repeat dose may be necessary) (BII); OR pyrantel pamoate 11 mg/kg (max 1 g/day) (BII) PO qd for 3 days	Perform repeat stool examination 2 weeks after treatment; re-treat if positive.
Hymenolepis nana	See TAPEWORMS.	
ISOSPORIASIS (*Isospora belli*)[1,23] (now also known as cystoisosporiasis)	TMP/SMX 10 mg TMP/kg/day PO div bid for 10 days; if still symptomatic, 5 mg TMP/kg/day PO div bid for an additional 1–3 wk; pyrimethamine may be effective (CII).	Infection often self-limited in immunocompetent hosts. Repeated stool examinations and special techniques (eg, modified AFB staining or UV microscopy) may be needed to detect low oocyst numbers. HIV-infected children may need longer courses of therapy (consider long-term maintenance therapy for multiple relapses).
LEISHMANIASIS,[57–62] including kala-azar		
Leishmania spp	Visceral: liposomal AmB 3 mg/kg/day on days 1–5, day 14, and day 21 (BII); OR sodium stibogluconate (from CDC) 20 mg/kg/day IM or IV for 28 days (or longer) (BIII); OR miltefosine 2.5 mg/kg/day PO (max 150 mg/day) for 28 days (BII); OR AmB 1 mg/kg/day IV daily for 15–20 days or every second day for 4–8 wk (BIII); OR paromomycin sulfate 15 mg/kg/day IM for 21 days (BII) Cutaneous: sodium stibogluconate 20 mg/kg/day IM or IV for 20 days (BIII); OR miltefosine (as above) (BII); OR pentamidine isethionate 2–3 mg/kg/day IM daily or qod for 10–14 days (BII) Mucosal: sodium stibogluconate 20 mg/kg/day IM or IV for 28 days; OR AmB 0.5–1 mg/kg/day IV daily for 15–20 days or qod for 4–8 wk; OR miltefosine (as above)	Consult with tropical medicine specialist if unfamiliar with leishmaniasis. Region where infection acquired affects therapeutic options; patients infected in south Asia (especially India, Nepal) should receive non-antimonial regimens because of high rates of resistance. Azoles (eg, fluconazole, ketoconazole) may be effective for cutaneous disease but should be avoided in treating mucosal or visceral disease. Topical paromomycin (15%) applied twice daily for 10–20 days may be considered for cutaneous leishmaniasis in areas where the potential for mucosal disease is extremely unlikely. For immunocompromised patients, FDA-approved dosing of liposomal amphotericin is 4 mg/kg on days 1–5, 10, 17, 24, 31, and 38, with further therapy on an individual basis.

LICE		
Pediculus capitis or *humanus*, *Phthirus pubis*[63,64]	Follow manufacturer's instructions for topical use: permethrin 1% OR pyrethrin (both preferred with piperonyl butoxide for children aged ≥2 y) (BII); OR 0.5% ivermectin lotion (BII); OR spinosad 0.9% topical suspension (BII); OR benzyl alcohol lotion 5% (BIII); OR malathion 0.5% (BIII); OR for topical therapies repeat in 1 wk; OR ivermectin 200 µg/kg PO once	Launder bedding and clothing; for eyelash infestation, use petrolatum; for head lice, remove nits with comb designed for that purpose. Use benzyl alcohol lotion and ivermectin lotion for children aged ≥6 mo, spinosad for aged ≥4 y, and malathion for aged ≥6 y. Benzyl alcohol can be irritating to skin; parasite resistance unlikely to develop. Consult health care professional before re-treatment with ivermectin lotion; re-treatment with spinosad topical suspension usually not needed unless live lice seen 1 wk after treatment. Administration of 3 doses of ivermectin (1 dose/wk separately by weekly intervals) may be needed to eradicate heavy infection.
MALARIA[65–70]		
Plasmodium falciparum, *Plasmodium vivax*, *Plasmodium ovale*, *Plasmodium malariae*	CDC Malaria Hotline 770/488-7788 or 855/856-4713 toll-free (Monday–Friday, 9:00 am–5:00 pm ET) or emergency consultation after hours 770/488-7100; online information at www.cdc.gov/malaria (accessed October 13, 2014). Consult tropical medicine specialist if unfamiliar with malaria.	No antimalarial drug provides absolute protection against malaria; fever after return from an endemic area should prompt an immediate evaluation. Emphasize personal protective measures (insecticides, bed nets, clothing, and avoidance of dusk–dawn mosquito exposures).

Disease/Organism	Treatment	Comments
Prophylaxis		
For areas with chloroquine-resistant *P falciparum* or *P vivax*	A-P: 5–8 kg, ½ pediatric tab/day; ≥9–10 kg, ¾ pediatric tab/day; ≥11–20 kg, 1 pediatric tab (62.5 mg atovaquone/25 mg proguanil); ≥21–30 kg, 2 pediatric tabs; ≥31–40 kg, 3 pediatric tabs; ≥40 kg, 1 adult tab (250 mg atovaquone/100 mg proguanil) PO daily starting 1–2 days before travel and continuing 7 days after last exposure; for children <5 kg, data on A-P limited (BII); OR mefloquine: for children <5 kg, 5 mg/kg; ≥5–9 kg, ⅛ tab; ≥10–19 kg, ≥¼ tab; 20–30 kg, ≥½ tab; ≥31–45 kg, ¾ tab; ≥45 kg (adult dose), 1 tab PO once weekly starting 1 wk before arrival in area and continuing for 4 wk after leaving area (BII); OR doxycycline (patients >7 y): 2 mg/kg (max 100 mg) PO daily starting 1–2 days before arrival in area and continuing for 4 wk after leaving area (BIII); OR primaquine (check for G6PD deficiency before administering): 0.5 mg/kg base daily starting 1 day before travel and continuing for 5 days after last exposure (BII)	Avoid mefloquine for persons with a history of seizures or psychosis, active depression, or cardiac conduction abnormalities. Avoid A-P in severe renal impairment (CrCl <30). *P falciparum* resistance to mefloquine exists along the borders between Thailand and Myanmar and Thailand and Cambodia, Myanmar and China, and Myanmar and Laos; isolated resistance has been reported in southern Vietnam. Take doxycycline with adequate fluids to avoid esophageal irritation and food to avoid GI side effects; use sunscreen and avoid excessive sun exposure.
For areas without chloroquine-resistant *P falciparum* or *P vivax*	Chloroquine phosphate 5 mg base/kg (max 300 mg base) PO once weekly, beginning 1 wk before arrival in area and continuing for 4 wk after leaving area (available in suspension outside the US and Canada) (AII). For heavy or prolonged (months) exposure to mosquitoes: consider treating with primaquine (check for G6PD deficiency before administering) 0.5 mg base/kg PO qd with final 2 wk of chloroquine for prevention of relapse with *P ovale* or *P vivax*.	
Treatment of disease		Consider exchange blood transfusion for >10% parasitemia, altered mental status, pulmonary edema, or renal failure.

– Chloroquine-resistant *P falciparum* or *P vivax*	Oral therapy: A-P: for children <5 kg, data limited; ≥5–8 kg, 2 pediatric tabs (62.5 mg atovaquone/25 mg proguanil) PO qd for 3 days; ≥9–10 kg, 3 pediatric tabs qd for 3 days; ≥11–20 kg, 1 adult tab (250 mg atovaquone/100 mg proguanil) qd for 3 days; ≥21–30 kg, 2 adult tabs qd for 3 days; 31–40 kg, 3 adult tabs qd for 3 days; ≥40 kg, 4 adult tabs qd for 3 days (BII); OR artemether/lumefantrine 6 doses over 3 days at 0, 8, 24, 36, 48, and 60 h; <15 kg, 1 tab/dose; ≥15–25 kg, 2 tabs/dose; ≥25–35 kg, 3 tabs/dose; ≥35 kg, 4 tabs/dose (BII); OR quinine 30 mg/kg/day (max 2 g/day) PO div tid for 3–7 days AND doxycycline (age >7 y) 4 mg/kg/day div bid for 7 days OR clindamycin 30 mg/kg/day div tid (max 900 mg tid) for 7 days. Parenteral therapy (check with CDC): quinidine 10 mg/kg (max 600 mg) IV (1 h infusion in normal saline) followed by continuous infusion of 0.02 mg/kg/min until oral therapy can be given (after 48-h therapy, decrease dose by ⅓ to ½) (BII); alternative: artesunate 2.4 mg/kg/dose IV for 3 days at 0, 12, 24, 48, and 72 h (from CDC) (B1) AND a second oral agent (A-P, clindamycin, or doxycycline for aged ≥7 y). For prevention of relapse with *P vivax, P ovale:* primaquine (check for G6PD deficiency before administering) 0.5 mg base/kg/day PO for 14 days.	Mild disease may be treated with oral antimalarial drugs; severe disease (impaired level of consciousness, convulsion, hypotension, or parasitemia >5%) should be treated parenterally. Avoid mefloquine for treatment of malaria if possible given higher dose and increased incidence of adverse events. Take clindamycin and doxycycline with plenty of liquids. Do not use primaquine during pregnancy; for relapses of primaquine-resistant *P vivax* or *P ovale,* consider retreating with primaquine 30 mg (base) for 28 days. Continuously monitor ECG, BP, and glucose in patients receiving quinidine. Avoid artemether/lumefantrine and mefloquine in patients with cardiac arrhythmias, and avoid concomitant use of drugs that prolong QT interval. Take A-P and artemether/lumefantrine with food or milk. Use artesunate for quinidine intolerance, lack of quinidine availability, or treatment failure; www.cdc.gov/malaria/resources/pdf/treatmenttable.pdf (accessed October 13, 2014); artemisinins should be used in combination with other drugs to avoid resistance.
– Chloroquine-susceptible *P falciparum,* chloroquine-susceptible *P vivax, P ovale, P malariae*	Oral therapy: chloroquine 10 mg/kg base (max 600 mg base) PO then 5 mg/kg 6, 24, and 48 h after initial dose. Parenteral therapy: quinidine, as above. See above for prevention of relapse due to *P vivax* and *P ovale.*	

Disease/Organism	Treatment	Comments
Paragonimus westermani	See FLUKES.	
PINWORMS (*Enterobius vermicularis*)[71]	Albendazole 10 mg/kg (max 400 mg) PO once (BII); OR pyrantel pamoate 11 mg/kg (max 1 g) PO once (BII); repeat treatment in 2 wk.	Treatment of entire household (and if this fails, consider close child care/school contacts) often recommended; re-treatment of contacts after 2 wk may be needed to prevent reinfection.
PNEUMOCYSTIS	See Chapter 8, Table 8B, *Pneumocystis jiroveci* (*carinii*) pneumonia.	
SCABIES (*Sarcoptes scabiei*)[72,73]	Permethrin 5% cream applied to entire body (including scalp in infants), left on for 8–14 h then bathe, repeat in 1 wk (BII); OR ivermectin 200 µg/kg PO once weekly for 1–2 doses (BII); OR crotamiton 10% applied topically overnight on days 1, 2, 3, and 8, bathe in am (BII).	Launder bedding and clothing. Reserve lindane for patients who do not respond to other therapy. Crotamiton treatment failure has been observed. Ivermectin safety not well established in children <15 kg and pregnant women.
SCHISTOSOMIASIS (*Schistosoma haematobium, Schistosoma japonicum, Schistosoma mansoni, Schistosoma mekongi, Schistosoma intercalatum*)[74–77]	Praziquantel 40 (for *S haematobium* and *S mansoni*) or 60 (for *S japonicum* and *S mekongi*) mg/kg/d PO div bid (if 40 mg/day) or tid (if 60 mg/d) for 1 day (AI); OR oxamniquine (not available in the US) 20 mg/kg PO div bid for 1 day (Brazil) or 40–60 mg/kg/day for 2–3 days (most of Africa) (BII)	Take praziquantel with food and liquids.
STRONGYLOIDIASIS (*Strongyloides stercoralis*)[78–82]	Ivermectin 200 µg/kg PO qd for 1–2 days (BI); OR albendazole 400 mg PO bid for 7 days (or longer for disseminated disease) (BII)	Albendazole is less effective but may be adequate if longer courses used. For immunocompromised patients (especially with hyperinfection syndrome), veterinary subcutaneous or enema formulations may be lifesaving. Safety of ivermectin in children <15 kg and pregnant women yet to be well established.
TAPEWORMS		
– *Cysticercus cellulosae*	See CYSTICERCOSIS.	
– *Echinococcus granulosus*	See ECHINOCOCCOSIS.	

– *Taenia saginata, Taenia solium, Hymenolepis nana, Diphyllobothrium latum, Dipylidium caninum*	Praziquantel 5–10 mg/kg PO once (25 mg/kg once for *H nana*) (BII); OR niclosamide tab 50 mg/kg PO once, chewed thoroughly (all but *H nana*)	Limited availability of niclosamide in US; may be available in compounding pharmacies. Nitazoxanide may be effective (published clinical data limited).
TOXOPLASMOSIS (*Toxoplasma gondii*)[83–85]	Pyrimethamine 2 mg/kg/day PO div bid for 2 days (max 100 mg) then 1 mg/kg/day (max 25 mg/day) PO daily AND sulfadiazine 120 mg/kg/day PO div qid (max 6 g/day); with supplemental folinic acid and leucovorin 10–25 mg with each dose of pyrimethamine (AI). See Chapter 5 for congenital infection. For treatment in pregnancy, spiramycin 50–100 mg/kg/day PO div qid (available as investigational therapy through the FDA at 301/796-0563) (CII).	Treatment continued for 2 wk after resolution of illness (approximately 3–6 wk); concurrent corticosteroids given for ocular or CNS infection. Prolonged therapy if HIV positive. Take pyrimethamine with food to decrease GI adverse effects; sulfadiazine should be taken on an empty stomach with water. Atovaquone or clindamycin plus pyrimethamine may be effective for patients intolerant of sulfa-containing drugs.
TRAVELER'S DIARRHEA[86–88]	Azithromycin 10 mg/kg qd for 3–5 days (BII); OR rifaximin 200 mg PO tid for 3 days (ages ≥12 y) (BIII); OR ciprofloxacin (BII); OR cefixime (CII)	Azithromycin preferable to ciprofloxacin for travelers to Southeast Asia given high prevalence of quinolone-resistant *Campylobacter*. Rifaximin may not be as efficacious for *Shigella* and other enterics in patients with bloody diarrhea and invasive infection.
TRICHINELLOSIS (*Trichinella spiralis*)[89]	Albendazole 20 mg/kg/day (max 400 mg/dose) PO div bid for 8–14 days (BII)	Therapy ineffective for larvae already in muscles. Anti-inflammatory drugs, steroids for CNS or cardiac involvement or severe symptoms.
TRICHOMONIASIS (*Trichomonas vaginalis*)[90]	Tinidazole 50 mg/kg (max 2 g) PO for 1 dose (BII) OR metronidazole 500 mg PO tid for 7 days (BII)	Treat sex partners simultaneously. Metronidazole resistance occurs and may be treated with higher-dose metronidazole or tinidazole.
Trichuris trichiura	See WHIPWORM.	

Disease/Organism	Treatment	Comments
TRYPANOSOMIASIS		
– Chagas disease[28,29] (*Trypanosoma cruzi*)	Nifurtimox PO (from CDC): age 1–10 y, 15–20 mg/kg/day div qid for 90 days; 11–16 y, 12.5–15 mg/kg/day div qid for 90 days; ≥17 y, 8–10 mg/kg/day div tid–qid for 90 days (BIII); OR benznidazole PO (from CDC): age <12 y, 10 mg/kg/day div bid for 60 days; ≥12 y, 5–7 mg/kg/day div bid for 60 d (BIII)	Therapy recommended for acute and congenital infection, reactivated infection, and chronic infection in children aged <18 y. Take benznidazole with meals to avoid GI adverse effects; benznidazole contraindicated in pregnancy. Interferon-γ in addition to nifurtimox may shorten acute disease duration or severity.
– Sleeping sickness[91–94] (*Trypanosoma brucei gambiense* [West African]; *T brucei rhodesiense* [East African]; acute [hemolymphatic] stage)	*Tb gambiense:* pentamidine isethionate 4 mg/kg/day (max 300 mg) IM or IV for 7 days (BII) *Tb rhodesiense:* suramin (from CDC) 2 mg/kg test dose IV, then 20 mg/kg (max 1.5 g) IV on days 1, 3, 5, 14, and 21 (BII)	Consult with tropical medicine specialist if unfamiliar with trypanosomiasis. Examination of the buffy coat of peripheral blood may be helpful. *Tb gambiense* may be found in lymph node aspirates.
Late (CNS) stage	*Tb gambiense:* eflornithine (from CDC) 400 mg/kg/day IV div q6h for 14 days (BIII); OR melarsoprol (from CDC) 2.2 mg/day (max 180 mg) IV for 10 days (BIII) *Tb rhodesiense:* melarsoprol, 2.2 mg/kg/day IV for 10 days; corticosteroids given with melarsoprol to decrease risk of CNS toxicity	CSF examination needed for management (double-centrifuge technique recommended); perform repeat CSF examinations every 6 mo for 2 y to detect relapse. Addition of nifurtimox for late stage *Tb gambiense* infection may shorten required duration of therapy and may be more effective vs standard melarsoprol regimens.
VISCERAL LARVA MIGRANS (TOXOCARIASIS)		
Toxocara canis; Toxocara cati	Albendazole 15 mg/kg/day (max 800 mg/day) PO bid for 5 days (BII), OR DEC (from CDC) 6 mg/kg/day PO div tid for 7–10 days	Some experts advocate longer therapy (eg, 20 days). Corticosteroids if severe or ocular involvement.
WHIPWORM (TRICHURIASIS)		
Trichuris trichiura[95]	Albendazole 400 mg PO for 3 days; OR ivermectin 200 µg/kg/day PO daily for 3 days (BII)	Stool reexamination after treatment usually not necessary
Wuchereria bancrofti	See FILARIASIS.	

11. Alphabetic Listing of Antimicrobials

NOTES

- Higher dosages in a dose range are generally indicated for illnesses that are more serious.
- For most antimicrobials, a maximum or upper adult limit dosage is provided, based on US Food and Drug Administration (FDA)-reviewed and approved clinical data. However, data may be published on higher dosages than originally approved by the FDA, particularly for generic drugs. Whenever possible, these dosages are also provided.
- In situations in which aggressive therapy is indicated, the benefits of using a high or adult-sized dose in an obese child may outweigh the unknown risks at that higher dosage. For information on dosing in obesity, see Chapter 12.
- Drugs with FDA-approved pediatric dosage, or dosages based on multiple randomized clinical trials, are given a Level of Evidence I. For dosages for which data are collected from adults, from non-comparative trials, or from small comparative trials, the Level of Evidence is II. For dosages that are based on expert or consensus opinion or case reports, the Level of Evidence given is III.
- Antiretroviral medications are not included. See Chapter 9.
- Commercially available dosage forms for children and adults are listed. If no oral liquid form is available, round the child's dose to the nearest value using a combination of commercially available solid dosage form strengths. Consult a pediatric pharmacist for recommendations on mixing with food (crushing tablets, emptying capsule contents) and the availability of an extemporaneously compounded liquid formulation.
- **Abbreviations:** AOM, acute otitis media; bid, twice daily; BSA, body surface area; CABP, community-acquired bacterial pneumonia; CA-MRSA, community-associated methicillin-resistant *Staphylococcus aureus;* cap, capsule or caplet; CMV, cytomegalovirus; CNS, central nervous system; CrCl, creatinine clearance; div, divided; DR, delayed-release; EC, enteric coated; ER, extended release; FDA, US Food and Drug Administration; hs, bedtime; HSV, herpes simplex virus; IBW, ideal body weight; IM, intramuscular; IV, intravenous; ivpb, iv piggyback (premixed bag); LD, loading dose; MAC, *Mycobacterium avium* complex; oint, ointment; ophth, ophthalmic; PCP, *Pneumocystis* pneumonia; PIP, piperacillin; PMA, post-menstrual age; PO, oral; pwd, powder; qd, once daily; qhs, every bedtime; qid, 4 times daily; SMX, sulfamethoxazole; soln, solution; SPAG-2, small particle aerosol generator model-2; SQ, subcutaneous; supp, suppository; susp, suspension; tab, tablet; TB, tuberculosis; TBW, total body weight; tid, 3 times daily; TMP, trimethoprim; top, topical; UTI, urinary tract infection; vag, vaginal; VZV, varicella-zoster virus.

A. SYSTEMIC ANTIMICROBIALS WITH DOSAGE FORMS AND USUAL DOSAGES

Generic and Trade Names	Dosage Form	Route	Dose (evidence level)	Interval
Acyclovir,[a] Zovirax	500-, 1,000-mg vial	IV	15–45 mg/kg/day (I) (See chapters 5 and 9.) 1,500 mg/m²/day	q8h
	200-mg/5-mL susp, 200-mg cap; 400-, 800-mg tab	PO	900 mg/m²/day (I) (See chapters 5 and 9.) 60–80 mg/kg/day (max 4 g/day) (I)	q8h q6–8h
Sitavig	50-mg tab	Buccal	Adults 50 mg, for herpes labialis	One time
Albendazole, Albenza	200-mg tab	PO	15 mg/kg/day (max 800 mg/day) (I)	q12h
Amikacin,[a] Amikin	500-mg/2-mL, 1,000-mg/4-mL vials	IV, IM	15–22.5 mg/kg/day (See Chapter 1 regarding q24h dosing.) (I)	q8–24h
		Intravesical	0.5 mg/mL in normal saline x 50–100 mL (III)	q12h
Amoxicillin,[a] Amoxil	125-, 200-, 250-, 400-mg/5-mL susp 125-, 250-mg chew tab 250-, 500-mg cap 500-, 875-mg tab	PO	Standard dose: 40–45 mg/kg/day (I) High dose: 80–90 mg/kg/day (I), max 4 g/day (III) 150 mg/kg/day div q8h for penicillin-resistant *S pneumoniae* otitis media (III) Adults 750–2,000 mg/day (I)	q8-12h q12h q8h
Amoxicillin extended release,[a] Moxatag	775-mg tab	PO	≥12 y and adults 775 mg/day	q24h

Amoxicillin/ clavulanate,[a] Augmentin	16:1 formulation (Augmentin XR): 1,000/62.5-mg tab	PO	16:1 formulation: ≥40 kg and adults 4,000 mg amoxicillin component/day (I)	q12h
	14:1 formulation (Augmentin ES): 600/42.9-mg/5-mL susp	PO	14:1 formulation: 90-mg amoxicillin component/kg/day (I), max 4,000 mg/day (III)	q12h
	7:1 formulation: 875/125-mg tab 200/28.5-, 400/57-mg chew tab; 200/28.5-, 400/57-mg/5-mL susp	PO	7:1 formulation: 25-45 mg amoxicillin component/kg/day (max 1,750 mg/day) (I)	q12h
	4:1 formulation: 500/125-mg tab 125/31.25-, 250/62.5-mg chew tab; 125/31.25-, 250/62.5-mg/5-mL susp	PO	4:1 formulation: 20–40 mg amoxicillin component/kg/day (max 1,500 mg/day) (I)	q8h
Amphotericin B deoxycholate,[a] Fungizone	50-mg vial	IV	1–1.5 mg/kg pediatric and adults (I), no max 0.5 mg/kg for *Candida* esophagitis or cystitis (II)	q24h
		Intravesical	50–100 µg/mL in sterile H_2O x 50–100 mL (III)	q8h
Amphotericin B, lipid complex, Abelcet	100-mg/20-mL vial	IV	5 mg/kg pediatric and adult dose (I) No max	q24h
Amphotericin B, liposomal, AmBisome	50-mg vial	IV	5 mg/kg pediatric and adult dose (I) No max	q24h
Ampicillin/ampicillin trihydrate[a]	250-, 500-mg cap 125-, 250-mg/5-mL susp	PO	50–100 mg/kg/day if <20 kg (I) ≥20 kg and adults 1–2 g/day (I)	q6h
Ampicillin sodium[a]	0.125-, 0.25-, 0.5-, 1-, 2-, 10-g vial	IV, IM	50–200 mg/kg/day (I)	q6h
			300–400 mg/kg/day endocarditis/meningitis (III) Adults 4–12 g/day (I)	q4–6h
Ampicillin and sulbactam,[a] Unasyn	1/0.5-, 2/1-, 10/5-g vial	IV/IM	200 mg/kg/day (ampicillin) if <40 kg (I) ≥40 kg and adults 4–8 g ampicillin/day (I)	q6h

A. SYSTEMIC ANTIMICROBIALS WITH DOSAGE FORMS AND USUAL DOSAGES (cont)

Generic and Trade Names	Dosage Form	Route	Dose (evidence grade)	Interval
Anidulafungin, Eraxis	50-, 100-mg vial	IV	1.5–3 mg/kg LD, then 0.75–1.5 mg/kg (II) Adults 100–200 mg LD, then 50-100 mg (I)	q24h
Atovaquone,[a] Mepron	750-mg/5-mL susp	PO	30 mg/kg/day if 1–3 mo or >24 mo (I) 45 mg/kg/day if 4–24 mo (I) Adolescents/adults 1,500 mg/day (I)	q12h q24h for prophylaxis
Atovaquone and proguanil,[a] Malarone	62.5/25-mg pediatric tab 250/100-mg adult tab	PO	Prophylaxis for malaria: 11–20 kg: 1 pediatric tab, 21–30 kg: 2 pediatric tabs, 31–40 kg: 3 pediatric tabs, >40 kg: 1 adult tab (I) Treatment: 5–8 kg: 2 pediatric tabs, 9–10 kg: 3 pediatric tabs, 11–20 kg: 1 adult tab, 21–30 kg: 2 adult tabs, 31–40 kg: 3 adult tabs, >40 kg: 4 adult tabs (I)	q24h
Azithromycin,[a] Zithromax, Zmax	250-, 500-, 600-mg tab 100-, 200-mg/5-mL susp 27-mg/mL ER susp (Zmax)	PO	Otitis: 10 mg/kg/day for 1 day, then 5 mg/kg for 4 days; or 10 mg/kg/day for 3 days; or 30 mg/kg once (I). Pharyngitis: 12 mg/kg/day for 5 days (I). Sinusitis: 10 mg/kg/day for 3 days (I). CABP: 10 mg/kg for 1 day, then 5 mg/kg/day for 4 days or 60 mg/kg once of ER (Zmax) susp (I). Adult single or total course dose 1.5–2 g (I). MAC/PCP prophylaxis: 5 mg/kg/day (I). See Chapter 6 for other specific disease dosing recommendations.	q24h
	500-mg vial	IV	10 mg/kg (II)	q24h
Aztreonam, Azactam	500-mg, 1-, 2-g vial,[a] 1-, 2-g ivpb	IV, IM	90–120 mg/kg/day (adults 3–6 g/day) (I)	q6–8h
Aztreonam inhalation, Cayston, Victrelis	75-mg vial	Inhaled	≥7 y: 75 mg/dose via Altera nebulizer (I)	q8h
Boceprevir	200-mg cap	PO	Adults 2,400 mg/day[b] (I)	q8h

Capreomycin, Capastat	1-g vial	IV, IM	15–30 mg/kg (III) Adults 1 g, max 20 mg/kg (I)	q24h
Caspofungin, Cancidas	50-, 70-mg vial	IV	70 mg/m^2 once, then 50 mg/m^2, max dose 70 mg (I)	q24h
Cefaclor,[a] Ceclor	125-, 187-, 250-, 375-mg/5-mL susp 250-, 500-mg cap 375-, 500-mg ER tab	PO	20–40 mg/kg/day, max 1 g/day (I)	q12h
Cefadroxil,[a] Duricef	250-, 500-mg/5-mL susp 500-mg cap, 1-g tab	PO	30 mg/kg/day (adults 1–2 g/day) (I)	q12–24h
Cefazolin,[a] Ancef	0.5-, 1-, 10-, 20-g vial, 1-, 2-g ivpb	IV, IM	25–100 mg/kg/day (adults 3–6 g/day) (I) For serious infections, up to 150 mg/kg/day (III)	q6–8h
Cefdinir,[a] Omnicef	125-, 250-mg/5-mL susp, 300-mg cap	PO	14 mg/kg/day, max 600 mg/day (I)	q24h
Cefditoren, Spectracef	200-, 400-mg tab	PO	≥12 y and adults, 400–800 mg/day (I)	q12h
Cefepime,[a] Maxipime	1-, 2-g vial 1-, 2-g ivpb	IV, IM	100 mg/kg/day (adults 2–4 g/day) (I)	q12h
			150 mg/kg/day empiric therapy of fever with neutropenia (adults 6 g/day) (I)	q8h
Cefixime, Suprax	100-, 200-, 500-mg/5-mL susp 100-, 150-, 200-mg chew tab 400-mg tab, cap	PO	8 mg/kg/day if <50 kg (adults 400 mg/day) (I) For convalescent oral therapy of serious infections, up to 20 mg/kg/day (III)	q12–24h
Cefotaxime,[a] Claforan	0.5-, 1-, 2-, 10-g vial	IV, IM	50–180 mg/kg/day (adults 3–8 g/day) (I)	q6–8h
			200–225 mg/kg/day for meningitis (adults 12 g/day) (I)	q6h
Cefotetan,[a] Cefotan	1-, 2-, 10-g vial 1-, 2-g ivpb	IV, IM	60–100 mg/kg/day (II)	q12h
			Adults 2–4 g/day (I)	q12h
Cefoxitin,[a] Mefoxin	1-, 2-, 10-g vial, 1-, 2-g ivpb	IV, IM	80–160 mg/kg/day, max 12 g/day (I)	q6–8h
Cefpodoxime,[a] Vantin	50-, 100-mg/5-mL susp 100-, 200-mg tab	PO	10 mg/kg/day, max 400 mg/day (I)	q12h
Cefprozil,[a] Cefzil	125-, 250-mg/5-mL susp 250-, 500-mg tab	PO	15–30 mg/kg/day (adults 0.5–1 g/d) (I)	q12h

A. SYSTEMIC ANTIMICROBIALS WITH DOSAGE FORMS AND USUAL DOSAGES (cont)

Generic and Trade Names	Dosage Form	Route	Dose (evidence grade)	Interval
Ceftaroline, Teflaro (Doses are investigational in children.)	400-, 600-mg vial	IV	<6 mo (II): 24 mg/kg/day for skin or CABP 30 mg/kg/day for complicated CABP ≥6 mo (II): 36 mg/kg/day for skin or CABP, max 1,200 mg/day 45 mg/kg/day for complicated CABP, max 1,800 mg/day	q8h
Ceftazidime,[a] Ceptaz, Fortaz	0.5-, 1-, 2-, 6-g vial 1-, 2-g ivpb	IV, IM	90–150 mg/kg/day (adults 3–6 g/day) (I)	q8h
		IV	200–300 mg/kg/day for serious *Pseudomonas* infection (max 8–12 g/day) (II)	q8h
Ceftibuten, Cedax	90-mg/5-mL susp 400-mg cap	PO	9 mg/kg/day (adults 400 mg/day) (I)	q24h
Ceftriaxone,[a] Rocephin	0.25-, 0.5-, 1-, 2-, 10-g vial 1-, 2-g ivpb	IV, IM	50 mg/kg, max 1 g, 1–3 doses IM for AOM (II) 50–75 mg/kg/day, max 2 g/day (I) 100 mg/kg/day for meningitis, max 4 g/day (I)	q24h q24h q12h
Cefuroxime axetil,[a] Ceftin	125-, 250-mg/5-mL susp 250-, 500-mg tab	PO	20–30 mg/kg/day (adults 0.5–1 g/day) (I) For bone and joint infections, up to 100 mg/kg/day (III)	q12h
Cefuroxime sodium,[a] Zinacef	0.75-, 1.5-g vial, ivpb	IV, IM	100–150 mg/kg/day (adults 1.5–3 g/day) (I)	q8h
Cephalexin,[a] Keflex	125-, 250-mg/5-mL susp 250-, 500-mg caps and tabs	PO	25–50 mg/kg/day, max 1 g/day (I)	q12h
			75–100 mg/kg/day for bone and joint, or severe infections (II) Adults 2–4 g/day (I)	q6–8h
Chloramphenicol sodium succinate,[a] Chloromycetin	1-g vial	IV	50–75 mg/kg/day 75–100 mg/kg/day for meningitis (I) Adults 50–100 mg/kg/day	q6h

Chloroquine phosphate,[a] Aralen	250-, 500-mg (150-, 300-mg base) tabs	PO	See Chapter 10.	
Cidofovir,[a] Vistide	375-mg/5-mL vial	IV	5 mg/kg (III); see also Chapter 9.	Weekly
Ciprofloxacin,[a] Cipro	250-, 500-mg/5-mL susp 100-, 250-, 500-, 750-mg tab	PO	20–40 mg/kg/day, max 1.5 g/day (I)	q12h
	200-, 400-mg vial, ivpb	IV	20–30 mg/kg/day, max 1.2 g/day (I)	q12h
Ciprofloxacin extended release,[a] Cipro XR	500-, 1,000-mg ER tab	PO	Adults 500–1,000 mg (I)	q24h
Clarithromycin,[a] Biaxin	125-, 250-mg/5-mL susp 250-, 500-mg tab	PO	15 mg/kg/day, max 1 g/day (I)	q12h
Clarithromycin extended release,[a] Biaxin XL[a]	500-, 1,000-mg ER tab	PO	Adults 1,000 mg (I)	q24h
Clindamycin,[a] Cleocin	75 mg/5-mL soln 75-, 150-, 300-mg cap	PO	10–25 mg/kg/day (adults 1.2–1.8 g/day) (I) 30–40 mg/kg/day for CA-MRSA, intra-abdominal infection, or AOM (III)	q8h
	0.3-, 0.6-, 0.9-g vial, ivpb	IV, IM	20–40 mg/kg/day (adults 1.8–2.7 g/day) (I)	q8h
Clotrimazole,[a] Mycelex	10-mg lozenge	PO	≥3 y and adults, dissolve lozenge in mouth (I).	5 times daily
Colistimethate,[a] Coly-Mycin M	150-mg (colistin base) vial 1-mg base = 2.7-mg colistimethate	IV, IM	2.5–5 mg base/kg/day based on IBW (I) Up to 5–7 mg base/kg/day (III)	q8h
Cycloserine, Seromycin	250-mg cap	PO	10–20 mg/kg/day (III) Adults max 1 g/day (I)	q12h
Dalbavancin, Dalvance	500-mg vial	IV	Adults 1 g one time then 500 mg in 1 wk	Once weekly
Dapsone[a]	25-, 100-mg tab	PO	2 mg/kg, max 100 mg (I)	q24h
			4 mg/kg, max 200 mg (I)	Once weekly

A. SYSTEMIC ANTIMICROBIALS WITH DOSAGE FORMS AND USUAL DOSAGES (cont)

Generic and Trade Names	Dosage Form	Route	Dose (evidence grade)	Interval
Daptomycin, Cubicin (Doses are investigational in children.)	500-mg vial	IV	2–5 y: 10 mg/kg (III) ≥6–11 y: 7 mg/kg (II) ≥12 y and adults: 4–6 mg/kg TBW (I)	q24h
Demeclocycline,[a] Declomycin	150-, 300-mg tab	PO	≥8 y: 7–13 mg/kg/day, max 600 mg/day (I)	q6h
Dicloxacillin,[a] Dynapen	125-, 250-, 500-mg cap	PO	12–25 mg/kg/day (adults 0.5–1 g/day) (I) For bone and joint infections, up to 100 mg/kg/day (III)	q6h
Doxycycline[a]	50-, 75-, 100-mg cap, tab 25-, 50-mg/5-mL susp	PO	≥8 y, ≤45 kg: 2–4 mg/kg/day (adults 100–200 mg/day) (I)	q12h
	100-mg vial	IV		
Ertapenem, Invanz	1-g vial	IV, IM	30 mg/kg/day, max 1 g/day (I) ≥13 y and adults: 1 g/day (I)	q12h q24h
Erythromycin base coated pellets, Eryc coated particles, PCE delayed release, Ery-Tab	250-, 500-mg tab 250-mg cap, EC 333-, 500-mg tabs EC particles 250-, 333-, 500-mg tab, EC	PO	50 mg/kg/day (adults 1–4 g/day) (I)	q6–8h
Erythromycin ethylsuccinate, EES, EryPed	200-, 400-mg/5-mL susp 400-mg tab	PO	50 mg/kg/day (adults 1–4 g/day) (I)	q6–8h
Erythromycin lactobionate,[a] Erythrocin	0.5-, 1-g vial	IV	20 mg/kg/day (adults 1–4 g/day) (I)	q6h
Erythromycin stearate	250-mg tab	PO	50 mg/kg/day (adults 1–4 g/day) (I)	q6–8h

Ethambutol,[a] Myambutol	100-, 400-mg tab	PO	15–25 mg/kg, max 2.5 g (I)	q24h
Ethionamide, Trecator	250-mg tab	PO	15–20 mg/kg/day, max 1 g/day (III)	q12h
Famciclovir,[a] Famvir	125-, 250-, 500-mg tab	PO	Adults 0.5–1.5 g/day (I)	q8–12h
Fluconazole,[a] Diflucan	50-, 100-, 150-, 200-mg tab 50-, 200-mg/5-mL susp	PO	3–12 mg/kg/day, max 600 mg/day (I). Max 800–1,000 mg/day may be used for some CNS fungal infections. See Chapter 8.	q24h
	100-, 200-, 400-mg vial, ivpb	IV		
Flucytosine,[a] Ancobon	250-, 500-mg cap	PO	50–150 mg/kg/day (III)	q6h
Foscarnet,[a] Foscavir	6-, 12-g vial	IV	CMV/VZV: 180 mg/kg/day (I)	q8h
			CMV suppression: 90–120 mg/kg (I)	q24h
			HSV: 120 mg/kg/day (I)	q8–12h
Ganciclovir,[a] Cytovene	500-mg vial	IV	CMV treatment: 10–15 mg/kg/day (I)	q12h
			CMV suppression: 5 mg/kg (I)	q24h
			VZV: 10 mg/kg/day (III)	q12h
Gemifloxacin, Factive	320-mg tab	PO	Adults 320 mg (I)	q24h
Gentamicin[a]	20-mg/2-mL pediatric vial 80-mg/2-mL, 800-mg/20-mL adult vial, numerous ivpb	IV, IM	3–7.5 mg/kg/day (cystic fibrosis 7–10); see Chapter 1 regarding q24h dosing.	q8–24h
		Intravesical	0.5 mg/mL in normal saline x 50–100 mL (III)	q12h
Griseofulvin microsized,[a] Grifulvin V	125-mg/5-mL susp 500-mg tab	PO	20–25 mg/kg (II) Adults 0.5–1 g (I)	q24h
Griseofulvin ultramicrosized,[a] Gris-PEG	125-, 250-mg tab	PO	10–15 mg/kg (II) Adults 0.375–0.75 g (I)	q24h

A. SYSTEMIC ANTIMICROBIALS WITH DOSAGE FORMS AND USUAL DOSAGES (cont)

Generic and Trade Names	Dosage Form	Route	Dose (evidence grade)	Interval
Imipenem/cilastatin,[a] Primaxin	250/250-, 500/500-mg vial	IV, IM	60–100 mg/kg/day (I) IM form not approved for <12 y	q6h
Interferon-PEG Alfa-2a, Pegasys Alfa-2b, PegIntron	Vials, prefilled syringes: 135-, 180-µg 50-, 80-, 120-, 150-µg	SQ	See Chapter 9, Hepatitis C virus.	Weekly
Iodoquinol,[a] Yodoxin	210-, 650-mg tab	PO	30–40 mg/kg/day, max 1.95 g/day (I)	q8h
Isoniazid,[a] Nydrazid	50-mg/5-mL syrup; 100-, 300-mg tab 1,000-mg vial	PO IV, IM	10–15 mg/kg/day, max 300 mg/day (I)	q12–24h
			With directly observed biweekly therapy, dosage is 20–30 mg/kg, max 900 mg/dose (I).	Twice weekly
Itraconazole, Sporanox	50-mg/5-mL soln 100-mg cap,[a] 200-mg tab	PO	10 mg/kg/day (III), max 200 mg/day	q12h
			5 mg/kg/day for chronic mucocutaneous *Candida* (III)	q24h
Ivermectin, Stromectol	3-mg tab	PO	150–200 µg/kg (I)	1 dose
Ketoconazole,[a] Nizoral	200-mg tab	PO	≥2 y: 3.3–6.6 mg/kg/day (II)	q24h
Levofloxacin,[a] Levaquin	125-mg/5-mL soln 250-, 500-, 750-mg tab, 500-, 750-mg vial 250-, 500-, 750-mg ivpb	PO, IV	16 mg/kg/day div q12h up to 50 kg body weight, then 500 mg qd for postexposure anthrax prophylaxis (I) For respiratory infections: <5 y: 20 mg/kg/day (II) ≥5 y: 10 mg/kg/day (II)	q12h q12h q24h

Linezolid, Zyvox	100-mg/5-mL susp 600-mg tab 200-mg ivpb	PO, IV	Pneumonia, complicated skin infections, vancomycin-resistant enterococci: Birth–11 y: 30 mg/kg/day (I) >11 y: 1,200 mg/day (I)	 q8h q12h
			Uncomplicated skin infections: Birth–5 y: 30 mg/kg/day (I) 5–11 y: 20 mg/kg/day (I) >11–18 y: 1,200 mg/day (I) Adults 800 mg/day (I)	 q8h q12h q12h q12h
Mefloquine,[a] Lariam	250-mg tab	PO	See Chapter 10 for detailed weight-based recommendations for malaria.	
Meropenem,[a] Merrem	0.5-, 1-g vial	IV	60 mg/kg/day, max 3 g/day (I) 120 mg/kg/day meningitis, max 6 g/day (I)	q8h q8h
Methenamine hippurate,[a] Hiprex	1-g tab	PO	6–12 y: 1–2 g/day (I) >12 y: 2 g/day (I)	q12h
Metronidazole,[a] Flagyl	250-, 500-mg tab, 375-mg cap	PO	30–50 mg/kg/day (adults 750–2,250 mg/day) (I)	q8h
	500-mg vial, ivpb	IV	22.5–40 mg/kg/day (II) Adults 1,500 mg/day (I)	q8h
Micafungin, Mycamine	50-, 100-mg vial	IV	2–4 mg/kg, max 150 mg (I) (100–150 mg if >40 kg)	q24h
Miconazole, Oravig	50-mg buccal tab	PO	≥16 y and adults: 50-mg buccal tab (I)	q24h
Miltefosine, Impavido	50-mg cap	PO	2.5 mg/kg/day (II) See Chapter 10. ≥12 y (I): 30–44 kg: 100 mg/day ≥45 kg: 150 mg/day	bid bid tid
Minocycline, Minocin	50-, 75-, 100-mg cap,[a] tab[a] 100-mg vial	PO, IV	≥8 y: 4 mg/kg/day (adults 200 mg/day) (I)	q12h
Moxifloxacin,[a] Avelox	400-mg tab, 400-mg ivpb	PO, IV	Adults 400 mg/day (I)	q24h

A. SYSTEMIC ANTIMICROBIALS WITH DOSAGE FORMS AND USUAL DOSAGES (cont)

Generic and Trade Names	Dosage Form	Route	Dose (evidence grade)	Interval
Nafcillin,[a] Nallpen	1-, 2-, 10-g vial, 1-, 2-g ivpb	IV, IM	150–200 mg/kg/day (II) Adults 3–6 g/day q4h (I)	q6h
Neomycin sulfate[a]	500-mg tab	PO	50–100 mg/kg/day (II)	q6–8h
Nitazoxanide, Alinia	500-mg tab; 100-mg/5-mL susp	PO	1–3 y: 200 mg/day (I) 4–11 y: 400 mg/day (I) ≥12 y: 1 g/day (I)	q12h
Nitrofurantoin,[a] Furadantin	25-mg/5-mL susp	PO	5–7 mg/kg/day (I)	q6h
			1–2 mg/kg for UTI prophylaxis (I)	q24h
Nitrofurantoin, macrocrystalline,[a] Macrodantin	25-, 50-, 100-mg cap	PO	Same as susp	
Nitrofurantoin monohydrate and macrocrystalline,[a] Macrobid	100-mg cap	PO	>12 y: 200 mg/day (I)	q12h
Nystatin,[a] Mycostatin	500,000-U/5-mL susp 500,000-U tabs	PO	Infants 2 mL/dose, children 4–6 mL/dose, to coat oral mucosa Tabs: 3–6 tabs/day	q6h tid
Ofloxacin, Floxin	300-mg tab	PO	Adults 600 mg/day	q12h

Oseltamivir, Tamiflu (See Chapter 9, Influenza virus.)	30-mg/5-mL susp 30-, 45-, 75-mg cap	PO	Preterm, <38 wk PMA (II): 1 mg/kg/dose PO bid Preterm, 38–40 wk PMA (II): 1.5 mg/kg/dose PO bid Preterm, >40 wk PMA (II), and term, birth–8 mo (I): 3 mg/kg/dose PO bid 9–11 mo (II): 3.5 mg/kg/dose PO bid ≥12 mo (I): ≤15 kg: 60 mg/day >15–23 kg: 90 mg/day >23–40 kg: 120 mg/day >40 kg: 150 mg/day	q12h
			Prophylaxis: give at the same mg/kg dose but only once a day rather than twice daily	q24h
Oxacillin,[a] Bactocill	1-, 2-, 10-g vial, 1-, 2-g ivpb	IV, IM	100 mg/kg/day (adults 4–12 g/day) (I) 150–200 mg/kg/day for meningitis (III)	q4–6h
Palivizumab, Synagis	50-, 100-mg vial	IM	15 mg/kg (I)	Monthly
Paromomycin,[a] Humatin	250-mg cap	PO	25–35 mg/kg/day (adult max 4 g/day) (I)	q8h
Penicillin G intramuscular				
– Penicillin G benzathine, Bicillin L-A	600,000 U/mL in 1-, 2-, 4-mL prefilled syringes	IM	50,000 U/kg for newborns and infants, children <60 lb: 300,000–600,000 U, children ≥60 lb: 900,000 U (I) (FDA approved in 1952 for dosing by pounds)	1 dose for treatment
– Penicillin G benzathine/procaine, Bicillin C-R, Bicillin C-R pediatric	1,200,000 IU per 2 mL prefilled syringe as 600,000 IU benzathine + 600,000 IU procaine per mL. Pediatric has a 1-inch needle.	IM	<30 lb: 600,000 U 30–60 lb: 900,000–1,200,000 U >60 lb: 2,400,000 U (I)	1 dose usually (may need repeat injections q 2–3 days)

A. SYSTEMIC ANTIMICROBIALS WITH DOSAGE FORMS AND USUAL DOSAGES (cont)

Generic and Trade Names	Dosage Form	Route	Dose (evidence grade)	Interval
– Penicillin G procaine[a]	600,000 U/mL in 1-, 2-mL prefilled syringes	IM	50,000 U/kg/day, max 1,200,000 U per dose (I)	q12–24h
Penicillin G intravenous				
– Penicillin G K,[a] Pfizerpen	5-, 20-million U vial 1-, 2-, 3-million U ivpb	IV, IM	100,000–250,000 U/kg/day (I). Max daily dose is 24 million U.	q4–6h
– Penicillin G sodium[a]	5-million U vial	IV, IM	100,000–250,000 U/kg/day (I). Max daily dose is 24 million U.	q4–6h
Penicillin V oral				
– Penicillin V K[a]	125-, 250-mg/5-mL soln 250-, 500-mg tab	PO	25–50 mg/kg/day (I)	q6h
Pentamidine,[a] Pentam Nebupent	300-mg vial	IV, IM	4 mg/kg/day (I)	q24h
	300-mg vial	Inhaled	300 mg q mo for prophylaxis (I)	q24h
Piperacillin/ tazobactam,[a] Zosyn	2/0.25-, 3/0.375-, 4/0.5-g vial ivpb 36/4.5-g vial	IV	≤40 kg: 240–300 mg PIP/kg/day (adults 12–16 g PIP/day q6h) (I)	q8h
Polymyxin B[a]	500,000 U vial 1 mg = 10,000 U	IV	2.5 mg/kg/day (I) Adults 2 mg/kg LD, then 2.5-3 mg/kg/day, dose based on TBW, no max (II)	q12h
Posaconazole, Noxafil	200-mg/5-mL susp	PO	≥13 y and adults (I): see Chapter 8. 100 mg q12h for 2 doses then 100 mg/day 600 mg/day for prophylaxis. 800 mg/day for refractory disease.	 q24h q8h q12h
	100-mg DR tab 300-mg/16.7-mL vial	PO IV	300 mg q12h for 2 doses then 300 mg/day	q24h
Praziquantel, Biltricide	600-mg triscored tab	PO	20–25 mg/kg (I)	q4–6h for 3 doses

Primaquine phosphate[a]	15-mg base tab	PO	0.3 mg (base)/kg for PCP, max 30 mg/day (with clindamycin) (III) See also Chapter 10.	q24h
Pyrantel,[a] Pin-X	250-mg chew tab 250-mg/5-mL susp	PO	11 mg/kg, max 1 g (I)	Once
Pyrazinamide[a]	500-mg tab	PO	15–30 mg/kg/day, max 2 g/day (I)	q24h
			Directly observed biweekly therapy, 40–50 mg/kg (I)	Twice weekly
Quinupristin/ dalfopristin, Synercid	150/350-mg vial (500 mg total)	IV	22.5 mg/kg/day (II) Adults 15–22.5 mg/kg/day (I)	q8h q8–12h
Raxibacumab	1,700-mg/35-mL vial	IV	≤15 kg: 80 mg/kg 15–50 kg: 60 mg/kg >50 kg: 40 mg/kg (I)	Once
Ribavirin,[a] Rebetol	200-mg cap/tab 400-, 500-, 600-mg tab 200-mg/5-mL soln	PO	15 mg/kg/day (With interferon, see Chapter 9.) (II)	q12h
Ribavirin, inhalation, Virazole	6-g vial	Inhaled	1 vial by SPAG-2; see Chapter 9, Respiratory Syncytial Virus.	q24h
Rifabutin,[a] Mycobutin	150-mg cap	PO	5 mg/kg for MAC prophylaxis (II) 10–20 mg/kg for MAC or TB treatment (I) Max 300 mg/day	q24h
Rifampin,[a] Rifadin	150-, 300-mg cap, 600-mg vial	PO, IV	10–20 mg/kg, max 600 mg for TB (I)	q24h
			With directly observed biweekly therapy, dosage is still 10–20 mg/kg/dose (max 600 mg).	Twice weekly
			20 mg/kg/day for 2 days for meningococcus prophylaxis, adult dose 1,200 mg/day (I)	q12h
Rifampin/isoniazid/ pyrazinamide, Rifater	120/50/300-mg tab	PO	Refer to individual agents.	

A. SYSTEMIC ANTIMICROBIALS WITH DOSAGE FORMS AND USUAL DOSAGES (cont)

Generic and Trade Names	Dosage Form	Route	Dose (evidence grade)	Interval
Rifapentine, Priftin	150-mg tab	PO	≥12 y and adults: 600 mg/dose (I)	Twice weekly
Rifaximin, Xifaxan	200-, 550-mg tab	PO	≥12 y and adults: 600 mg/day (I)	q8h
Simeprevir, Olysio	150-mg cap	PO	Adults 150 mg[b] (I)	q24h
Sofosbuvir, Sovaldi	400-mg tab	PO	Adults 400 mg[b] (I)	q24h
Streptomycin[a]	1-g vial	IM, IV	20–30 mg/kg/day, max 1 g/day (I)	q12h
Sulfadiazinea	500-mg tab	PO	120–150 mg/kg/day, max 4–6 g/day (I)	q6h
			Rheumatic fever secondary prophylaxis 500 mg once daily if ≤27 kg, 1,000 mg once daily if >27 kg (II)	q24h
			See also Chapter 10.	
Tedizolid, Sivextro	200-mg tab, vial	PO, IV	Adults 200 mg (I)	q24h
Telaprevir, Incivek	375-mg tab	PO	Adults 750 mg PO tid[b] (I)	q8h
Telbivudine, Tyzeka	600-mg tab	PO	≥16 y and adults: 600 mg/day (I)	q24h
Telithromycin, Ketek	300-, 400-mg tab	PO	Adults 800 mg/day (I)	q24h
Terbinafine, Lamisil	125-, 187.5-mg oral granules 250-mg tab[a]	PO	>4 y <25 kg: 125 mg/day 25–35 kg: 187.5 mg/day >35 kg: 250 mg/day (I)	q24h
Tetracycline[a]	250-, 500-mg cap, tab	PO	≥8 y: 25–50 mg/kg/day (I)	q6h
Ticarcillin/clavulanate, Timentin	3/0.1-g vial, ivpb, 30/1-g vial	IV	200–300 mg ticarcillin/kg/day (adults 12–18 g/day) (I)	q4–6h
Tinidazole,[a] Tindamax	250-, 500-mg tab	PO	50 mg/kg, max 2 g (I) See also Chapter 10.	q24h

Tobramycin,[a] Nebcin	20-mg/2-mL pediatric vial 80-mg/2-mL, 1.2-g vial	IV, IM	3–7.5 mg/kg/day (cystic fibrosis 7–10); see Chapter 1 regarding q24h dosing.	q8–24h
Tobraycin inhalation,[a] Tobi	300-mg ampule	Inhaled	≥6 y: 600 mg/day (I)	q12h
Tobi Podhaler	28-mg caps for inhalation	Inhaled	≥6 y: 224 mg/day via Podhaler device (I)	q12h
Trimethoprim/ sulfamethoxazole,[a] Bactrim, Septra	80-mg TMP/400-mg SMX tab (single strength) 160-mg TMP/800-mg SMX tab (double strength) 40-mg TMP/200-mg SMX per 5-mL susp 16-mg TMP/80-mg SMX per mL inject soln in 5-, 10-, 30-mL vials	PO, IV	8–10 mg TMP/kg/day (I)	q12h
			2 mg TMP/kg/day for UTI prophylaxis (I)	q24h
			15–20 mg TMP/kg/day for PCP treatment (I)	q6–8h
			150 mg TMP/m^2/day, OR 5 mg TMP/kg/day for PCP prophylaxis (I)	q12h 3 times a week OR q24h
Valacyclovir,[a] Valtrex	500-mg, 1-g tab	PO	VZV: ≥3 mo: 60 mg/kg/day (I, II) HSV: ≥3 mo: 40 mg/kg/day (II) Max single dose 1 g (I)	q8h q12h
Valganciclovir, Valcyte	250-mg/5-mL soln 450-mg tab	PO	Congenital CMV treatment: 32 mg/kg/day (II). CMV prophylaxis: 7 x BSA x CrCl (using the modified Schwartz formula for CrCl). Max 900 mg (I). See also Chapter 9.	q12h q24h
			Adults 900–1,800 mg/day (I)	q12–24h

A. SYSTEMIC ANTIMICROBIALS WITH DOSAGE FORMS AND USUAL DOSAGES (cont)

Generic and Trade Names	Dosage Form	Route	Dose (evidence grade)	Interval
Vancomycin,[a] Vancocin	125-, 250-mg cap	PO	40 mg/kg/day (I), max 500 mg/day (III)	q6h
	0.5-, 0.75-, 1-, 5-, 10-g vial 0.5-, 0.75-, 1-g ivpb	IV	30–40 mg/kg/day (adjusted based on therapeutic drug monitoring) (I) For life-threatening invasive MRSA infection, 60–70 mg/kg/day adjusted to achieve area under the curve >400 mg·h/L (II)	q6–8h
Voriconazole,[a] Vfend (See Chapter 8.)	200-mg vial	IV	2–12 y: 18 mg/kg/day LD for 1 day, then 16 mg/kg/day (II) >12 y: 12 mg/kg/day LD for 1 day, then 8 mg/kg/day (max 600 mg/day) (I)	q12h
	200-mg/5-mL susp 50-, 200-mg tab	PO	18 mg/kg/day (II) Adults 400–600 mg/day (I)	
Zanamivir, Relenza	5-mg blister cap for inhalation	Inhaled	Prophylaxis: ≥5 y: 10 mg (I)	q24h
			Treatment: ≥7 y: 10 mg (I)	q12h

[a]Available in a generic formulation.
[b]Given as a cocktail with ribavirin ± interferon-PEG.

B. TOPICAL ANTIMICROBIALS (SKIN, EYE, EAR)

Generic and Trade Names	Dosage Form	Route	Dose	Interval
Acyclovir + hydrocortisone, Xerese	5% + 1 % cream			
Azithromycin, AzaSite	1% ophth soln	Ophth	1 drop	bid for 2 days then qd for 5 days
Bacitracin[a]	Ophth oint	Ophth	Apply to affected eye.	q3–4h
	Oint[b]	Top	Apply to affected area.	bid–qid
Benzyl alcohol, Ulesfia	5% lotion	Top	Apply to scalp and hair.	Once; repeat in 7 days.
Besifloxacin, Besivance	0.6% ophth susp	Ophth	≥1 y: 1 drop to affected eye	tid
Butenafine, Mentax	1% cream	Top	≥12 y: to affected area	qd
Butoconazole, Gynazole-1	2% prefilled cream	Vag	Adults 1 applicatorful	One time
Ciclopirox,[b] Loprox, Penlac	0.77% cream, gel, lotion	Top	≥10 y: apply to affected area.	bid
	1% shampoo		≥16 y: apply to scalp.	Twice weekly
	8% nail lacquer		≥12 y: apply to infected nail.	qd
Ciprofloxacin,[a] Cetraxal	0.2% otic soln	Otic	≥1 y: apply 3 drops to affected ear.	bid for 7 days
Ciprofloxacin,[a] Ciloxan	0.3% ophth soln	Ophth	≥12 y: apply to affected eye.	q2h for 2 days then q4h for 5 days
	0.3% ophth oint			q8h for 2 days then q12h for 5 days
Ciprofloxacin + dexamethasone, Ciprodex	0.3% + 0.1% otic soln	Otic	≥6 mo: apply 4 drops to affected ear.	bid for 7 days
Ciprofloxacin + hydrocortisone, Cipro HC	0.2% + 1% otic soln	Otic	≥1 y: apply 3 drops to affected ear.	bid for 7 days

B. TOPICAL ANTIMICROBIALS (SKIN, EYE, EAR) (cont)

Generic and Trade Names	Dosage Form	Route	Dose	Interval
Clindamycin				
Clindesse	2% cream	Vag	Adolescents and adults: 1 applicatorful	One time
Cleocin	100-mg ovule		1 ovule	qhs for 3 days
	2% cream[a]		1 applicatorful	qhs for 3–7 days
Cleocin-T[a]	1% soln, gel, lotion	Top	Apply to affected area.	qd–bid
Evoclin	1% foam			qd
Clindamycin + benzoyl peroxide,[a] Benzaclin	1% gel	Top	≥12 y: apply to affected area.	bid
Acanya	1.2% gel	Top	Apply small amount to face.	q24h
Clindamycin + tretinoin, Ziana, Veltin	1.2% gel	Top	Apply small amount to face.	hs
Clotrimazole,[a,b] Lotrimin	1% cream, lotion, soln	Top	Apply to affected area.	bid
Gyne-Lotrimin-7[a,b]	1% cream	Vag	≥12 y: 1 applicatorful	qhs for 7–14 days
Gyne-Lotrimin-3[a,b]	2% cream			qhs for 3 days
Clotrimazole + betamethasone,[a] Lotrisone	1% + 0.05% cream, lotion	Top	≥12 y: apply to affected area.	bid
Colistin + neomycin + hydrocortisone, Coly-Mycin S, Cortisporin TC otic	0.3% otic susp	Otic	Apply 3–4 drops to affected ear canal; may use with wick.	q6–8h
Cortisporin; bacitracin + neomycin + polymyxin B + hydrocortisone	Oint	Top	Apply to affected area.	bid–qid

Cortisporin; neomycin + polymyxin B + hydrocortisone	Otic soln,[a] susp	Otic	3 drops to affected ear	bid–qid
	Cream	Top	Apply to affected area.	bid–qid
Dapsone, Aczone	5% gel	Top	Apply to affected area.	bid
Econazole,[a] Spectazole	1% cream	Top	Apply to affected area.	qd–bid
Efinaconazole, Jublia	10% soln	Top	Apply to toenail.	qd for 48 wk
Erythromycin	0.5% ophth oint[a]	Ophth	Apply to affected eye.	q4h
Eryderm, Erygel	2% soln,[a] gel[a]	Top	Apply to affected area.	bid
Ery Pads	2% pledgets[a]			
Akne-Mycin	2% oint			
Erythromycin + benzoyl peroxide,[a] Benzamycin	3% gel	Top	≥12 y: apply to affected area.	qd–bid
Ganciclovir, Zirgan	0.15% ophth gel	Ophth	≥2 y: 1 drop in affected eye	q3h while awake (5 times/day) until healed then tid for 7 days
Gatifloxacin, Zymaxid	0.5% ophth soln	Ophth	Apply to affected eye.	q2h for 1 day then q6h
Gentamicin,[a] Garamycin	0.1% cream, oint	Top	Apply to affected area.	tid–qid
	0.3% ophth soln, oint	Ophth	Apply to affected eye.	q1–4h (soln) q4–8h (oint)
Gentamicin + prednisolone, Pred-G	0.3% ophth soln, oint	Ophth	Adults: apply to affected eye.	q1–4h (soln)
				qd–tid (oint)
Ivermectin, Sklice	0.5% lotion	Top	≥6 mo: thoroughly coat hair and scalp, rinse after 10 minutes.	Once

B. TOPICAL ANTIMICROBIALS (SKIN, EYE, EAR) (cont)

Generic and Trade Names	Dosage Form	Route	Dose	Interval
Ketoconazole		Top	≥12 y: apply to affected area.	
Nizoral	2% shampoo[a]			qd
	2% cream[a]			qd–bid
Nizoral A-D[a]	1% shampoo			bid
Extina, Xolegel	2% foam,[a] gel			bid
Levofloxacin,[a] Quixin	0.5% ophth soln	Ophth	Apply to affected eye.	q1–4h
Luliconazole, Luzu	1% cream	Top	Adults: apply to affected area.	q24h for 1–2 wk
Mafenide, Sulfamylon	8.5% cream	Top	Apply to burn.	qd–bid
	5-g pwd for reconstitution		To keep burn dressing wet	q4–8h as needed
Malathion, Ovide	0.5% soln	Top	≥6 y: apply to hair and scalp.	Once
Maxitrol[a]; neomycin + polymyxin B + dexamethasone	Susp, oint	Ophth	Apply to affected eye.	q4h (oint) q1–4h (susp)
Metronidazole[a]	0.75% cream, gel, lotion	Top	Adults: Apply to affected area.	bid
MetroGel-Vaginal[a]	0.75% vag gel	Vag	Adults: 1 applicatorful	qd–bid
Noritate, MetroGel	1% cream, gel	Top	Adults: apply to affected area.	qd
Miconazole				
Micatin[a,b] and others	2% cream, pwd, oint, spray, lotion, gel	Top	Apply to affected area.	qd–bid
Fungoid[a]	2% tincture	Top	Apply to affected area.	bid
Vusion	0.25% oint	Top	To diaper dermatitis	Each diaper change for 7 days

Monistat-1[a,b]	1.2-g ovule + 2% cream	Vag	≥12 y: insert one ovule (plus cream to external vulva bid as needed).	Once
Monistat-3[a,b]	200-mg ovule, 4% cream			qhs for 3 days
Monistat-7[a,b]	100-mg ovule, 2% cream			qhs for 7 days
Moxifloxacin, Vigamox	0.5% ophth soln	Ophth	Apply to affected eye.	tid
Mupirocin, Bactroban	2% oint,[a] cream,[a] nasal oint	Top	Apply to infected skin or nasal mucosa.	tid
Naftifine, Naftin	2% cream, gel	Top	Adults: apply to affected area.	qd
Natamycin, Natacyn	5% ophth soln	Ophth	Adults: apply to affected eye.	q1–4h
Neosporin[a]				
bacitracin + neomycin	Ophth oint	Ophth	Apply to affected eye.	q4h
+ polymyxin B	Top oint[a]	Top	Apply to affected area.	bid–qid
gramicidin + neomycin + polymyxin B	Ophth soln	Ophth	Apply to affected eye.	q4h
Nystatin,[a] Mycostatin	100,000 U/g cream, oint, pwd	Top	Apply to affected area.	bid–qid
Nystatin + triamcinolone,[a] Mycolog II	100,000 U/g + 0.1% cream, oint	Top	Apply to affected area.	bid
Ofloxacin,[a] Floxin Otic	0.3% otic soln	Otic	5–10 drops to affected ear	qd–bid
Ocuflox	0.3% ophth soln	Ophth	Apply to affected eye.	q1–6h
Oxiconazole, Oxistat	1% cream, lotion	Top	Apply to affected area.	qd–bid
Penciclovir, Denavir	1% top cream	Top	See Chapter 9.	Not recommended
Permethrin, Nix[a,b]	1% cream	Top	Apply to hair/scalp.	Once for 10 min
Elimite[a]	5% cream		Apply to all skin surfaces.	Once for 8–14 h
Piperonyl butoxide + pyrethrins,[a,b] Rid	4% + 0.3% shampoo, gel	Top	Apply to affected area.	Once for 10 min

B. TOPICAL ANTIMICROBIALS (SKIN, EYE, EAR) (cont)

Generic and Trade Names	Dosage Form	Route	Dose	Interval
Polysporin,[a] polymyxin B + bacitracin	Ophth oint	Ophth	Apply to affected eye.	qd–tid
	Oint[a], pwd[a]	Top	Apply to affected area.	
Polytrim,[a] polymyxin B + trimethoprim	Ophth soln	Ophth	Apply to affected eye.	q3–4h
Retapamulin, Altabax	1% oint	Top	Apply thin layer to affected area.	bid for 5 days
Selenium sulfide,[a] Selsun	2.5% susp/lotion	Top	Lather into scalp or affected area.	Twice weekly then every 1–2 wk
Selsun Blue[a,b]	1% shampoo	Top		qd
Sertaconazole, Ertaczo	2% cream	Top	≥12 y: apply to affected area.	bid
Silver sulfadiazine,[a] Silvadene	1% cream	Top	Apply to affected area.	qd–bid
Spinosad, Natroba	0.9% susp	Top	Apply to scalp and hair.	Once; may repeat in 7 days.
Sulconazole, Exelderm	1% soln, cream	Top	Adults: apply to affected area.	qd–bid
Sulfacetamide sodium[a]	10%, 15%, 30% soln	Ophth	Apply to affected eye.	q1–3h
	10% ophth oint			q4-6h
	10% top lotion	Top	≥12 y: apply to affected area.	bid–qid
Sulfacetamide sodium + fluorometholone, FML-S	10% ophth soln	Ophth	Apply to affected eye.	qid
Sulfacetamide sodium + prednisolone, Blephamide	10% ophth oint, soln	Ophth	Apply to affected eye.	tid–qid
Tavaborole, Kerydin	5% soln	Top	Adults: apply to toenail.	qd for 48 wk
Terbinafine, Lamisil-AT[b]	1% cream, spray, gel	Top	Apply to affected area.	qd–bid

Terconazole,[a] Terazol-7	0.4% cream	Vag	Adults: 1 applicatorful or 1 supp	qhs for 7 days
Terazol-3	0.8% cream, 80 mg supp	Vag		qhs for 3 days
Tioconazole[a,b]	6.5% ointment	Vag	≥12 y: 1 applicatorful	One time
Tobramycin,[a] Tobrex	0.3% ophth soln, oint	Ophth	Apply to affected eye.	q1–4h (soln) q4–8h (oint)
Tobramycin + dexamethasone, Tobradex	0.3% ophth soln,[a] oint	Ophth	Apply to affected eye.	q2–6h (soln) q6–8h (oint)
Tolnaftate,[a,b] Tinactin	1% cream, soln, pwd, spray	Top	Apply to affected area.	bid
Trifluridine,[a] Viroptic	1% ophth soln	Ophth	1 drop (max 9 drops/day)	q2h

[a]Generic available.
[b]Over the counter.

12. Antibiotic Therapy for Obese Children

When prescribing an antimicrobial for an overweight child, selecting a dose based on mg per kg of total body weight (TBW) may expose the child to supratherapeutic plasma concentrations if the drug doesn't freely distribute into fat tissue. The beta-lactams and aminoglycosides are examples of such potentially problematic antibiotics because they are hydrophilic and their distribution volumes are correlated with extracellular fluid. In general, these and other hydrophilic compounds may be dosed appropriately using a weight adjustment of 30% to 50% of the difference between TBW and expected body weight (EBW); see Dosing Recommendations.

For aminoglycosides in obese adults, a 40% adjustment in dosing weight (40% of the difference between TBW and EBW) has been recommended.

Example

A 9-year-old boy with measurements of 37 kg and 135 cm has a calculated body mass index of 20 kg/m^2 (>90th percentile). He requires amoxicillin 90 mg/kg/day divided every 12 hours for treatment of acute bacterial sinusitis. Based on his TBW, a dose of 1,700 mg twice daily would be chosen. Using his EBW of about 30 kg, the difference between his EBW and TBW is 7 kg, so his adjusted dosing weight is 32 kg (30% of 7 kg, added to his EBW). His new dosage is 1,400 mg twice daily. Performing the adjustment reduced the daily potentially unnecessary exposure by 600 mg.

When performing this empiric dosing with aminoglycosides in obese children, we recommend closely following serum concentrations with early sampling to confirm predictions.

In the setting of cephalosporins for surgical prophylaxis (see Chapter 14), adult studies of obese patients have generally found that distribution to the subcutaneous fat tissue target is subtherapeutic when standard adult doses are used. Given the wide safety margin of these agents in the short-term setting of surgical prophylaxis, maximum doses are recommended in obese adults (eg, cefazolin 2 g instead of the standard 1 g) with re-dosing at 4-hour intervals for longer cases. Based on the adult data, we recommend dosing cephalosporins based on TBW up to the adult maximum for that drug, for surgical prophylaxis.

Vancomycin is usually dosed based on TBW in obese patients. Newer data suggest that this approach may result in supratherapeutic concentrations in children, and adjustments using body surface area may be more appropriate. As with aminoglycosides, we recommend early and frequent serum measurement to confirm empiric dosing predictions.

Listed in the Table are the major classes of antimicrobials and our suggestion on how to calculate the most appropriate dose. The level of evidence to support these recommendations is Level II–III (mostly based on adult studies and expert opinion). Whenever a dose is used that is greater than one prospectively investigated for efficacy and safety, the clinician must weigh the benefits with potential risks. Data are not available on all agents.

	DOSING RECOMMENDATIONS		
Drug Class	**By EBW[a]**	**Intermediate Dosing**	**By TBW[b]**
ANTIBACTERIALS			
Beta-lactams		EBW + 0.3 (TBW-EBW)	
Penicillins		X	
Cephalosporins		X	X (surgical prophylaxis)
Carbapenems		X	
Macrolides			
Erythromycin	X		
Azithromycin	X (for gastrointestinal infections)		X
Clarithromycin	X		
Lincosamides			
Clindamycin			X
Glycopeptides			
Vancomycin		1,500–2,000 mg/m²/day	X
Aminoglycosides		EBW + 0.4 (TBW-EBW)	
Gentamicin		X	
Tobramycin		X	
Amikacin		X	
Fluoroquinolones		EBW + 0.45 (TBW-EBW)	
Ciprofloxacin		X	
Levofloxacin		X	
Rifamycins			
Rifampin	X		
Miscellaneous			
TMP/SMX			X
Metronidazole	X		
Linezolid	X		
Daptomycin			X

Drug Class	By EBW[a]	Intermediate Dosing	By TBW[b]
	DOSING RECOMMENDATIONS		
ANTIFUNGALS			
Amphotericin B (conventional and lipid formulations)			X
Echinocandins			
Caspofungin			X
Micafungin		X	
Azoles			
Fluconazole			X
Voriconazole	X		
Flucytosine	X		
ANTIVIRALS (non-HIV)			
Nucleoside analogues (acyclovir, ganciclovir)	X		
Oseltamivir	X		
ANTIMYCOBACTERIALS			
Isoniazid	X		
Rifampin	X		
Pyrazinamide	X		
Ethambutol	X		

Abbreviations: BMI, body mass index; EBW, expected body weight; HIV, human immunodeficiency virus; TBW, total body weight; TMP/SMX, trimethoprim/sulfamethoxazole.

[a]EBW (kg) = BMI 50th percentile for age × actual height (m)^2; from Le Grange D, et al. *Pediatrics.* 2012;129:e438–e446.

[b]Actual measured body weight.

Bibliography

Camaione L, et al. *Pharmacotherapy.* 2013;33(12):1278–1287

Heble DE Jr, et al. *Pharmacotherapy.* 2013;33(12):1273–1277

Pai MP, et al. *Antimicrob Agents Chemother.* 2011;55(12):5640–5645

Payne KD, et al. *Expert Rev Anti Infect Ther.* 2014;12(7):829–854

Sampson M, et al. *GaBi J.* 2013;2(2):76–81

13. Sequential Parenteral-Oral Antibiotic Therapy (Oral Step-down Therapy) for Serious Infections

Bacterial pneumonias, bone and joint infections,[1–3] deep-tissue abscesses, and appendicitis,[4,5] as well as cellulitis or pyelonephritis,[6] may require initial parenteral therapy to control the growth and spread of pathogens and minimize injury to tissues. However, intravenous (IV) therapy carries risks of catheter-related complications that are unpleasant for the child whether therapy is provided in the hospital or on an outpatient basis. For the beta-lactam class of antibiotics, absorption of orally administered antibiotics in standard dosages provides peak serum concentrations that are routinely only 5% to 20% of those achieved with IV or intramuscular administration. However, clindamycin and many newer antibiotics of the fluoroquinolone class (ciprofloxacin, levofloxacin)[7] and oxazolidinone class (linezolid, tedizolid) have excellent absorption of their oral formulations and provide virtually the same tissue antibiotic exposure at a particular mg/kg dose, compared with the exposure when the antibiotic is given at that dose IV. Following initial parenteral therapy of serious infections, it may be possible to provide oral antibiotic therapy to achieve the tissue antibiotic exposure that is required for cure. One must also assume that the parent and child are compliant with the administration of each antibiotic dose and that the parents will seek medical care if the clinical course does not continue to improve for their child.

High-dose oral beta-lactam antibiotic therapy of osteoarticular infections, associated with achieving a particular level of bactericidal activity in serum, has been associated with treatment success since 1978.[1] While most hospital laboratories no longer offer bactericidal assays, the need to achieve bactericidal activity with high-dose oral therapy, explained below, remains important. Comparable mg/kg dosages of parenteral and oral beta-lactam medications often result in comparable tissue concentrations 4 to 6 hours after a dose (although the high mg/kg doses given orally may not always be well tolerated). The momentary high serum concentrations that occur during IV administration of beta-lactam antibiotics may provide for better tissue penetration; however, killing of bacteria by beta-lactam antibiotics is not dependent on the height of the antibiotic concentration but on the time that the antibiotic is present at the site of infection at concentrations above the minimum inhibitory concentration of the antibiotic for that pathogen.

For abscesses in soft tissues, joints, and bones, most organisms are removed by surgical drainage and killed by the initial parenteral therapy. When the signs and symptoms of infection begin to resolve, usually within 1 to 4 days, continuing IV therapy may not be required as a normal host response begins to assist in clearing the infection. Following objective laboratory markers such as C-reactive protein (CRP) or procalcitonin (PCT) during the hospitalization may help the clinician better assess the response to therapy, particularly in the infant or child who is difficult to examine.[8,9]

Large-dosage oral beta-lactam therapy (based on in vitro susceptibilities) provides the tissue antibiotic exposure required to eradicate the remaining pathogens at the infection site as the tissue perfusion improves. For beta-lactams, begin with a dosage 2 to 3 times the normal dosage (eg, 75–100 mg/kg/day of amoxicillin or 100 mg/kg/day of cephalexin). High-dose prolonged oral beta-lactam therapy may be associated with reversible neutropenia; checking for hematologic toxicity every few weeks during therapy should be considered.

Monitor the child clinically for a continued response on oral therapy; follow CRP or PCT after the switch to oral therapy if there are concerns about continued response to make sure that the antibiotic and dosage you selected are appropriate.

14. Antimicrobial Prophylaxis/Prevention of Symptomatic Infection

This chapter provides a summary of recommendations for prophylaxis of infections, defined as providing therapy prior to the onset of clinical signs or symptoms of infection. Prophylaxis can be considered in several clinical scenarios.

A. Postexposure Prophylaxis

Given for a short, specified period after exposure to specific pathogens/organisms, where the risks of acquiring the infection are felt to justify antimicrobial treatment to eradicate the pathogen or prevent symptomatic infection in situations in which the child (healthy or with increased susceptibility to infection) is likely to have been inoculated (eg, asymptomatic child closely exposed to meningococcus; a neonate born to a mother with active genital herpes simplex virus).

B. Long-term Symptomatic Disease Prophylaxis

Given to a particular, defined population of children who are of relatively high risk of acquiring a severe infection (eg, a child postsplenectomy; a child with documented rheumatic heart disease to prevent subsequent streptococcal infection), with prophylaxis provided during the period of risk, potentially months or years.

C. Preemptive Treatment/Latent Infection Treatment ("Prophylaxis of Symptomatic Infection")

Where a child has a documented but asymptomatic infection and targeted antimicrobials are given to prevent the development of symptomatic disease (eg, latent tuberculosis infection or therapy of a stem cell transplant patient with documented cytomegalovirus viremia but no symptoms of infection or rejection). Treatment period is usually defined, but certain circumstances, such as reactivation of a herpesvirus, may require re-treatment.

D. Surgical/Procedure Prophylaxis

A child receives a surgical/invasive catheter procedure, planned or unplanned, where the risk of infection postoperatively or post-procedure may justify prophylaxis to prevent an infection from occurring (eg, prophylaxis to prevent infection following spinal rod placement). Treatment is usually short-term, beginning just prior to the procedure and ending at the conclusion of the procedure, or within 24 to 48 hours.

E. Travel-Related Exposure Prophylaxis

Not discussed in this chapter; please refer to information on specific disease entities (eg, traveler's diarrhea, Chapter 6) or pathogens (eg, malaria, Chapter 10). Updated, current information for travelers about prophylaxis and current worldwide infection risks can be found on the Centers for Disease Control and Prevention Web site at www.cdc.gov/travel (accessed October 14, 2014).

NOTE

- **Abbreviations:** AHA, American Heart Association; amox/clav, amoxicillin/clavulanate; ARF, acute rheumatic fever; bid, twice daily; CDC, Centers for Disease Control and Prevention; div, divided; DOT, directly observed therapy; GI, gastrointestinal; HSV, herpes simplex virus; IGRA, interferon-gamma release assay; IM, intramuscular; INH, isoniazid; IV, intravenous; MRSA, methicillin-resistant *Staphylococcus aureus;* PCR, polymerase chain reaction; PO, orally; PPD, purified protein derivative; qd, once daily; qid, 4 times daily; spp, species; TB, tuberculosis; tid, 3 times daily; TIG, tetanus immune globulin; TMP/SMX, trimethoprim/sulfamethoxazole; UTI, urinary tract infection.

A. POSTEXPOSURE PROPHYLAXIS

Prophylaxis Category	Therapy (evidence grade)	Comments
Bacterial		
Bites, animal and human[1–4] (*Pasteurella multocida* [animal], *Eikenella corrodens* [human], *Staphylococcus* spp, and *Streptococcus* spp)	Amox/clav 45 mg/kg/day PO div tid (amox/clav 7:1, see Chapter 1) for 3–5 days (AII) OR ampicillin and clindamycin (BII). For penicillin allergy, consider ciprofloxacin (for *Pasteurella*) plus clindamycin (BIII).	Recommended for children who are (1) immunocompromised; (2) asplenic; (3) have moderate to severe injuries, especially to the hand or face; or (4) have injuries that may have penetrated the periosteum or joint capsule (AII).[3] Consider rabies prophylaxis for animal bites (AI); consider tetanus prophylaxis. Human bites have a very high rate of infection (do not close open wounds routinely). Cat bites have a higher rate of infection than dog bites. *Staphylococcus aureus* coverage is only fair with amox/clav and provides no coverage for MRSA.
Endocarditis Prophylaxis[5]**:** Given that (1) endocarditis is rarely caused by dental/GI procedures and (2) prophylaxis for procedures prevents an exceedingly small number of cases, the risks of antibiotics most often outweigh benefits. However, some "highest risk" conditions are currently recommended for prophylaxis: (1) prosthetic heart valve (or prosthetic material used to repair a valve); (2) previous endocarditis; (3) cyanotic congenital heart disease that is unrepaired (or palliatively repaired with shunts and conduits); (4) congenital heart disease that is repaired but with defects at the site of repair adjacent to prosthetic material; (5) completely repaired congenital heart disease using prosthetic material, for the first 6 months after repair; or (6) cardiac transplant patients with valvulopathy. Routine prophylaxis no longer is required for children with native valve abnormalities. Follow-up data suggest that following these new guidelines, no increase in endocarditis has been detected.[6]		
– In highest-risk patients: dental procedures that involve manipulation of the gingival or periodontal region of teeth	Amoxicillin 50 mg/kg PO 1 h before procedure OR ampicillin or ceftriaxone or cefazolin, all at 50 mg/kg IM/IV 30–60 min before procedure	If penicillin allergy: clindamycin 20 mg/kg PO (60 min before) or IV (30 min before); OR azithromycin 15 mg/kg or clarithromycin 15 mg/kg, 1 h before
– Genitourinary and gastrointestinal procedures	None	No longer recommended

A. POSTEXPOSURE PROPHYLAXIS (cont)

Prophylaxis Category	Therapy (evidence grade)	Comments
Bacterial (cont)		
Meningococcus (*Neisseria meningitidis*)[7]	For prophylaxis of close contacts, including household members, child care center contacts, and anyone directly exposed to the patient's oral secretions (eg, through kissing, mouth-to-mouth resuscitation, endotracheal intubation, endotracheal tube management) in the 7 days before symptom onset Rifampin Children <1 mo: 5 mg/kg PO q12h for 4 doses Children >1 mo: 10 mg/kg PO q12h for 4 doses (max 600 mg/dose) OR Ceftriaxone Children <15 y: 125 mg IM once Children ≥16 y: 250 mg IM once OR Ciprofloxacin 500 mg PO once (adolescents and adults)	A single dose of ciprofloxacin should not present a significant risk of cartilage damage, but no prospective data exist in children for prophylaxis of meningococcal disease. For a child, an equivalent exposure for ciprofloxacin to that in adults would be 15–20 mg/kg as a single dose (max 500 mg). A few ciprofloxacin-resistant strains have now been reported. Insufficient data to recommend azithromycin at this time.
Pertussis[8,9]	Azithromycin 10 mg/kg/day qd for 5 days OR clarithromycin (for infants >1 mo) 15 mg/kg/day div bid for 7 days OR erythromycin (estolate preferable) 40 mg/kg/day PO div qid for 14 days (AII) Alternative: TMP/SMX (8 mg/kg/day) div bid for 14 days (BIII)	Prophylaxis to family members; contacts defined by CDC: persons within 21 days of exposure to an infectious pertussis case, who are at high risk of severe illness or who will have close contact with a person at high risk of severe illness (including infants, pregnant women in their third trimester, immunocompromised persons, contacts who have close contact with infants <12 mo). Community-wide prophylaxis is not currently recommended. Azithromycin and clarithromycin are better tolerated than erythromycin (see Chapter 5); azithromycin is preferred in exposed young infants to reduce pyloric stenosis risk.

Tetanus
(*Clostridium tetani*)[10,11]

NEED FOR TETANUS VACCINE OR TIG[a]

Number of past tetanus vaccine doses	Clean Wound: Need for tetanus vaccine	Clean Wound: Need for TIG 250 U IM	Contaminated Wound: Need for tetanus vaccine	Contaminated Wound: Need for TIG 250 U IM
<3 doses	Yes	No	Yes	Yes
≥3 doses	No (if <10 y[b]) Yes (if ≥10 y[b])	No	No (if <5 y[b]) Yes (if ≥5 y[b])	No

For deep, contaminated wounds, wound debridement is essential. For wounds that cannot be fully debrided, consider metronidazole 30 mg/kg/day PO div q8h until wound healing is underway and anaerobic conditions no longer exist, as short as 3–5 days (BIII).

[a]Intravenous immune globulin should be used when TIG is not available.

[b]Years since last tetanus-containing vaccine dose.

Tuberculosis
(*Mycobacterium tuberculosis*)
Exposed infant <4 y, or immunocompromised patient (high risk of dissemination)[12,13]
For treatment of latent TB infection, see Table 14C.

Scenario 1: Previously uninfected child becomes exposed to a person with active disease.

Exposed infant <4 y, or immunocompromised patient (high risk of dissemination): INH 10–15 mg/kg PO daily for 2–3 mo after last exposure AND with repeat skin test or IGRA test negative (AIII).

For older children, may also begin prophylaxis postexposure, but if exposure is questionable, can wait 2–3 mo after exposure; start INH, if repeat PPD/IGRA at 2–3 mo is positive at that time.

If PPD or IGRA remains negative at 2–3 mo and child remains well, consider stopping empiric therapy. However, tests at 2–3 mo may not be reliable in immunocompromised patients.

This regimen is to prevent infection in a compromised host after exposure, rather than to treat latent asymptomatic infection.

Scenario 2: Asymptomatic child is found to have a positive skin test/IGRA test for TB, documenting latent TB Infection.

INH 10–15 mg/kg PO daily for 9 mo (≥12 mo for an immunocompromised child), OR

INH 20–30 mg/kg PO directly observed therapy twice weekly for 9 mo

Other options

For INH intolerance or INH resistance if a direct contact can be tested: rifampin 10 mg/kg PO daily for 4 mo

For children ≥12 y, can use once weekly DOT with INH AND rifapentine for 12 wk; much less data for children 2–12 y[14]

A. POSTEXPOSURE PROPHYLAXIS (cont)

Prophylaxis Category	Therapy (evidence grade)	Comments
Viral		
Herpes Simplex Virus		
During pregnancy	For women with recurrent genital herpes: acyclovir 400 mg PO bid; valacyclovir 500 mg PO qd OR 1 g PO qd from 36 wk gestation until delivery (CII)[15]	Unfortunately, development of neonatal HSV disease after maternal suppression has been documented.
Neonatal: Primary maternal infection, infant exposed at delivery[16]	Asymptomatic, exposed infant: at 24 h of life, culture mucosal sites (see Comments), obtain plasma PCR for HSV, and start prophylactic acyclovir IV (60 mg/kg/day div q8h) for 10 days (AII). Some experts would evaluate at birth and start therapy.	These recommendations also to apply to women with first symptomatic episode of genital HSV. Mucosal sites for culture: conjunctivae, mouth, nasopharynx, rectum. Any symptomatic baby, at any time, requires a full evaluation for invasive infection and IV acyclovir therapy for 14–21 days.
Neonatal: Recurrent maternal infection, infant exposed at delivery[16]	Asymptomatic, exposed infant: at 24 h of life, culture mucosal sites, obtain plasma PCR for HSV. Hold on therapy unless cultures or PCR are positive, at which time IV acyclovir (60 mg/kg/day div q8h) for 10 days should be administered (AIII).	Any symptomatic baby, at any time, requires a full evaluation for invasive infection and IV acyclovir therapy. Risk of neonatal HSV infection following inoculation (even if not documented by newborn evaluation) lasts 6–8 wk.
Neonatal: Following symptomatic disease, to prevent recurrence during first year of life[16]	300 mg/m^2/dose PO tid for 6 mo following cessation of IV acyclovir treatment of acute disease (AI)	Follow absolute neutrophil counts at 2 and 4 wk, then monthly during prophylactic/suppressive therapy. It is not known if 12 mo of suppression would provide additional benefit compared with 6 mo.
Keratitis (ocular) in otherwise healthy children	Suppressive therapy for frequent recurrence (no pediatric data): 20 mg/kg/dose bid (up to 400 mg) for 6–12 mo; then reevaluate need (AIII)	Based on data from adults. Anecdotally, some children may require tid dosing to prevent recurrences. Check for acyclovir resistance for those who relapse while on appropriate therapy. Watch for severe recurrence at conclusion of suppression.

Influenza virus (A or B)[17]	Oseltamivir (AI) 3–≤8 mo: 3.0 mg/kg/dose qd for 10 days 9–11 mo: 3.5 mg/kg/dose PO bid qd for 10 days[18] Based on body weight for children ≥12 mo ≤15 kg: 30 mg qd for 10 days >15–23 kg: 45 mg qd for 10 days >23–40 kg: 60 mg qd for 10 days >40 kg: 75 mg qd for 10 days	Amantadine and rimantadine are not recommended for prophylaxis. Not recommended for infants 0 to ≤3 mo unless situation judged critical because of limited data on use in this age group.
	Zanamivir (AI) Children ≥5 y: 10 mg (two 5-mg inhalations) qd for as long as 28 days (community outbreaks) or 10 days (household settings)	
Rabies virus[19]	Rabies immune globulin, 20 IU/kg, infiltrate around wound, with remaining volume injected IM (AII). Rabies immunization should be provided postexposure (AII).	For dog, cat, or ferret bite from symptomatic animal, immediate rabies immune globulin and immunization; otherwise, can wait 10 days for observation of animal, if possible, prior to rabies immune globulin or vaccine. Bites of squirrels, hamsters, guinea pigs, gerbils, chipmunks, rats, mice and other rodents, rabbits, hares, and pikas almost never require antirabies prophylaxis. For bites of bats, skunks, raccoons, foxes, most other carnivores, and woodchucks, immediate rabies immune globulin and immunization (regard as rabid unless geographic area is known to be free of rabies or until animal proven negative by laboratory tests).

A. POSTEXPOSURE PROPHYLAXIS (cont)		
Prophylaxis Category	**Therapy (evidence grade)**	**Comments**
Fungal		
– ***Pneumocystis jiroveci*** (previously ***Pneumocystis carinii***)[20,21]	TMP/SMX as 5 mg TMP/kg/day PO, divided in 2 doses, q12h, either daily or 3 times/wk on consecutive days (AI); OR TMP/SMX 5 mg TMP/kg/day PO as a single dose, qd, given 3 times/wk on consecutive days (AI) (once-weekly regimens have also been successful) OR dapsone 2 mg/kg (max 100 mg) PO qd, or 4 mg/kg (max 200 mg) once weekly; OR atovaquone: 30 mg/kg/day for infants 1–3 mo; 45 mg/kg/day for infants 4–24 mo; and 30 mg/kg/day for infants >24 mo until no longer immunocompromised, based on oncology or transplant treatment regimen	Prophylaxis in specific populations based on degree of immunosuppression

B. LONG-TERM SYMPTOMATIC DISEASE PROPHYLAXIS

Prophylaxis Category	Therapy (evidence grade)	Comments
Bacterial otitis media[22,23]	Amoxicillin or other antibiotics can be used in half the therapeutic dose qd or bid to prevent infections if the benefits outweigh the risks of (1) development of resistant organisms for that child and (2) the risk of antibiotic side effects.	To prevent recurrent infections, also consider the risks and benefits of placing tympanostomy tubes to improve middle ear ventilation. Studies have demonstrated that amoxicillin, sulfisoxazole, and TMP/SMX are effective. However, antimicrobial prophylaxis may alter the nasopharyngeal flora and foster colonization with resistant organisms, compromising long-term efficacy of the prophylactic drug. Continuous PO-administered antimicrobial prophylaxis should be reserved for control of recurrent acute otitis media, only when defined as ≥3 distinct and well-documented episodes during a period of 6 mo or ≥4 episodes during a period of 12 mo. Although prophylactic administration of an antimicrobial agent limited to a period when a person is at high risk of otitis media has been suggested (eg, during acute viral respiratory tract infection), this method has not been evaluated critically.
Acute rheumatic fever	For >27.3 kg (>60 lb): 1.2 million U penicillin G benzathine, q4wk (q3wk for high-risk children) For <27.3 kg: 600,000 U penicillin G benzathine, q4wk (q3wk for high-risk children) OR Penicillin V (phenoxymethyl) oral, 250 mg PO bid	AHA policy statement at http://circ.ahajournals.org/content/119/11/1541.full.pdf (accessed October 14, 2014). Doses studied many years ago, with no new data; ARF an uncommon disease currently in the US. Alternatives to penicillin include sulfisoxazole or macrolides, including erythromycin, azithromycin, and clarithromycin.
Urinary tract infection, recurrent[24–27]	TMP/SMX 3 mg/kg/dose TMP PO qd OR nitrofurantoin 1–2 mg/kg PO qd at bedtime; more rapid resistance may develop using beta-lactams (BII).	Only for those with grade III–V reflux or with recurrent febrile UTI: prophylaxis no longer recommended for patients with grade I–II (some also exclude grade III) reflux and no evidence of renal damage. Early treatment of new infections is recommended for these children. Resistance eventually develops to every antibiotic; follow resistance patterns for each patient.

C. PREEMPTIVE TREATMENT/LATENT INFECTION TREATMENT ("PROPHYLAXIS OF SYMPTOMATIC INFECTION")

Tuberculosis[12,13] (latent TB infection [asymptomatic infection], defined by a positive skin test or IGRA, with no clinical or x-ray evidence of active disease)	INH 10–15 mg/kg/day (max 300 mg) PO daily for 9 mo (12 mo for immunocompromised patients) (AII); treatment with INH at 20–30 mg twice weekly for 9 mo is also effective (AIII).	Single drug therapy if no clinical or radiographic evidence of active disease. For exposure to known INH-resistant but rifampin-susceptible strains, use rifampin 10 mg/kg PO daily for 6 mo (AIII). For children ≥12 y, can use once weekly DOT with INH AND rifapentine for 12 wk; much less data for children 2–12 y.[14] For exposure to multidrug-resistant strains, consult with TB specialist.

D. SURGICAL/PROCEDURE PROPHYLAXIS[28–35]

The CDC and National Healthcare Safety Network use a classification of surgical procedure-related wound infections based on an estimation of the load of bacterial contamination: Class I, clean; Class II, clean-contaminated; Class III, contaminated; and Class IV, dirty/infected.[27,31] Other major factors creating risk for postoperative surgical site infection include the duration of surgery (a longer-duration operation, defined as one that exceeded the 75th percentile for a given procedure) and the medical comorbidities of the patient, as determined by an American Society of Anesthesiologists score of III, IV, or V (presence of severe systemic disease that results in functional limitations, is life-threatening, or is expected to preclude survival from the operation). The virulence/pathogenicity of bacteria inoculated and the presence of foreign debris/devitalized tissue/surgical material in the wound are also considered risk factors for infection.

For all categories of surgical prophylaxis, dosing recommendations are derived from (1) choosing agents based on the organisms likely to be responsible for inoculation of the surgical site; (2) giving the agents shortly before starting the operation to achieve appropriate serum and tissue exposures at the time of incision through the end of the procedure; (3) providing additional doses during the procedure at times based on the standard dosing guideline for that agent; and (4) stopping the agents at the end of the procedure but no longer than 24 to 48 h after the procedure.[30–32,34,35]

Procedure/Operation	Recommended Agents	Preoperative Dose	Re-dosing Interval (h) for Prolonged Surgery
Cardiovascular			
Cardiothoracic *Staphylococcus epidermidis, Staphylococcus aureus, Corynebacterium* spp	Cefazolin, OR	30 mg/kg	4
	Vancomycin, if MRSA likely	15 mg/kg	8

Vascular *S epidermidis, S aureus, Corynebacterium* spp, gram-negative enteric bacilli, particularly for procedures in the groin	Cefazolin, OR	30 mg/kg	4
	Vancomycin, if MRSA likely	15 mg/kg	8
Gastrointestinal			
Gastroduodenal Enteric gram-negative bacilli, respiratory tract gram-positive cocci	Cefazolin	30 mg/kg	4
Biliary Procedure, Open Enteric gram-negative bacilli, enterococci, *Clostridia*	Cefazolin, OR	30 mg/kg	4
	Cefoxitin	40 mg/kg	2
Appendectomy, non-perforated	Cefoxitin, OR	40 mg/kg	2
	Cefazolin and metronidazole	30 mg/kg cefazolin and 10 mg/kg metronidazole	4 for cefazolin 8 for metronidazole
Complicated appendicitis or other ruptured viscus Enteric gram-negative bacilli, enterococci, anaerobes. May require additional therapy for treatment of infection.	Cefoxitin, OR	40 mg/kg	2
	Cefazolin and metronidazole, OR	30 mg/kg cefazolin and 10 mg/kg metronidazole	4 for cefazolin 8 for metronidazole
	Meropenem, OR	20 mg/kg	4
	Imipenem, OR	20 mg/kg	4
	Ertapenem	30 mg/kg	8

D. SURGICAL/PROCEDURE PROPHYLAXIS[28–35] (cont)

Procedure/Operation	Recommended Agents	Preoperative Dose	Re-dosing Interval (h) for Prolonged Surgery
Genitourinary			
Cystoscopy (only requires prophylaxis for children with suspected active UTI or those having foreign material placed) Enteric gram-negative bacilli, enterococci	Cefazolin, OR	30 mg/kg	4
	TMP/SMX (if low local resistance), OR Select a 3rd-generation cephalosporin (cefotaxime) or fluoroquinolone (ciprofloxacin) if the child is colonized with cefazolin-resistant, TMP/SMX-resistant strains.	4–5 mg/kg	N/A
Open or laparoscopic surgery Enteric gram-negative bacilli, enterococci	Cefazolin	30 mg/kg	4
Head and Neck Surgery			
Assuming incision through respiratory tract mucosa Anaerobes, enteric gram-negative bacilli, *S aureus*	Clindamycin, OR	10 mg/kg	6
	Cefazolin and metronidazole	30 mg/kg cefazolin and 10 mg/kg metronidazole	4 for cefazolin 8 for metronidazole
Neurosurgery			
Craniotomy, ventricular shunt placement *S epidermidis, S aureus*	Cefazolin, OR	30 mg/kg	4
	Vancomycin, if MRSA likely	15 mg/kg	8
Orthopedic			
Internal fixation of fractures, spinal rod placement,[33] prosthetic joints *S epidermidis, S aureus*	Cefazolin, OR	30 mg/kg	4
	Vancomycin, if MRSA likely	15 mg/kg	8

Trauma			
Exceptionally varied; agents should focus on skin flora (*S epidermidis, S aureus*) as well as the flora inoculated into the wound, based on the trauma exposure, that may include enteric gram-negative bacilli, anaerobes (including *Clostridia* spp), and fungi. Cultures at time of wound exploration are critical to focus therapy.	Cefazolin (for skin) OR	30 mg/kg	4
	Vancomycin (for skin), if MRSA likely, OR	15 mg/kg	8
	Meropenem OR imipenem (for anaerobes, including *Clostridia* spp, and non-fermenting gram-negative bacilli) OR	20 mg/kg for either	4
	Gentamicin and metronidazole (for anaerobes, including *Clostridia* spp, and non-fermenting gram-negative bacilli), OR	2.5 mg/kg gentamicin and 10 mg/kg metronidazole	6 for gentamicin 8 for metronidazole
	Piperacillin/tazobactam	100 mg/kg piperacillin component	2

15. Adverse Reactions to Antimicrobial Agents

A good rule of clinical practice is to be suspicious of an adverse drug reaction when a patient's clinical course deviates from the expected. This section focuses on reactions that may require close observation or laboratory monitoring because of their frequency or severity. For more detailed listings of reactions, review the US Food and Drug Administration (FDA)-approved package labels available at the National Library of Medicine (NLM) (http://dailymed.nlm.nih.gov, accessed October 14, 2014) with more recently approved agents actually having adverse events listed for the new agent and the comparator agent from the phase 3 prospective clinical trials. This allows one to assign drug-attributable side effects for specific drugs such as oseltamivir, used for influenza, when influenza and the antiviral may cause nausea. The NLM also provides an online drug information service for patients (MedlinePlus) at www.nlm.nih.gov/medlineplus/druginformation.html.

Antibacterial Drugs

Aminoglycosides. Any of the aminoglycosides can cause serious nephrotoxicity and ototoxicity. Monitor all patients receiving aminoglycoside therapy for more than a few days for renal function with periodic determinations of blood urea nitrogen and creatinine to assess potential problems of drug accumulation with deteriorating renal function. Common practice has been to measure the peak serum concentration 0.5 to 1 hour after a dose to make sure one is in a safe and therapeutic range and to measure a trough serum concentration immediately preceding a dose to assess for drug accumulation and pending toxicity. Monitoring is especially important in patients with any degree of renal insufficiency. Elevated trough concentrations (>2 mg/mL for gentamicin and tobramycin; >10 mg/mL for amikacin) suggest drug accumulation and should be a warning to decrease the dose, even if the peak is not yet elevated. Renal toxicity may be related to the total exposure of the kidney to the aminoglycoside over time. With once-daily administration regimens, peak values are 2 to 3 times greater, and trough values are usually very low. Nephrotoxicity seems to be less common in adults with once-daily (as opposed to 3 times daily) dosing regimens, but data are generally lacking in children.[1] In cystic fibrosis patients with pulmonary exacerbations, once-daily aminoglycosides appear less toxic and equally effective.[2]

The "loop" diuretics (furosemide and bumetanide) potentiate the ototoxicity of the aminoglycosides. Aminoglycosides potentiate botulinum toxin neuromuscular junction dysfunction and are to be avoided in young infants with infant botulism.

Minor side effects, such as allergies, rashes, and drug fever, are rare.

Beta-lactam Antibiotics. The most feared reaction to penicillins, anaphylactic shock, is extremely rare, and no absolutely reliable means of predicting its occurrence exists. For most infections, alternative therapy to penicillin or beta-lactams exists. However, in certain situations, the benefits of penicillin or a beta-lactam may outweigh the risk of anaphylaxis, requiring that skin testing and desensitization be performed in a medically supervised environment. The commercially available skin testing material, benzylpenicilloyl polylysine (Pre-Pen, AllerQuest), contains the major determinants thought to be primarily responsible for urticarial reactions but does not contain the minor determinants that are more often associated with anaphylaxis. No commercially available minor determinant mixture is available. For adults, the Centers for Disease Control and Prevention (CDC) suggests using a dilute solution of freshly prepared benzyl penicillin G as the skin test material in place of a standardized mixture of minor determinants (www.cdc.gov/std/treatment/2010/penicillin-allergy.htm, accessed October 14, 2014). Testing should be performed on children with a credible history of a possible reaction to a penicillin before these drugs are used in oral or parenteral formulations. Anaphylaxis has been reported in adults receiving penicillin skin testing. Recent reviews provide more in-depth discussion,[3,4] with additional information on desensitization available at the CDC Web site noted above. Cross-reactions between classes of beta-lactam antibiotics (penicillins, cephalosporins, carbapenems, and monobactams) occur at a rate of less than 5% to 20%, with the rate of reaction to cephalosporins in patients without a serious reaction to penicillin of 0.1%.[5] No commercially available skin testing reagent has been developed for beta-lactam antibiotics other than penicillin.

Amoxicillin and other aminopenicillins are associated with minor adverse effects. Diarrhea, oral or diaper area candidiasis, morbilliform, and blotchy rashes are not uncommon. The kinds of non-urticarial rashes that may occur while a child is receiving amoxicillin are not known to predispose to anaphylaxis and may not actually be caused by amoxicillin itself; they do not represent a routine contraindication to subsequent use of amoxicillin or any other penicillins. Rarely, beta-lactams cause serious, life-threatening pseudomembranous enterocolitis due to suppression of normal bowel flora and overgrowth of toxin-producing strains of *Clostridium difficile*. Drug-related fever may occur; serum sickness is uncommon. Reversible neutropenia and thrombocytopenia may occur with any of the beta-lactams and seem to be related to dose and duration of therapy but do not appear to carry the same risk of bacterial superinfection that is present with neutropenia in oncology patients.

The cephalosporins have been a remarkably safe series of antibiotics. The third-generation cephalosporins cause profound alteration of normal flora on mucosal surfaces, and all have caused pseudomembranous colitis on rare occasions. Ceftriaxone commonly causes loose stools, but it is rarely severe enough to require stopping therapy. Ceftriaxone in high dosages may cause fine "sand" (a calcium complex of ceftriaxone) to develop in the gallbladder. In adults, and rarely in children, these deposits may cause biliary tract symptoms; these are not gallstones, and the deposits are reversible after stopping the drug. In neonates receiving calcium-containing hyperalimentation concurrent with intravenous (IV) ceftriaxone, precipitation of ceftriaxone-calcium in the bloodstream resulting in death has been reported,[6] leading to an FDA warning against the concurrent use of ceftriaxone and parenteral calcium in neonates younger than 28 days (http://1.usa.gov/1Av2N5t, accessed October 14, 2014). As ceftriaxone may also displace bilirubin from albumin-binding sites and increase free bilirubin in serum, the antibiotic is not routinely used in neonatal infections until the normal physiologic jaundice is resolving after the first few weeks of life. Cefotaxime is the preferred IV third-generation cephalosporin for neonates.

Imipenem/cilastatin, meropenem, and ertapenem have rates of adverse effects on hematopoietic, hepatic, and renal systems that are similar to other beta-lactams. However, children treated with imipenem for bacterial meningitis were noted to have an increase in probable drug-related seizures not seen with meropenem therapy in controlled studies.[7] For children requiring carbapenem therapy, meropenem is preferred for those with any underlying central nervous system inflammatory condition.

Fluoroquinolones (FQs). All quinolone antibiotics (nalidixic acid, ciprofloxacin, levofloxacin, gatifloxacin, and moxifloxacin) cause cartilage damage to weight-bearing joints in toxicity studies in various immature animals; however, no conclusive data indicate similar toxicity in young children. Studies to evaluate cartilage toxicity and failure to achieve predicted growth have not consistently found statistically significant differences between those children treated with FQs and controls, although in an FDA-requested, blinded, prospective study of complicated urinary tract infections, the number of muscular/joint/tendon events was greater in the ciprofloxacin-treated group than in the comparator (www.fda.gov/downloads/Drugs/DevelopmentApprovalProcess/DevelopmentResources/UCM162536.pdf, accessed October 14, 2014). This continues to be an area of active investigation by the pediatric infectious disease community as well as the FDA. Fluoroquinolone toxicities in adults, which vary in incidence considerably between individual agents, include cardiac dysrhythmias, hepatotoxicity, and photodermatitis; other reported side effects include gastrointestinal symptoms, dizziness, headaches, tremors, confusion, seizures, and alterations of glucose metabolism producing hyperglycemia and hypoglycemia. The American Academy of Pediatrics published a clinical report on the use of fluoroquinolones and, based on the best available evidence, concluded that IV fluoroquinolones should be used when safer IV antibiotic alternatives were not available and that oral fluoroquinolones should be used if no other safe and effective oral therapy existed, even if effective alternative IV therapy existed.[8]

Lincosamides. Clindamycin can cause nausea, vomiting, and diarrhea. Pseudomembranous colitis due to suppression of normal flora and overgrowth of *C difficile* is uncommon, especially in children, but potentially serious. Urticaria, glossitis, pruritus, and skin rashes occur occasionally. Serum sickness, anaphylaxis, and photosensitivity are rare, as are hematologic and hepatic abnormalities. Extensive use of clindamycin since 2000 for treatment of community-associated methicillin-resistant *Staphylococcus aureus* infections has not been accompanied by reports of significantly increasing rates of *C difficile*–mediated colitis in children.

Macrolides. Erythromycin is one of the safest antimicrobial agents but has largely been replaced by azithromycin because of substantially decreased epigastric distress and nausea. Alteration of normal flora is generally not a problem, but oral or perianal candidiasis occasionally develops. Intravenous erythromycin lactobionate causes phlebitis and should be administered slowly (1–2 hours); the gastrointestinal side effects seen with oral administration also accompany IV use. However, IV azithromycin is better tolerated than IV erythromycin and has been evaluated for pharmacokinetics in limited numbers of children.[9]

Erythromycin therapy has been associated with pyloric stenosis in newborns and young infants; due to this toxicity and with limited data on safety of azithromycin in the first months of life, azithromycin is now the preferred macrolide for treatment of pertussis in neonates and young infants.[10]

Oxazolidinones. Linezolid represents the first oxazolidinone antibiotic approved for all children, including neonates, by the FDA. Toxicity is primarily hematologic, with thrombocytopenia and neutropenia that is dependent on dosage and duration of therapy, occurring most often with treatment courses of 2 weeks or longer. Routine monitoring for bone marrow toxicity every 1 to 2 weeks is recommended for children on long-term therapy. Peripheral neuropathy and optic neuritis may also occur with long-term therapy.[11]

Sulfonamides and Trimethoprim. The most common adverse reaction to sulfonamides is a hypersensitivity rash. Stevens-Johnson syndrome, a life-threatening systemic reaction characterized by immune-mediated injury to the skin and mucous membranes, occurs in approximately 3 of 100,000 exposed people. Neutropenia, anemia, and thrombocytopenia occur occasionally. Sulfa drugs can precipitate hemolysis in patients with glucose-6-phosphate dehydrogenase deficiency. Drug fever and serum sickness are infrequent hypersensitivity reactions. Hepatitis with focal or diffuse necrosis is rare. A rare idiosyncratic reaction to sulfa drugs is acute aseptic meningitis.

Tetracyclines. Tetracyclines are used infrequently in pediatric patients because the major indications are uncommon diseases (rickettsial infections, brucellosis, Lyme disease), with the exception of acne. Tetracyclines are deposited in growing bones and teeth, with depression of linear bone growth, dental staining, and defects in enamelization in deciduous and permanent teeth. This effect is dose related, and the risk extends up to 8 years of age. A single treatment course of tetracyclines has not been found to cause dental staining, leading to the recommendation for tetracyclines as the drugs of choice in children for a number of uncommon pathogens. Doxycycline is likely to produce less dental staining than tetracycline. A parenteral tetracycline approved for adults in 2005, tigecycline, produces the same "staining" of bones in experimental animals as seen with other tetracyclines.

Side effects include minor gastrointestinal disturbances, photosensitization, angioedema, glossitis, pruritus ani, and exfoliative dermatitis. Potential adverse drug reactions from tetracyclines involve virtually every organ system. Hepatic and pancreatic injuries have occurred with accidental overdosage and in patients with renal failure. (Pregnant women are particularly at risk for hepatic injury.)

Vancomycin. Vancomycin can cause phlebitis if the drug is injected rapidly or in concentrated form. Vancomycin has the potential for ototoxicity and nephrotoxicity, and serum concentrations should be monitored for children on more than a few days of therapy. Hepatic toxicity is rare. Neutropenia has been reported. If the drug is infused too rapidly, a transient rash of the upper body with itching may occur from histamine release (red man syndrome). It is not a contraindication to continued use and the rash is less likely to occur if the infusion rate is increased to 60 to 120 minutes and the children are pretreated with oral or IV antihistamines.

Antituberculous Drugs

Isoniazid (INH) is generally well tolerated and hypersensitivity reactions are rare. Peripheral neuritis (preventable or reversed by pyridoxine administration) and mental aberrations from euphoria to psychosis occur more often in adults than in children. Mild elevations of alanine transaminase in the first weeks of therapy, which disappear or remain stable with continued administration, are common. Rarely, hepatitis develops but is reversible if INH is stopped; if INH is not stopped, liver failure may develop in these children. Monitoring of liver functions is not routinely required in children receiving INH single drug therapy for latent tuberculosis as long as the children can be followed closely and liver functions can be drawn if the children develop symptoms of hepatitis.

Rifampin can also cause hepatitis; it is more common in patients with preexisting liver disease or in those taking large dosages. The risk of hepatic damage increases when rifampin and INH are taken together in dosages of more than 15 mg/kg/day of each. Gastrointestinal, hematologic, and neurologic side effects of various types have been observed on occasion. Hypersensitivity reactions are rare.

Pyrazinamide also can cause hepatic damage, which again seems to be dosage related. Ethambutol has the potential for optic neuritis, but this toxicity seems to be rare in children at currently prescribed dosages. Young children who cannot comment to examiners regarding color blindness or other signs of optic neuritis should have an ophthalmologic examination every few months on therapy. Optic neuritis is usually reversible.

Antifungal Drugs

Amphotericin B (deoxycholate) causes chills, fever, flushing, and headaches, the most common of the many adverse reactions. Some degree of decreased renal function occurs in virtually all patients given amphotericin B. Anemia is common and, rarely, hepatic toxicity and neutropenia occur. Patients should be monitored for hyponatremia and hypokalemia. However, much better tolerated (but more costly) lipid formulations of amphotericin B are now commonly used (see Chapter 2). For reasons of safety and tolerability, the lipid formulations should be used whenever possible.

Fluconazole is usually very well tolerated from clinical and laboratory standpoints. Gastrointestinal symptoms, rash, and headache occur occasionally. Transient, asymptomatic elevations of hepatic enzymes have been reported but are rare.

Voriconazole, a new antifungal suspension, may interfere with metabolism of other drugs the child may be receiving due to hepatic P450 metabolism. However, a poorly understood visual field abnormality has been described, usually at the beginning of a course of therapy and uniformly self-resolving, in which objects appear to glow. There is no pain and no known anatomic or biochemical correlate of this side effect; no lasting effects on vision have yet been reported. Hepatic toxicity has also been reported but is not so common as to preclude the use of voriconazole for serious fungal infections.

Caspofungin, micafungin, and anidulafungin (echinocandins) are very well tolerated as a class. Fever, rash, headache, and phlebitis at the site of infection have been reported in adults. Uncommon hepatic side effects have also been reported.

Flucytosine (5-FC) is seldom used due to the availability of safer, equally effective therapy. The major toxicity is bone marrow depression, which is dosage related, especially in patients treated concomitantly with amphotericin B. Renal function should be monitored.

Antiviral Drugs

After extensive clinical use, acyclovir has proved to be an extremely safe drug with only rare serious adverse effects. Renal dysfunction with IV acyclovir has occurred mainly with too rapid infusion of the drug. Neutropenia has been associated with administration of parenteral and oral acyclovir but is responsive to granulocyte colony-stimulating factor use and resolves spontaneously following temporary halting of the drug. At very high doses, parenteral acyclovir can cause neurologic irritation, including seizures. Rash, headache, and gastrointestinal side effects are uncommon. There has been little controlled experience in children with famciclovir and valacyclovir.

Ganciclovir causes hematologic toxicity that is dependent on the dosage and duration of therapy. Gastrointestinal disturbances and neurologic damage are rarely encountered. Oral valganciclovir can have these same toxicities as parenteral ganciclovir, but neutropenia is seen much less frequently following oral valganciclovir compared with IV ganciclovir.

Oseltamivir is well tolerated except for nausea with or without vomiting, which may be more likely to occur with the first few doses but usually resolves within a few days while still on therapy. Neuropsychiatric events have been reported, primarily from Japan, in patients with influenza treated with oseltamivir (a rate of approximately 1:50,000), but also are seen in patients on all of the other influenza antivirals and in patients with influenza receiving no antiviral therapy. It seems that these spontaneously reported side effects may be a function of influenza itself, oseltamivir itself, possibly a genetic predisposition to this clinical event, or a combination of all 3 factors.

Foscarnet can cause renal dysfunction, anemia, and cardiac rhythm disturbances. Alterations in plasma minerals and electrolytes occur, and any clinically significant metabolic changes should be corrected. Patients who experience mild (eg, perioral numbness or paresthesia) or severe (eg, seizures) symptoms of electrolyte abnormalities should have serum electrolyte and mineral levels assessed as close in time to the event as possible.

16. Drug Interactions

NOTES

- Antimicrobial drug-drug interactions that are known to be clinically significant and likely to be encountered in children are listed in this chapter. Interactions involving probenecid, synergy-antagonism, and in vitro physical incompatibilities are not listed. Interactions involving antiretrovirals can be found at www.aidsinfo.nih.gov (accessed October 14, 2014). Interactions involving QT interval prolongation can be found at www.crediblemeds.org (accessed October 14, 2014). Common antimicrobials with an increased risk of QT interval prolongation include azole antifungals, macrolides, fluoroquinolones, and trimethoprim/sulfamethoxazole. Cited references at the end of this section provide more extensive details of all reported and theoretical interactions, including antimicrobial drug-disease interactions.
- Erythromycin, clarithromycin, and the azole antifungals inhibit cytochrome P450 (CYP) enzyme activity and interact with numerous drugs. Cytochrome P450 inhibition can increase the concentration of the interacting drug and cause toxicity. Fluconazole and posaconazole are relatively weak CYP inhibitors within this notorious group, but even they have many significant interactions. Drug transporter protein inhibition is another source of some azole interactions. Conversely, enzyme-inducing antiepileptic drugs and rifamycins are inducers of CYP activity and can reduce an interacting drug's concentration and efficacy.
- **Abbreviations:** ACE, angiotensin-converting enzyme; conc, concentration; CYP, cytochrome P450; decr, decreased; EIAED, enzyme-inducing antiepileptic drug; incr, increased; INR, international normalized ratio; IV, intravenous; MAO, monoamine oxidase; NSAID, nonsteroidal anti-inflammatory drug; PGP, p-glycoprotein; PO, orally; PPI, proton pump inhibitors; TMP/SMX, trimethoprim/sulfamethoxazole.

Anti-infective Agent	Interacting Drug(s)	Adverse Effect
Acyclovir/valacyclovir	Nephrotoxins[a]	Additive nephrotoxicity
Amantadine	Anticholinergics,[b] trimethoprim	Neurotoxicity
Aminoglycosides[c] (parenteral)	Nephrotoxins[a]	Additive nephrotoxicity
	Neuromuscular blocking agents	Incr neuromuscular blockade
	Indomethacin, ibuprofen	Incr aminoglycoside conc
	Carboplatin/cisplatin	Additive ototoxicity
Amphotericin B	Nephrotoxins[a]	Additive nephrotoxicity
	Cisplatin, corticosteroids, diuretics	Additive hypokalemia
Atovaquone	Metoclopramide, rifamycins, tetracycline	Decr atovaquone conc
Carbapenems	Valproic acid	Decr valproic acid conc
Caspofungin	Cyclosporine	Incr caspofungin conc, hepatotoxicity
	Tacrolimus, sirolimus	Decr conc of interacting drug
	Rifampin, EIAEDs[d]	Decr caspofungin conc
Cefdinir	Iron, antacids	Decr cefdinir oral absorption
Cefpodoxime, cefuroxime PO	Antacids, H_2 antagonists, PPI	Decr anti-infective oral absorption
Ceftriaxone, IV	Calcium, IV	Precipitation, cardiopulmonary embolism
Ciprofloxacin	Caffeine, theophylline, sildenafil, warfarin	Incr conc of interacting drug
	Phenytoin	Decr conc of phenytoin
	Antacids, bismuth, calcium, iron, sucralfate, zinc	Decr ciprofloxacin oral absorption[e]
Clindamycin	Neuromuscular blocking agents	Incr neuromuscular blockade
Doxycycline	Antacids, bismuth, calcium, iron, sucralfate, zinc	Decr doxycycline oral absorption[e]
	EIAEDs,[d] rifamycins	Decr doxycycline conc
Erythromycin, clarithromycin	CYP 3A4 substrates[f]	Incr conc of interacting drug
	Rifamycins	Decr anti-infective conc

Anti-infective Agent	Interacting Drug(s)	Adverse Effect
Fluconazole[g]	Cyclosporine, cyclophosphamide, fentanyl, alfentanil, methadone, midazolam, NSAIDs, omeprazole, phenytoin, sirolimus, tacrolimus, warfarin	Incr conc of interacting drug
	EIAEDs,[d] rifampin	Decr fluconazole conc
Griseofulvin	EIAEDs[d]	Decr griseofulvin conc
Isoniazid	Acetaminophen, carbamazepine	Hepatotoxicity
	Antacids	Decr isoniazid conc
	Carbamazepine, phenytoin, valproic acid, warfarin	Incr conc of interacting drug
	Antidepressants, linezolid, sympathomimetics	MAO inhibition toxicity, hypertensive reaction
Itraconazole, ketoconazole[h]	CYP 3A4 substrates[f]	Incr conc of interacting drug
	Antacids, H_2 antagonists, PPI	Decr azole absorption, itraconazole oral solution less affected, voriconazole not affected
	EIAEDs,[d] rifamycins	Decr azole conc
	Digoxin (with itraconazole)	Incr digoxin conc (inhibition of PGP transport)
Linezolid	Antidepressants, isoniazid, sympathomimetics	MAO inhibition toxicity, hypertensive reaction
Metronidazole	Busulfan, 5-fluorouacil, phenytoin, warfarin	Incr conc of interacting drug
	EIAEDs[d]	Decr metronidazole conc
Nafcillin	Warfarin	Decr warfarin effect, decr INR
Penicillins	Methotrexate	Incr methotrexate conc
Posaconazole	Antacids, H_2 antagonists, PPI	Decr absorption of oral posaconazole
	Midazolam, sirolimus, tacrolimus, vincristine	Incr conc of interacting drug
	EIAEDs[d]	Decr posaconazole conc
Rifampin, rifabutin	Numerous CYP and transporter substrates	Decr conc of interacting drug

Anti-infective Agent	Interacting Drug(s)	Adverse Effect
Terbinafine	Antidepressants, β-blockers	Incr conc of interacting drug
Tetracycline	Isotretinoin	Intracranial hypertension
TMP/SMX	Amantadine, methotrexate, phenytoin, warfarin	Incr conc of interacting drug
	ACE inhibitors, spironolactone	Additive hyperkalemia
Vancomycin	Indomethacin, ibuprofen	Incr vancomycin conc
Voriconazole[i]	See fluconazole.[j]	
	EIAEDs,[d] rifamycins	Decr voriconazole conc

[a]Examples of nephrotoxic drugs: ACE inhibitors, acyclovir, aminoglycosides, cidofovir, contrast agents, cyclosporine, diuretics, foscarnet, NSAIDs, pentamidine, polymyxins, tacrolimus, vancomycin.
[b]Examples of anticholinergics: atropine, belladonna, dicyclomine, diphenhydramine, glycopyrrolate, hyoscyamine, promethazine, scopolamine.
[c]Gentamicin, tobramycin, amikacin, streptomycin.
[d]EIAEDs: carbamazepine, phenobarbital, phenytoin, and primidone.
[e]Class-wide effect; interaction will also occur with other fluoroquinolones (levofloxacin, moxifloxacin) and tetracyclines (minocycline).
[f]CYP 3A4 substrates: alfentanil, antineoplastics (known interactions with busulfan, cyclophosphamide, docetaxel, irinotecan and vinca alkaloids, many others possible; see Ruggiero et al), benzodiazepines (CYP 3A4 oxidized benzodiazepines: alprazolam, chlordiazepoxide, clonazepam, clorazepate, diazepam, midazolam, and triazolam), bosentan, carbamazepine, cyclosporine, dexamethasone, erythromycin/clarithromycin, fentanyl, loratadine, methadone, methylprednisolone, sildenafil, sirolimus, tacrolimus, tiagabine.
[g]Fluconazole interactions mediated mainly by CYP 2C9, 2C19, and some 3A4 inhibition.
[h]Ketoconazole is also known to have or may potentially have the same interactions as fluconazole due to similar inhibition of CYP 2C9 and CYP 2C19 drug metabolism.
[i]Potent CYP 3A4 inhibitor; may inhibit CYP 3A4 substrates (see footnote f).
[j]Interaction profile is similar to fluconazole due to similar CYP inhibition.

Bibliography

Baciewicz AM, et al. *Curr Med Res Opin.* 2013;29(1):1-12 PMID: 23136913
Hansten PD, et al. *Drug Interactions Analysis and Management 2013.* 2013
Indiana University Division of Clinical Pharmacology. P450 drug interaction table: abbreviated "clinically relevant" table. http://medicine.iupui.edu/clinpharm/ddis/clinical-table. Accessed October 14, 2014
Perucca E. *Br J Clin Pharmacol.* 2006;61(3):246–255 PMID:16487217
Piscitelli SC, et al, eds. *Drug Interactions in Infectious Diseases.* 3rd ed. 2011
Ruggiero A, et al. *Eur J Clin Pharmacol.* 2013;69(1):1–10 PMID: 22660443

Appendix

Nomogram for Determing Body Surface Area

Based on the nomogram shown below, a straight line joining the patient's height and weight will intersect the center column at the calculated body surface area (BSA). For children of normal height and weight, the child's weight in pounds is used, then the examiner reads across to the corresponding BSA in meters. Alternatively, Mosteller's formula can be used.

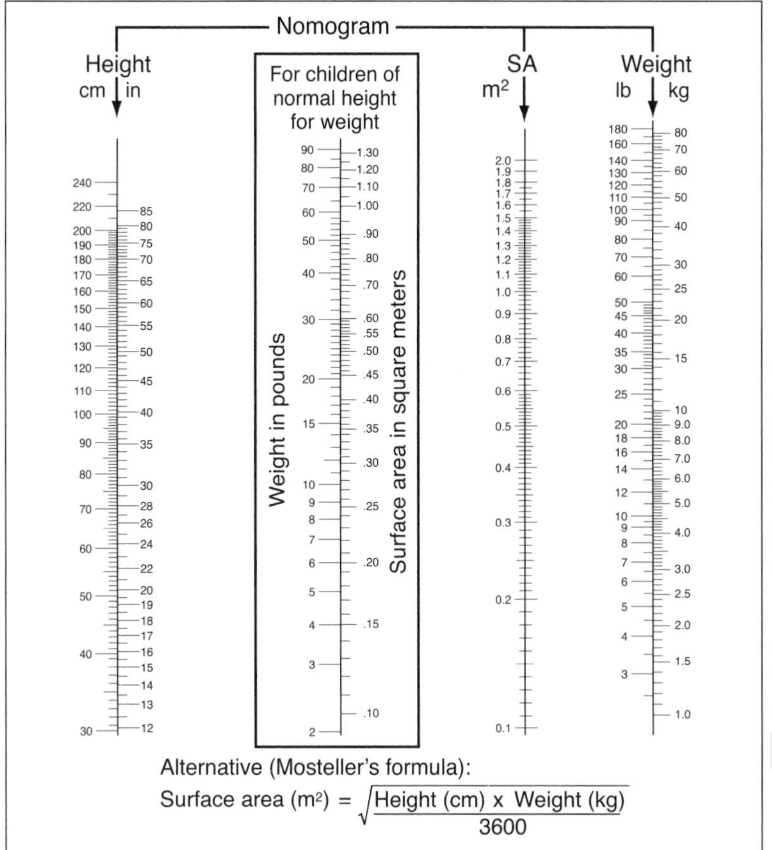

$$\text{Surface area (m}^2) = \sqrt{\frac{\text{Height (cm)} \times \text{Weight (kg)}}{3600}}$$

Nomogram and equation to determine body surface area. (From Tschudy MM, Arcara KM, eds. *The Harriet Lane Handbook*. 19th ed. St Louis, MO: Mosby; 2012. Reprinted with permission from Elsevier.)

References

Chapter 2

1. Cornely OA, et al. *Clin Infect Dis.* 2007;44(10):1289–1297 PMID: 17443465
2. Piper L, et al. *Pediatr Infect Dis J.* 2011;30(5):375–378 PMID: 21085048
3. Friberg LE, et al. *Antimicrob Agents Chemother.* 2012;56(6):3032–3042 PMID: 22430956
4. Smith PB, et al. *Pediatr Infect Dis J.* 2009;28(5):412–415 PMID: 19319022
5. Hope WW, et al. *Antimicrob Agents Chemother.* 2010;54(6):2633–2637 PMID: 20308367
6. Benjamin DK Jr, et al. *Clin Pharmacol Ther.* 2010;87(1):93–99 PMID: 19890251
7. Cohen-Wolkowiez M, et al. *Clin Pharmacol Ther.* 2011;89(5):702–707 PMID: 21412233

Chapter 4

1. Liu C, et al. *Clin Infect Dis.* 2011;52(3):e18–e55 PMID: 21208910
2. Le J, et al. *Pediatr Infect Dis J.* 2013;32(4):e155–e163 PMID: 23340565
3. Huang JT, et al. *Pediatrics.* 2009;123(5):e808–e814 PMID: 19403473

Chapter 5

1. Fox E, et al. Drug therapy in neonates and pediatric patients. In: Atkinson AJ, et al, eds. *Principles of Clinical Pharmacology.* 2007:359–373
2. Wagner CL, et al. *J Perinatol.* 2000;20(6):346–350 PMID: 11002871
3. Intravenous ceftriaxone (marketed as Rocephin and generics) and calcium drug-drug interaction: potential risk for cardiovascular adverse events in neonates. US Food and Drug Administration. http://www.fda.gov/Drugs/DrugSafety/DrugSafetyNewsletter/ucm189806.htm#IntravenousCeftriaxoneMarketedasRocephinandGenericsandCalciumDrug-DrugInteraction:PotentialRiskforCardiovascularAdverseEventsinNeonates. Accessed October 14, 2014
4. Martin E, et al. *Eur J Pediatr.* 1993;152(6):530–534 PMID: 8335024
5. Rours IG, et al. *Pediatrics.* 2008;121(2):e321–e326 PMID: 18245405
6. American Academy of Pediatrics. Chlamydial infections. In: Pickering LK, et al, eds. *Red Book: 2012 Report of the Committee on Infectious Diseases.* 2012:272–281
7. Hammerschlag MR, et al. *Pediatr Infect Dis J.* 1998;17(11):1049–1050 PMID: 9849993
8. Zar HJ. *Paediatr Drugs.* 2005;7(2):103–110 PMID: 15871630
9. Honein MA, et al. *Lancet.* 1999;354(9196):2101–2105 PMID: 10609814
10. Laga M, et al. *N Engl J Med.* 1986;315(22):1382–1385 PMID: 3095641
11. Workowski KA, et al. *MMWR Recomm Rep.* 2010;59(RR-12):1–110 PMID: 21160459
12. Newman LM, et al. *Clin Infect Dis.* 2007;44(S3):S84–S101 PMID: 17342672
13. MacDonald N, et al. *Adv Exp Med Biol.* 2008;609:108–130 PMID: 18193661
14. American Academy of Pediatrics. Gonococcal infections. In: Pickering LK, et al, eds. *Red Book: 2012 Report of the Committee on Infectious Diseases.* 2012:336–344
15. Cimolai N. *Am J Ophthalmol.* 2006;142(1):183–184 PMID: 16815280
16. Marangon FB, et al. *Am J Ophthalmol.* 2004;137(3):453–458 PMID: 15013867
17. American Academy of Pediatrics. Staphylococcal infections. In: Pickering LK, et al, eds. *Red Book: 2012 Report of the Committee on Infectious Diseases.* 2012:653–668
18. Brito DV, et al. *Braz J Infect Dis.* 2003;7(4):234–235 PMID: 14533982
19. Chen CJ, et al. *Am J Ophthalmol.* 2008;145(6):966–970 PMID: 18378213
20. Shah SS, et al. *J Perinatol.* 1999;19(6pt1):462–465 PMID: 10685281
21. Kimberlin DW, et al. *J Pediatr.* 2003;143(1):16–25 PMID: 12915819
22. Kimberlin DW, et al. *J Infect Dis.* 2008;197(6):836–845 PMID: 18279073
23. American Academy of Pediatrics. Cytomegalovirus infection. In: Pickering LK, et al, eds. *Red Book: 2012 Report of the Committee on Infectious Diseases.* 2012:300–305

24. Kimberlin DW, et al, for the NIAID Collaborative Antiviral Study Group (CASG). Six months versus six weeks of oral valganciclovir for infants with symptomatic congenital cytomegalovirus (CMV) disease with and without central nervous system (CNS) involvement: results of a Phase III, randomized, double-blind, placebo-controlled, multinational study. IDWeek 2013, San Francisco, CA, October 5, 2013; Late-Breaker Abstract #43178
25. American Academy of Pediatrics. Candidiasis. In: Pickering LK, et al, eds. *Red Book: 2012 Report of the Committee on Infectious Diseases.* 2012:265–269
26. Hundalani S, et al. *Expert Rev Anti Infect Ther*. 2013;11(7):709–721 PMID: 23829639
27. Saez-Llorens X, et al. *Antimicrob Agents Chemother.* 2009;53(3):869–875 PMID: 19075070
28. Benjamin DK Jr, et al. *JAMA*. 2014;311(17):1742–1749 PMID: 24794367
29. Smith PB, et al. *Pediatr Infect Dis J.* 2009;28(5):412–415 PMID: 19319022
30. Wurthwein G, et al. *Antimicrob Agents Chemother.* 2005;49(12):5092–5098 PMID: 16304177
31. Heresi GP, et al. *Pediatr Infect Dis J.* 2006;25(12):1110–1115 PMID: 17133155
32. Kawaguchi C, et al. *Pediatr Int.* 2009;51(2):220–224 PMID: 19405920
33. Hsieh E, et al. *Early Hum Dev*. 2012;88(S2):S6–S10 PMID: 22633516
34. Piper L, et al. *Pediatr Infect Dis J.* 2011;30(5):375–378 PMID: 21085048
35. Santos RP, et al. *Pediatr Infect Dis J.* 2007;26(4):364–366 PMID: 17414408
36. Frankenbusch K, et al. *J Perinatol.* 2006;26(8):511–514 PMID: 16871222
37. Thomas L, et al. *Expert Rev Anti Infect Ther.* 2009;7(4):461–472 PMID: 19400765
38. Shah D, et al. *Cochrane Database Syst Rev*. 2012;8:CD007448 PMID: 22895960
39. Brook I. *Am J Perinatol.* 2008;25(2):111–118 PMID: 18236362
40. Wang Q, et al. *J Pediatr Surg*. 2012;47(1):241–248 PMID: 22244424
41. Lin PW, et al. *Lancet.* 2006;368(9543):1271–1283 PMID: 17027734
42. Cohen-Wolkowiez M, et al. *Clin Infect Dis*. 2012;55(11):1495–1502 PMID: 22955430
43. Jost T, et al. *PLoS One*. 2012;7(8):e44595 PMID: 22957008
44. American Academy of Pediatrics. *Salmonella* infections. In: Pickering LK, et al, eds. *Red Book: 2012 Report of the Committee on Infectious Diseases.* 2012:635–640
45. Pinninti SG, et al. *Pediatr Clin North Am*. 2013;60(2):351–365 PMID: 23481105
46. American Academy of Pediatrics. Herpes simplex. In: Pickering LK, et al, eds. *Red Book: 2012 Report of the Committee on Infectious Diseases.* 2012:398–408
47. Jones CA, et al. *Cochrane Database Syst Rev.* 2009;(3):CD004206 PMID: 19588350
48. Kimberlin DW, et al. *N Engl J Med*. 2011;365(14):1284–1292 PMID: 21991950
49. Sampson MR, et al. *Pediatr Infect Dis J.* 2014;33(1):42–49 PMID: 24346595
50. Panel on Antiretroviral Therapy and Medical Management of HIV-Infected Children. Guidelines for the use of antiretroviral agents in pediatric HIV infection. http://aidsinfo.nih.gov/ContentFiles/PediatricGuidelines.pdf. Updated February 12, 2014. Accessed October 14, 2014
51. Panel on Treatment of HIV-Infected Pregnant Women and Prevention of Perinatal Transmission. Recommendations for use of antiretroviral drugs in pregnant HIV-1-infected women for maternal health and interventions to reduce perinatal HIV transmission in the United States. http://aidsinfo.nih.gov/guidelines/html/3/perinatal-guidelines/0/. Updated March 28, 2014. Accessed October 14, 2014
52. Nielsen-Saines K, et al. *N Engl J Med*. 2012;366(25):2368–2379 PMID: 22716975
53. American Academy of Academy Committee on Infectious Diseases. *Pediatrics.* 2013;132(4):e1089–e1104 PMID: 23999962
54. Acosta EP, et al. *J Infect Dis.* 2010;202(4):563–566 PMID: 20594104
55. Kimberlin DW, et al. *J Infect Dis*. 2013;207(5):709–720 PMID: 23230059
56. Fraser N, et al. *Acta Paediatr.* 2006;95(5):519–522 PMID: 16825129
57. Ulloa-Gutierrez R, et al. *Pediatr Emerg Care.* 2005;21(9):600–602 PMID: 16160666
58. Sawardekar KP. *Pediatr Infect Dis J.* 2004;23(1):22–26 PMID: 14743041
59. Bingol-Kologlu M, et al. *J Pediatr Surg.* 2007;42(11):1892–1897 PMID: 18022442
60. Brook I. *J Perinat Med.* 2002;30(3):197–208 PMID: 12122901
61. Kaplan SL. *Adv Exp Med Biol.* 2009;634:111–120 PMID: 19280853
62. Korakaki E, et al. *Jpn J Infect Dis.* 2007;60(2-3):129–131 PMID: 17515648
63. Dessi A, et al. *J Chemother.* 2008;20(5):542–550 PMID: 19028615

64. Berkun Y, et al. *Arch Dis Child.* 2008;93(8):690–694 PMID: 18337275
65. Greenberg D, et al. *Paediatr Drugs.* 2008;10(2):75–83 PMID: 18345717
66. Ismail EA, et al. *Pediatr Int.* 2013;55(1):60–64 PMID: 23039834
67. Engle WD, et al. *J Perinatol.* 2000;20(7):421–426 PMID: 11076325
68. Brook I. *Microbes Infect.* 2002;4(12):1271–1280 PMID: 12467770
69. Darville T. *Semin Pediatr Infect Dis.* 2005;16(4):235–244 PMID: 16210104
70. Waites KB, et al. *Semin Fetal Neonatal Med.* 2009;14(4):190–199 PMID: 19109084
71. Morrison W. *Pediatr Infect Dis J.* 2007;26(2):186–188 PMID: 17259889
72. American Academy of Pediatrics. Pertussis. In: Pickering LK, et al, eds. *Red Book: 2012 Report of the Committee on Infectious Diseases.* 2012:553–566
73. Foca MD. *Semin Perinatol.* 2002;26(5):332–339 PMID: 12452505
74. American Academy of Pediatrics Committee on Infectious Diseases and Bronchiolitis Guidelines Committee. *Pediatrics.* 2014;134(2):415–420 PMID: 25070315
75. Vergnano S, et al. *Pediatr Infect Dis J.* 2011;30(10):850–854 PMID: 21654546
76. Nelson MU, et al. *Semin Perinatol.* 2012;36(6):424–430 PMID: 23177801
77. Lyseng-Williamson KA, et al. *Paediatr Drugs.* 2003;5(6):419–431 PMID: 12765493
78. American Academy of Pediatrics. Group B streptococcal infections. In: Pickering LK, et al, eds. *Red Book: 2012 Report of the Committee on Infectious Diseases.* 2012:680–685
79. Schrag S, et al. *MMWR Recomm Rep.* 2002;51(RR-11):1–22 PMID: 12211284
80. American Academy of Pediatrics. *Ureaplasma urealyticum* infections. In: Pickering LK, et al, eds. *Red Book: 2012 Report of the Committee on Infectious Diseases.* 2012:772–774
81. American Academy of Pediatrics. *Escherichia coli* and other gram-negative bacilli. In: Pickering LK, et al, eds. *Red Book: 2012 Report of the Committee on Infectious Diseases.* 2012:321–324
82. Venkatesh MP, et al. *Expert Rev Anti Infect Ther.* 2008;6(6):929–938 PMID: 19053905
83. American Academy of Pediatrics. *Listeria monocytogenes* infections (listeriosis). In: Pickering LK, et al, eds. *Red Book: 2012 Report of the Committee on Infectious Diseases.* 2012:471–474
84. Fortunov RM, et al. *Pediatrics.* 2006;118(3):874–881 PMID: 16950976
85. Fortunov RM, et al. *Pediatrics.* 2007;120(5):937–945 PMID: 17974729
86. Stauffer WM, et al. *Pediatr Emerg Care.* 2003;19(3):165–166 PMID: 12813301
87. Dehority W, et al. *Pediatr Infect Dis J.* 2006;25(11):1080–1081 PMID: 17072137
88. American Academy of Pediatrics. Syphilis. In: Pickering LK, et al, eds. *Red Book: 2012 Report of the Committee on Infectious Diseases.* 2012:690–702
89. American Academy of Pediatrics. Tetanus. In: Pickering LK, et al, eds. *Red Book: 2012 Report of the Committee on Infectious Diseases.* 2012:707–712
90. American Academy of Pediatrics. *Toxoplasma gondii* infections. In: Pickering LK, et al, eds. *Red Book: 2012 Report of the Committee on Infectious Diseases.* 2012:720–728
91. Petersen E. Toxoplasmosis. *Semin Fetal Neonatal Med.* 2007;12(3):214–223 PMID: 17321812
92. Beetz R. *Curr Opin Pediatr.* 2012;24(2):205–211 PMID: 22227782
93. RIVUR Trial Investigators, et al. *N Engl J Med.* 2014;370(25):2367–2376 PMID: 24795142
94. Roberts SW, et al. Placental transmission of antibiotics. In: *Glob Libr Women's Med.* DOI 10.3843/GLOWM.10174
95. Nanovskaya TN, et al. *J Matern Fetal Neonatal Med.* 2012;25(11):2312–2315 PMID: 22590979
96. Nanovskaya T, et al. *Am J Obstet Gynecol.* 2012;207(4):331.e1–331.e6 PMID: 22867688
97. Sachs HC, et al. *Pediatrics.* 2013;132(3):e796–e809 PMID: 23979084
98. Hale TW. *Medication and Mothers' Milk: A Manual of Lactational Pharmacology.* 15th ed. 2012

Chapter 6

1. Stevens DL, et al. *Clin Infect Dis.* 2014;59(2):147–159 PMID: 24947530
2. Liu C, et al. *Clin Infect Dis.* 2011;52(3):e18–e55 PMID: 21208910
3. Elliott DJ, et al. *Pediatrics.* 2009;123(6):e959–e966 PMID: 19470525
4. Inman JC, et al. *Laryngoscope.* 2008;118(12):2111–2114 PMID: 18948832
5. Martinez-Aguilar G, et al. *Pediatr Infect Dis J.* 2003;22(7):593–598 PMID: 12867833

6. American Academy of Pediatrics. Staphylococcal infections. In: Pickering LK, et al, eds. *Red Book: 2012 Report of the Committee on Infectious Diseases.* 2012:653–668
7. American Academy of Pediatrics. Group A streptococcal infections. In: Pickering LK, et al, eds. *Red Book: 2012 Report of the Committee on Infectious Diseases.* 2012:668–675
8. Bass JW, et al. *Pediatr Infect Dis J.* 1998;17(6):447–452 PMID: 9655532
9. Timmerman MK, et al. *Clin Otolaryngol.* 2008;33(6):546–552 PMID: 19126128
10. Lindeboom JA. *J Oral Maxillofac Surg.* 2012;70(2):345–348 PMID: 21741739
11. Griffith DE, et al. *Am J Respir Crit Care Med.* 2007;175(4):367–416 PMID: 17277290
12. Lindeboom JA. *Clin Infect Dis.* 2011;52(2):180–184 PMID: 21288841
13. American Thoracic Society, et al. *MMWR Recomm Rep.* 2003;52(RR-11):1–77 PMID: 12836625
14. American Academy of Pediatrics. Tuberculosis. In: Pickering LK, et al, eds. *Red Book: 2012 Report of the Committee on Infectious Diseases.* 2012:736–759
15. Bradley JS, et al. *Pediatrics.* 2014;133(5):e1411–e1436 PMID: 24777226
16. Talan DA, et al. *Clin Infect Dis.* 2003;37(11):1481–1489 PMID: 14614671
17. Oehler RL, et al. *Lancet Infect Dis.* 2009;9(7):439–447 PMID: 19555903
18. Thomas N, et al. *Expert Rev Anti Infect Ther.* 2011;9(2):215–226 PMID: 21342069
19. Lion C, et al. *Int J Antimicrob Agents.* 2006;27(4):290–293 PMID: 16564680
20. American Academy of Pediatrics. Rabies. In: Pickering LK, et al, eds. *Red Book: 2012 Report of the Committee on Infectious Diseases.* 2012:600–607
21. Hyun DY, et al. *Pediatr Infect Dis J.* 2009;28(1):57–59 PMID: 19057459
22. American Academy of Pediatrics. *Haemophilus influenzae* infections. In: Pickering LK, et al, eds. *Red Book: 2012 Report of the Committee on Infectious Diseases.* 2012:345–352
23. Yang LP, et al. *Am J Clin Dermatol.* 2008;9(6):411–413 PMID: 18973410
24. Bass JW, et al. *Pediatr Infect Dis J.* 1997;16(7):708–710 PMID: 9239775
25. Lin HW, et al. *Clin Pediatr (Phila).* 2009;48(6):583–587 PMID: 19286617
26. Pannaraj PS, et al. *Clin Infect Dis.* 2006;43(8):953–960 PMID: 16983604
27. Smith-Slatas CL, et al. *Pediatrics.* 2006;117(4):e796–e805 PMID: 16567392
28. Jamal N, et al. *Pediatr Emerg Care.* 2011;27(12):1195–1199 PMID: 22158285
29. Stevens DL. *Annu Rev Med.* 2000;51:271–288 PMID: 10774464
30. Abuhammour W, et al. *Pediatr Emerg Care.* 2006;22(1):48–51 PMID: 16418613
31. Daum RS. *N Engl J Med.* 2007;357(4):380–390 PMID: 17652653
32. Lee MC, et al. *Pediatr Infect Dis J.* 2004;23(2):123–127 PMID: 14872177
33. Karamatsu ML, et al. *Pediatr Emerg Care.* 2012;28(2):131–135 PMID: 22270497
34. Elliott SP. *Clin Microbiol Rev.* 2007;20(1):13–22 PMID: 17223620
35. Berk DR, et al. *Pediatr Ann.* 2010;39(10):627–633 PMID: 20954609
36. Kaplan SL. *Adv Exp Med Biol.* 2009;634:111–120 PMID: 19280853
37. Peltola H, et al. *Clin Infect Dis.* 2009;48(9):1201–1210 PMID: 19323633
38. Bradley JS. *Clin Infect Dis.* 2009;48(9):1211–1212 PMID: 19323629
39. Saphyakhajon P, et al. *Pediatr Infect Dis J.* 2008;27(8):765–767 PMID: 18600193
40. Faust SN, et al. *Arch Dis Child.* 2012;97(6):545–553 PMID: 22440930
41. Arnold JC, et al. *Pediatrics.* 2012;130(4):e821–e828 PMID: 22966033
42. Workowski KA, et al. *MMWR Recomm Rep.* 2010;59(RR-12):1–110 PMID: 21160459
43. American Academy of Pediatrics. Gonococcal infections. In: Pickering LK, et al, eds. *Red Book: 2012 Report of the Committee on Infectious Diseases.* 2012:336–344
44. Saavedra-Lozano J, et al. *J Pediatr Orthop.* 2008;28(5):569–575 PMID: 18580375
45. Martinez-Aguilar G, et al. *Pediatr Infect Dis J.* 2004;23(8):701–706 PMID: 15295218
46. Messina AF, et al. *Pediatr Infect Dis J.* 2011;30(12):1019–1021 PMID: 21817950
47. Howard-Jones AR, et al. *J Paediatr Child Health.* 2013;49(9):760–768 PMID: 23745943
48. Pääkkönen M, et al. *N Engl J Med.* 2014;370(14):1365–1366 PMID: 24693913
49. Ceroni D, et al. *J Pediatr Orthop.* 2010;30(3):301–304 PMID: 20357599
50. Chen CJ, et al. *Pediatr Infect Dis J.* 2007;26(11):985–988 PMID: 17984803
51. Chachad S, et al. *Clin Pediatr (Phila).* 2004;43(3):213–216 PMID: 15094944
52. Bradley JS, et al. *Pediatrics.* 2011;128(4):e1034–e1045 PMID: 21949152
53. Vaska VL, et al. *Pediatr Infect Dis J.* 2011;30(11):1003–1006 PMID: 21681121

54. Seltz LB, et al. *Pediatrics.* 2011;127(3):e566–e572 PMID: 21321025
55. Peña MT, et al. *JAMA Otolaryngol Head Neck Surg.* 2013;139(3):223–227 PMID: 23429877
56. Bedwell J, et al. *Curr Opin Otolaryngol Head Neck Surg.* 2011;19(6):467–473 PMID: 22001661
57. Wald ER. *Pediatr Rev.* 2004;25(9):312–320 PMID: 15342822
58. Sheikh A, et al. *Cochrane Database Syst Rev.* 2012;9:CD001211 PMID: 22972049
59. Williams L, et al. *J Pediatr.* 2013;162(4):857–861 PMID: 23092529
60. Pichichero ME. *Clin Pediatr (Phila).* 2011;50(1):7–13 PMID: 20724317
61. Wilhelmus KR. *Cochrane Database Syst Rev.* 2010;(12):CD002898 PMID: 21154352
62. Liu S, et al. *Ophthalmology.* 2012;119(10):2003–2008 PMID: 22796308
63. Young RC, et al. *Arch Ophthalmol.* 2010;128(9):1178–1183 PMID: 20837803
64. Thordsen JE, et al. *Retina.* 2008;28(3suppl):S3–S7 PMID: 18317341
65. Soheilian M, et al. *Arch Ophthalmol.* 2007;125(4):460–465 PMID: 17420365
66. Riddell J 4th, et al. *Clin Infect Dis.* 2011;52(5):648–653 PMID: 21239843
67. Kedhar SR, et al. *Herpes.* 2007;14(3):66–71 PMID: 18371289
68. Nassetta L, et al. *J Antimicrob Chemother.* 2009;63(5):862–867 PMID: 19287011
69. Kimberlin DW, et al. *J Pediatr.* 2003;143(1):16–25 PMID: 12915819
70. Rosenfeld RM, et al. *Otolaryngol Head Neck Surg.* 2014;150(1Suppl):S1–S24 PMID: 24491310
71. Dohar JE. *Pediatr Infect Dis J.* 2003;22(4):299–308 PMID: 12690268
72. Carfrae MJ, et al. *Otolaryngol Clin North Am.* 2008;41(3):537–549 PMID: 18435997
73. Kaushik V, et al. *Cochrane Database Syst Rev.* 2010;(1):CD004740 PMID: 20091565
74. Hoberman A, et al. *N Engl J Med.* 2011;364(2):105–115 PMID: 21226576
75. Tähtinen PA, et al. *N Engl J Med.* 2011;364(2):116–126 PMID: 21226577
76. Lieberthal AS, et al. *Pediatrics.* 2013;131(3):e964–e999 PMID: 23439909
77. Rovers MM, et al. *Lancet.* 2006;368(9545):1429–1435 PMID: 17055944
78. Leach AJ, et al. *Cochrane Database Syst Rev.* 2006;(4):CD004401 PMID: 17054203
79. Hoberman A, et al. *Clin Pediatr (Phila).* 2011;50(2):114–120 PMID: 21098526
80. Pichichero ME. *Pediatr Clin North Am.* 2013;60(2):391–407 PMID: 23481107
81. Macfadyen CA, et al. *Cochrane Database Syst Rev.* 2006;(1):CD005608 PMID: 16437533
82. Marchisio P, et al. *Otolaryngol Head Neck Surg.* 2013;148(4Suppl):e102–e121 PMID: 23536528
83. Haynes DS, et al. *Otolaryngol Clin North Am.* 2007;40(3):669–683 PMID: 17544701
84. Groth A, et al. *Int J Pediatr Otorhinolaryngol.* 2012;76(10):1494–1500 PMID: 22832239
85. Stahelin-Massik J, et al. *Eur J Pediatr.* 2008;167(5):541–548 PMID: 17668240
86. Ongkasuwan J, et al. *Pediatrics.* 2008;122(1):34–39 PMID: 18595984
87. Wald ER, et al. *Pediatrics.* 2009;124(1):9–15 PMID: 19564277
88. Wald ER, et al. *Pediatrics.* 2013;132(1):e262–e280 PMID: 23796742
89. Whitby CR, et al. *Int J Pediatr Otorhinolaryngol.* 2011;75(1):118–121 PMID: 21074863
90. Chow AW, et al. *Clin Infect Dis.* 2012;54(8):e72–e112 PMID: 22438350
91. Ellison SJ. *Br Dent J.* 2009;206(7):357–362 PMID: 19357666
92. Siqueira JF Jr, et al. *Clin Microbiol Rev.* 2013;26(2):255–273 PMID: 23554416
93. American Academy of Pediatrics. Diphtheria. In: Pickering LK, et al, eds. *Red Book: 2012 Report of the Committee on Infectious Diseases.* 2012:307–311
94. Wheeler DS, et al. *Pediatr Emerg Care.* 2008;24(1):46–49 PMID: 18212612
95. Sobol SE, et al. *Otolaryngol Clin North Am.* 2008;41(3):551–566 PMID: 18435998
96. Nasser M, et al. *Cochrane Database Syst Rev.* 2008;(4):CD006700 PMID: 18843726
97. Amir J, et al. *BMJ.* 1997;314(7097):1800–1803 PMID: 9224082
98. Kimberlin DW, et al. *Clin Infect Dis.* 2010;50(2):221–228 PMID: 20014952
99. Riordan T. *Clin Microbiol Rev.* 2007;20(4):622–659 PMID: 17934077
100. Kizhner V, et al. *J Laryngol Otol.* 2013;127(7):721–723 PMID: 23701713
101. Baldassari CM, et al. *Otolaryngol Head Neck Surg.* 2011;144(4):592–595 PMID: 21493241
102. Shulman ST, et al. *Clin Infect Dis.* 2012;55(10):e86–e102 PMID: 22965026
103. Lennon DR, et al. *Arch Dis Child.* 2008;93(6):474–478 PMID: 18337284
104. Spinks A, et al. *Cochrane Database Syst Rev.* 2013;11:CD000023 PMID: 24190439
105. Casey JR, et al. *Diagn Microbiol Infect Dis.* 2007;57(3Suppl):39S–45S PMID: 17292576
106. Altamimi S, et al. *Cochrane Database Syst Rev.* 2012;8:CD004872 PMID: 22895944

107. Abdel-Haq N, et al. *Pediatr Infect Dis J.* 2012;31(7):696–699 PMID: 22481424
108. Cheng J, et al. *Otolaryngol Head Neck Surg.* 2013;148(6):1037–1042 PMID: 23520072
109. Hopkins A, et al. *Pediatrics.* 2006;118(4):1418–1421 PMID: 17015531
110. Tebruegge M, et al. *Scand J Infect Dis.* 2009;41(8):548–557 PMID: 19401934
111. Lemaître C, et al. *Pediatr Infect Dis J.* 2013;32(10):1146–1149 PMID: 23722529
112. Bender JM, et al. *Clin Infect Dis.* 2008;46(9):1346–1352 PMID: 18419434
113. Brook I. *Adv Exp Med Biol.* 2011;697:117–152 PMID: 21120724
114. Agarwal R, et al. *Clin Exp Allergy.* 2013;43(8):850–873 PMID: 23889240
115. Schuh S. *Curr Opin Pediatr.* 2011;23(1):110–114 PMID: 21157348
116. Mogayzel PJ Jr, et al. *Am J Respir Crit Care Med.* 2013;187(7):680–689 PMID: 23540878
117. Plummer A, et al. *Cochrane Database Syst Rev.* 2013;5:CD006682 PMID: 23728662
118. Bhatt JM. *Eur Respir Rev.* 2013;22(129):205–216 PMID: 23997047
119. Mayer-Hamblett N, et al. *Pediatr Pulmonol.* 2013;48(10):943–953 PMID: 23818295
120. Blumer JL, et al. *Chest.* 2005;128(4):2336–2346 PMID: 16236892
121. Ryan G, et al. *Cochrane Database Syst Rev.* 2012;12:CD008319 PMID: 23235659
122. Saiman L. *Paediatr Respir Rev.* 2007;8(3):249–255 PMID: 17868923
123. Waters V, et al. *Cochrane Database Syst Rev.* 2008;(3):CD006961 PMID: 18646176
124. Cheer SM, et al. *Drugs.* 2003;63(22):2501–2520 PMID: 14609360
125. Hutchinson D, et al. *Expert Opin Pharmacother.* 2013;14(15):2115–2124 PMID: 23992352
126. Döring G, et al. *J Cyst Fibros.* 2012;11(6):461–479 PMID: 23137712
127. Southern KW, et al. *Cochrane Database Syst Rev.* 2012;11:CD002203 PMID: 23152214
128. Moskowitz SM, et al. *Pediatr Pulmonol.* 2008;43(9):874–881 PMID: 18668689
129. American Academy of Pediatrics. Pertussis. In: Pickering LK, et al, eds. *Red Book: 2012 Report of the Committee on Infectious Diseases.* 2012:553–566
130. Altunaiji S, et al. *Cochrane Database Syst Rev.* 2007;(3):CD004404 PMID: 17636756
131. Pavia AT. *Clin Infect Dis.* 2011;52(S4):S284–S289 PMID: 21460286
132. Bradley JS, et al. *Clin Infect Dis.* 2011;53(7):e25–e76 PMID: 21880587
133. Esposito S, et al. *Pediatr Infect Dis J.* 2012;31(6):e78–e85 PMID: 22466326
134. Queen MA, et al. *Pediatrics.* 2014;133(1):e23–e29 PMID: 24324001
135. Ambroggio L, et al. *J Pediatr.* 2012;161(6):1097–1103 PMID: 22901738
136. Bradley JS, et al. *Pediatr Infect Dis J.* 2007;26(10):868–878 PMID: 17901791
137. Hidron AI, et al. *Lancet Infect Dis.* 2009;9(6):384–392 PMID: 19467478
138. Wunderink RG, et al. *Clin Infect Dis.* 2012;54(5):621–629 PMID: 22247123
139. St Peter SD, et al. *J Pediatr Surg.* 2009;44(1):106–111 PMID: 19159726
140. Islam S, et al. *J Pediatr Surg.* 2012;47(11):2101–2110 PMID: 23164006
141. Aziz A, et al. *Surg Infect (Larchmt).* 2008;9(3):317–323 PMID: 18570573
142. Sonnappa S, et al. *Am J Respir Crit Care Med.* 2006;174(2):221–227 PMID: 16675783
143. Freifeld AG, et al. *Clin Infect Dis.* 2011;52(4):e56–e93 PMID: 21258094
144. American Thoracic Society, et al. *Am J Respir Crit Care Med.* 2005;171(4):388–416 PMID: 15699079
145. Foglia E, et al. *Clin Microbiol Rev.* 2007;20(3):409–425 PMID: 17630332
146. Srinivasan R, et al. *Pediatrics.* 2009;123(4):1108–1115 PMID: 19336369
147. Boselli E, et al. *Intensive Care Med.* 2007;33(9):1519–1523 PMID: 17530217
148. Kollef MH, et al. *Curr Opin Infect Dis.* 2013;26(6):538–544 PMID: 24126716
149. American Academy of Pediatrics. Chlamydial infections. In: Pickering LK, et al, eds. *Red Book: 2012 Report of the Committee on Infectious Diseases.* 2012:272–281
150. American Academy of Pediatrics. Cytomegalovirus infection. In: Pickering LK, et al, eds. *Red Book: 2012 Report of the Committee on Infectious Diseases.* 2012:300–305
151. Kotton CN, et al. *Transplantation.* 2013;96(4):333–360 PMID: 23896556
152. American Academy of Pediatrics. Tularemia. In: Pickering LK, et al, eds. *Red Book: 2012 Report of the Committee on Infectious Diseases.* 2012:768–769
153. Levy ER, et al. *Clin Infect Dis.* 2013;56(11):1573–1578 PMID: 23463636
154. American Academy of Pediatrics. Coccidioidomycosis. In: Pickering LK, et al, eds. *Red Book: 2012 Report of the Committee on Infectious Diseases.* 2012:289–291

155. American Academy of Pediatrics. Histoplasmosis. In: Pickering LK, et al, eds. *Red Book: 2012 Report of the Committee on Infectious Diseases.* 2012:409–411
156. Wheat LJ, et al. *Clin Infect Dis.* 2007;45(7):807–825 PMID: 17806045
157. American Academy of Pediatrics Committee on Infectious Diseases. *Pediatrics.* 2007;119(4):852–860 PMID: 17403862
158. American Academy of Academy Committee on Infectious Diseases. *Pediatrics.* 2013;132(4):e1089–e1104 PMID: 23999962
159. Kimberlin DW, et al. *J Infect Dis.* 2013;207(5):709–720 PMID: 23230059
160. Yang K, et al. *Ann Pharmacother.* 2007;41(9):1427–1435 PMID: 17666573
161. Badal RE, et al. *Pediatr Infect Dis J.* 2013;32(6):636–640 PMID: 23838732
162. Mulholland S, et al. *Cochrane Database Syst Rev.* 2012;9:CD004875 PMID: 22972079
163. Cardinale F, et al. *J Clin Microbiol.* 2013;51(2):723–724 PMID: 23224091
164. Mofenson LM, et al. *MMWR Recomm Rep.* 2009;58(RR-11):1–166 PMID: 19730409
165. Caselli D, et al. *J Pediatr.* 2014;164(2):389.e1–392.e1 PMID: 24252793
166. Michalopoulos A, et al. *Crit Care Clin.* 2008;24(2):377–391 PMID: 18361952
167. Micek ST, et al. *Medicine (Baltimore).* 2011;90(6):390–395 PMID: 22033455
168. American Academy of Pediatrics. Respiratory syncytial virus. In: Pickering LK, et al, eds. *Red Book: 2012 Report of the Committee on Infectious Diseases.* 2012:609–619
169. Centers for Disease Control and Prevention. *MMWR Morb Mortal Wkly Rep.* 2011;60(48):1650–1653 PMID: 22157884
170. Meehan WP III, et al. *Pediatr Emerg Care.* 2010;26(12):875–880 PMID: 21088637
171. Biondi E, et al. *Pediatrics.* 2013;132(6):990–996 PMID: 24218461
172. Byington CL, et al. *Pediatrics.* 2003;111(5pt1):964–968 PMID: 12728072
173. Lee GM, et al. *Pediatrics.* 2001;108(4):835–844 PMID: 11581433
174. Ishimine P. *Emerg Med Clin North Am.* 2013;31(3):601–626 PMID: 23915596
175. Joffe MD, et al. *Pediatr Emerg Care.* 2010;26(6):448–457 PMID: 20531134
176. Hakim H, et al. *Am J Infect Control.* 2007;35(2):102–105 PMID: 17327189
177. Luthander J, et al. *Acta Paediatr.* 2013;102(2):182–186 PMID: 23121094
178. Russell CD, et al. *J Med Microbiol.* 2014;63(Pt6):841–848 PMID: 24623637
179. Carrillo-Marquez MA, et al. *Pediatr Infect Dis J.* 2010;29(5):410–414 PMID: 20431380
180. Baddour LM, et al. *Circulation.* 2005;111(23):e394–e434 PMID: 15956145
181. Johnson JA, et al. *Mayo Clin Proc.* 2012;87(7):629–635 PMID: 22766082
182. Russell HM, et al. *Ann Thorac Surg.* 2013;96(1):171–174 PMID: 23602067
183. Wilson W, et al. *Circulation.* 2007;116(15):1736–1754 PMID: 17446442
184. Silberbach M. *Pediatr Rev.* 2008;29(5):169–170 PMID: 18450838
185. Ridgway JM, et al. *Am J Otolaryngol.* 2010;31(1):38–45 PMID: 19944898
186. Goldenberg NA, et al. *Pediatrics.* 2005;116(4):e543–e548 PMID: 16147971
187. Parikh SV, et al. *Medicine (Baltimore).* 2009;88(1):52–65 PMID: 19352300
188. Demmler GJ. *Pediatr Infect Dis J.* 2006;25(2):165–166 PMID: 16462296
189. Denno DM, et al. *Clin Infect Dis.* 2012;55(7):897–904 PMID: 22700832
190. Pfeiffer ML, et al. *J Infect.* 2012;64(4):374–386 PMID: 22266388
191. Goldwater PN. *Expert Rev Anti Infect Ther.* 2007;5(4):653–663 PMID: 17678428
192. Bennish ML, et al. *Clin Infect Dis.* 2006;42(3):356–362 PMID: 16392080
193. Smith KE, et al. *Pediatr Infect Dis J.* 2012;31(1):37–41 PMID: 21892124
194. Tribble DR, et al. *Clin Infect Dis.* 2007;44(3):338–346 PMID: 17205438
195. Ang JY, et al. *Pediatr Ann.* 2008;37(12):814–820 PMID: 19143332
196. Paredes-Paredes M, et al. *Curr Gastroenterol Rep.* 2011;13(5):402–407 PMID: 21773708
197. DuPont HL. *Clin Infect Dis.* 2007;44(3):347–349 PMID: 17205439
198. DuPont HL, et al. *J Travel Med.* 2009;16(3):149–160 PMID: 19538575
199. Ouyang-Latimer J, et al. *Antimicrob Agents Chemother.* 2011;55(2):874–878 PMID: 21115800
200. O'Ryan M, et al. *Expert Rev Anti Infect Ther.* 2010;8(6):671–682 PMID: 20521895
201. Koo HL, et al. *Curr Opin Gastroenterol.* 2010;26(1):17–25 PMID: 19881343
202. Riddle MS, et al. *Clin Infect Dis.* 2008;47(8):1007–1014 PMID: 18781873
203. Butler T. *Clin Infect Dis.* 2008;47(8):1015–1016 PMID: 18781871

204. Janda JM, et al. *Clin Microbiol Rev.* 2010;23(1):35–73 PMID: 20065325
205. American Academy of Pediatrics. *Campylobacter* infections. In: Pickering LK, et al, eds. *Red Book: 2012 Report of the Committee on Infectious Diseases.* 2012:262–264
206. Fullerton KE, et al. *Pediatr Infect Dis J.* 2007;26(1):19–24 PMID: 17195700
207. Kirkpatrick BD, et al. *Curr Opin Gastroenterol.* 2011;27(1):1–7 PMID: 21124212
208. Leibovici-Weissman Y, et al. *Cochrane Database Syst Rev.* 2014;6:CD008625 PMID: 24944120
209. Pant C, et al. *Curr Med Res Opin.* 2013;29(8):967–984 PMID: 23659563
210. American Academy of Pediatrics. *Clostridium difficile.* In: Pickering LK, et al, eds. *Red Book: 2012 Report of the Committee on Infectious Diseases.* 2012:285–287
211. Kelly CP, et al. *N Engl J Med.* 2008;359(18):1932–1940 PMID: 18971494
212. Hill DR, et al. *Curr Opin Infect Dis.* 2010;23(5):481–487 PMID: 20683261
213. Rimbara E, et al. *Nat Rev Gastroenterol Hepatol.* 2011;8(2):79–88 PMID: 21293508
214. McColl KE. *N Engl J Med.* 2010;362(17):1597–1604 PMID: 20427808
215. Bontems P, et al. *J Pediatr Gastroenterol Nutr.* 2011;53(6):646–650 PMID: 21701406
216. American Academy of Pediatrics. *Helicobacter pylori* infections. In: Pickering LK, et al, eds. *Red Book: 2012 Report of the Committee on Infectious Diseases.* 2012:354–356
217. Haeusler GM, et al. *Adv Exp Med Biol.* 2013;764:13–26 PMID: 23654054
218. Onwuezobe IA, et al. *Cochrane Database Syst Rev.* 2012;11:CD001167 PMID: 23152205
219. Trivedi NA, et al. *J Postgrad Med.* 2012;58(2):112–118 PMID: 22718054
220. Frenck RW Jr, et al. *Clin Infect Dis.* 2004;38(7):951–957 PMID: 15034826
221. Effa EE, et al. *Cochrane Database Syst Rev.* 2008;(4):CD006083 PMID: 18843701
222. Effa EE, et al. *Cochrane Database Syst Rev.* 2011;(10):CD004530 PMID: 21975746
223. Shiferaw B, et al. *Clin Infect Dis.* 2012;54(Suppl5):S458–S463 PMID: 22572670
224. Basualdo W, et al. *Pediatr Infect Dis J.* 2003;22(4):374–377 PMID: 12712971
225. American Academy of Pediatrics. *Shigella* infections. In: Pickering LK, et al, eds. *Red Book: 2012 Report of the Committee on Infectious Diseases.* 2012:645–647
226. Abdel-Haq NM, et al. *Pediatr Infect Dis J.* 2000;19(10):954–958 PMID: 11055595
227. Abdel-Haq NM, et al. *Int J Antimicrob Agents.* 2006;27(5):449–452 PMID: 16621458
228. Fallon SC, et al. *J Surg Res.* 2013;185(1):273–277 PMID: 23835072
229. Lee SL, et al. *J Pediatr Surg.* 2010;45(11):2181–2185 PMID: 21034941
230. Chen CY, et al. *Surg Infect (Larchmt).* 2012;13(6):383–390 PMID: 23231389
231. Solomkin JS, et al. *Clin Infect Dis.* 2010;50(2):133–164 PMID: 20034345
232. Bradley JS, et al. *Pediatr Infect Dis J.* 2001;20(1):19–24 PMID: 11176562
233. Fraser JD, et al. *J Pediatr Surg.* 2010;45(6):1198–1202 PMID: 20620320
234. Cruz AT, et al. *Int J Tuberc Lung Dis.* 2013;17(2):169–74 PMID: 23317951
235. Hlavsa MC, et al. *Clin Infect Dis.* 2008;47(2):168–175 PMID: 18532886
236. Brook I, et al. *Pediatrics.* 1980;66(2):282–284 PMID: 7402814
237. Chadha V, et al. *Pediatr Nephrol.* 2010;25(3):425–440 PMID: 19190935
238. Warady BA, et al. *Perit Dial Int.* 2012;32(Suppl2):S32–S86 PMID: 22851742
239. Preece ER, et al. *ANZ J Surg.* 2012;82(4):283–284 PMID: 22510192
240. Workowski K. *Ann Intern Med.* 2013;158(3):ITC2-1 PMID: 23381058
241. Santillanes G, et al. *Pediatr Emerg Care.* 2011;27(3):174–178 PMID: 21346680
242. Klin B, et al. *Isr Med Assoc J.* 2001;3(11):833–835 PMID: 11729579
243. Smith JC, et al. *Adv Exp Med Biol.* 2013;764:219–239 PMID: 23654071
244. Centers for Disease Control and Prevention. *MMWR Morb Mortal Wkly Rep.* 2012;61(31):590–594 PMID: 22874837
245. Centers for Disease Control and Prevention. *MMWR Morb Mortal Wkly Rep.* 2007;56(14):332–336 PMID: 17431378
246. James SH, et al. *Clin Pharmacol Ther.* 2010;88(5):720–724 PMID: 20881952
247. Fife KH, et al. *Sex Transm Dis.* 2008;35(7):668–673 PMID: 18461016
248. Mitchell C, et al. *Infect Dis Clin North Am.* 2013;27(4):793–809 PMID: 24275271
249. Cohen SE, et al. *Infect Dis Clin North Am.* 2013;27(4):705–722 PMID: 24275265
250. O'Brien G. *Pediatr Rev.* 2008;29(6):209–211 PMID: 18515339
251. das Neves J, et al. *Drugs.* 2008;68(13):1787–1802 PMID: 18729533

252. Bumbulienė Ž, et al. *Postgrad Med J.* 2014;90(1059):8–12 PMID: 24191064
253. Jasper JM, et al. *Pediatr Emerg Care.* 2006;22(8):585–586 PMID: 16912629
254. Hansen MT, et al. *J Pediatr Adolesc Gynecol.* 2007;20(5):315–317 PMID: 1786890
255. Yogev R, et al. *Pediatr Infect Dis J.* 2004;23(2):157–159 PMID: 14872183
256. Frazier JL, et al. *Neurosurg Focus.* 2008;24(6):e8 PMID: 18518753
257. Tunkel AR, et al. *Clin Infect Dis.* 2008;47(3):303–327 PMID: 18582201
258. Long SS. *Adv Exp Med Biol.* 2011;697:153–173 PMID: 21120725
259. Kotton CN, et al. *Transplantation.* 2010;89(7):779–795 PMID: 20224515
260. Doja A, et al. *J Child Neurol.* 2006;21(5):384–391 PMID: 16901443
261. Whitley RJ. *Adv Exp Med Biol.* 2008;609:216–232 PMID: 18193668
262. Brouwer MC, et al. *Cochrane Database Syst Rev.* 2013;6:CD004405 PMID: 23733364
263. Fritz D, et al. *Neurology.* 2012;79(22):2177–2179 PMID: 23152589
264. Peltola H, et al. *Clin Infect Dis.* 2007;45(10):1277–1286 PMID: 17968821
265. Molyneux EM, et al. *Pediatr Infect Dis J.* 2014;33(2):214–216 PMID: 24136368
266. Tunkel AR, et al. *Clin Infect Dis.* 2004;39(9):1267–1284 PMID: 15494903
267. Prasad K, et al. *Cochrane Database Syst Rev.* 2008;(1):CD002244 PMID: 18254003
268. Kandasamy J, et al. *Childs Nerv Syst.* 2011;27(4):575–581 PMID: 20953871
269. Al-Dabbagh M, et al. *Adv Exp Med Biol.* 2011;719:105–115 PMID: 22125038
270. National Institute for Health and Care Excellence. Urinary tract infection in children: diagnosis, treatment and long-term management. http://www.nice.org.uk/guidance/CG54. Reviewed October 2013. Accessed October 14, 2014
271. Montini G, et al. *N Engl J Med.* 2011;365(3):239–250 PMID: 21774712
272. Yang CC, et al. *J Microbiol Immunol Infect.* 2010;43(3):207–214 PMID: 21291848
273. Cheng CH, et al. *Pediatr Infect Dis J.* 2010;29(7):624–628 PMID: 20234330
274. Hodson EM, et al. *Cochrane Database Syst Rev.* 2007;(4):CD003772 PMID: 17943796
275. Bocquet N, et al. *Pediatrics.* 2012;129(2):e269–e275 PMID: 22291112
276. American Academy of Pediatrics Subcommittee on Urinary Tract Infection, Steering Committee on Quality Improvement and Management. *Pediatrics.* 2011;128(3):595–610 PMID: 21873693
277. Craig JC, et al. *N Engl J Med.* 2009;361(18):1748–1759 PMID: 19864673
278. Williams GJ, et al. *Adv Exp Med Biol.* 2013;764:211–218 PMID: 23654070
279. RIVUR Trial Investigators, et al. *N Engl J Med.* 2014;370(25):2367–2376 PMID: 24795142
280. American Academy of Pediatrics. Actinomycosis. In: Pickering LK, et al, eds. *Red Book: 2012 Report of the Committee on Infectious Diseases.* 2012:219–220
281. Brook I. *South Med J.* 2008;101(10):1019–1023 PMID: 18791528
282. Thomas RJ, et al. *Expert Rev Anti Infect Ther.* 2009;7(6):709–722 PMID: 19681699
283. Bradley JS, et al. *Pediatrics.* 2014;133(5):e1411–e1436 PMID: 24777226
284. American Academy of Pediatrics. Brucellosis. In: Pickering LK, et al, eds. *Red Book: 2012 Report of the Committee on Infectious Diseases.* 2012:256–258
285. Shen MW. *Pediatrics.* 2008;121(5):e1178–e1183 PMID: 18450861
286. Mile B, et al. *Trop Doct.* 2012:42(1):13–17 PMID: 22290107
287. Franco MP, et al. *Lancet Infect Dis.* 2007;7(12):775–786 PMID: 18045560
288. Florin TA, et al. *Pediatrics.* 2008;121(5):e1413–e1425 PMID: 18443019
289. Massei F, et al. *Infect Dis Clin North Am.* 2005;19(3):691–711 PMID: 16102656
290. Klassen TP, et al. *Cochrane Database Syst Rev.* 2005;(4):CD002980 PMID: 16235308
291. Kimberlin DW, et al. *Clin Infect Dis.* 2010;50(2):221–228 PMID: 20014952
292. Saez-Llorens X, et al. *Antimicrob Agents Chemother.* 2009;53(5):1912–1920 PMID: 19273678
293. Ismail N, et al. *Clin Lab Med.* 2010;30(1):261–292 PMID: 20513551
294. Schutze GE, et al. *Pediatr Infect Dis J.* 2007;26(6):475–479 PMID: 17529862
295. Wormser GP, et al. *Clin Infect Dis.* 2006;43(9):1089–1134 PMID: 17029130
296. Thomas RJ, et al. *Expert Rev Anti Infect Ther.* 2009;7(6):709–722 PMID: 19681699
297. Freifeld AG, et al. *Clin Infect Dis.* 2011;52(4):e56–e93 PMID: 21258094
298. Arnon SS. *Pediatrics.* 2007;119(4):785–789 PMID: 17403850
299. Newburger JW, et al. *Circulation.* 2004;110(17):2747–2771 PMID: 15505111
300. Newburger JW, et al. *N Engl J Med.* 2007;356(7):663–675 PMID: 17301297

301. Kobayashi T, et al. *Lancet.* 2012;379(9826):1613–1620 PMID: 22405251
302. Son MB, et al. *J Pediatr.* 2011;158(4):644–649 PMID: 21129756
303. Son MB, et al. *Pediatr Rev.* 2013;34(4):151–162 PMID: 23547061
304. American Academy of Pediatrics. Leprosy. In: Pickering LK, et al, eds. *Red Book: 2012 Report of the Committee on Infectious Diseases.* 2012:466–469
305. Griffith ME, et al. *Curr Opin Infect Dis.* 2006;19(6):533–537 PMID: 17075327
306. American Academy of Pediatrics. Leptospirosis. In: Pickering LK, et al, eds. *Red Book: 2012 Report of the Committee on Infectious Diseases.* 2012:469–471
307. American Academy of Pediatrics. Lyme disease. In: Pickering LK, et al, eds. *Red Book: 2012 Report of the Committee on Infectious Diseases.* 2012:474–479
308. Wiersinga WJ, et al. *N Engl J Med.* 2012;367(11):1035–1044 PMID: 22970946
309. Cheng AC, et al. *Am J Trop Med Hyg.* 2008;78(2):208–209 PMID: 18256414
310. Cheng AC, et al. *Antimicrob Agents Chemother.* 2009;53(10):4193–4199 PMID: 19620336
311. Cruz AT, et al. *Pediatr Infect Dis J.* 2010;29(8):772–774 PMID: 20661106
312. Wilson JW. *Mayo Clin Proc.* 2012;87(4):403–407 PMID: 22469352
313. American Academy of Pediatrics. Nocardiosis. In: Pickering LK, et al, eds. *Red Book: 2012 Report of the Committee on Infectious Diseases.* 2012:521–522
314. Koirala J. *Infect Dis Clin North Am.* 2006;20(2):273–287 PMID: 16762739
315. Stenseth NC, et al. *PLoS Med.* 2008;5(1):e3 PMID: 18198939
316. American Academy of Pediatrics. Plague. In: Pickering LK, et al, eds. *Red Book: 2012 Report of the Committee on Infectious Diseases.* 2012:569–571
317. Kersh GJ. *Expert Rev Anti Infect Ther.* 2013;11(11):1207–1214 PMID: 24073941
318. Anderson A, et al. *MMWR Recomm Rep.* 2013;62(RR-03):1–30 PMID: 23535757
319. Woods CR. *Pediatr Clin North Am.* 2013;60(2):455–470 PMID: 23481111
320. American Academy of Pediatrics. Rocky Mountain spotted fever. In: Pickering LK, et al , eds. *Red Book: 2012 Report of the Committee on Infectious Diseases.* 2012:623–625
321. American Academy of Pediatrics. Tetanus. In: Pickering LK, et al, eds. *Red Book: 2012 Report of the Committee on Infectious Diseases.* 2012:707–712
322. Brook I. *Expert Rev Anti Infect Ther.* 2008;6(3):327–336 PMID: 18588497
323. Lappin E, et al. *Lancet Infect Dis.* 2009;9(5):281–290 PMID: 19393958
324. Dellinger RP, et al. *Crit Care Med.* 2013;41(2):580–637 PMID: 23353941
325. Nigrovic LE, et al. *Infect Dis Clin North Am.* 2008;22(3):489–504 PMID: 18755386

Chapter 7

1. Vila J, et al. *Expert Opin Pharmacother.* 2012;13(16):2319–2336 PMID: 23035697
2. Fishbain J, et al. *Clin Infect Dis.* 2010;51(1):79–84 PMID: 20504234
3. Hsu AJ, et al. *Clin Infect Dis.* 2014;58(10):1439–1448 PMID: 24501388
4. Bonnin RA, et al. *Expert Rev Anti Infect Ther.* 2013;11(6):571–583 PMID: 23750729
5. Brook I. *South Med J.* 2008;101(10):1019–1023 PMID: 18791528
6. Janda JM, et al. *Clin Microbiol Rev.* 2010;23(1):35–73 PMID: 20065325
7. Paturel L, et al. *Clin Microbiol Infect.* 2004;10(2):98–118 PMID: 14759235
8. Thomas RJ, et al. *Expert Rev Anti Infect Ther.* 2009;7(6):709–722 PMID: PMC2739015
9. Ismail N, et al. *Clin Lab Med.* 2010;30(1):261–292 PMID: 20513551
10. Therriault BL, et al. *Ann Pharmacother.* 2008;42(11):1697–1702 PMID: 18812563
11. Bradley JS, et al. *Pediatrics.* 2014;133(5):e1411–e1436 PMID: 24777226
12. American Academy of Pediatrics. *Bacillus cereus* infections. In: Pickering LK, et al, eds. *Red Book: 2012 Report of the Committee on Infectious Diseases.* 2012:245–247
13. Bottone EJ. *Clin Microbiol Rev.* 2010;23(2):382–398 PMID: 20375358
14. Wexler HM. *Clin Microbiol Rev.* 2007;20(4):593–621 PMID: 17934076
15. Snydman DR, et al. *Clin Infect Dis.* 2010;50(S1):S26–S33 PMID: 20067390
16. Florin TA, et al. *Pediatrics.* 2008;121(5):e1413–e1425 PMID: 18443019
17. Massei F, et al. *Infect Dis Clin North Am.* 2005;19(3):691–711 PMID: 16102656
18. Foucault C, et al. *Emerg Infect Dis.* 2006;12(2):217–223 PMID: 16494745
19. Tiwari T, et al. *MMWR Recomm Rep.* 2005;54(RR-14):1–16 PMID: 16340941

20. American Academy of Pediatrics. Pertussis. In: Pickering LK, et al, eds. *Red Book: 2012 Report of the Committee on Infectious Diseases.* 2012:553–566
21. Feder HM Jr. *Infect Dis Clin North Am.* 2008;22(2):315–326 PMID: 18452804
22. American Academy of Pediatrics. Lyme disease. In: Pickering LK, et al, eds. *Red Book: 2012 Report of the Committee on Infectious Diseases.* 2012:474–479
23. Wormser GP, et al. *Clin Infect Dis.* 2006;43(9):1089–1134 PMID: 17029130
24. American Academy of Pediatrics. *Borrelia* infections. In: Pickering LK, et al, eds. *Red Book: 2012 Report of the Committee on Infectious Diseases.* 2012:254–256
25. Dworkin MS, et al. *Infect Dis Clin North Am.* 2008;22(3):449–468 PMID: 18755384
26. American Academy of Pediatrics. Brucellosis. In: Pickering LK, et al, eds. *Red Book: 2012 Report of the Committee on Infectious Diseases.* 2012:256–258
27. Shen MW. *Pediatrics.* 2008;121(5):e1178–e1183 PMID: 18450861
28. Mile B, et al. *Trop Doct.* 2012;42(1):13–17 PMID: 22290107
29. American Academy of Pediatrics. *Burkholderia* infections. In: Pickering LK, et al, eds. *Red Book: 2012 Report of the Committee on Infectious Diseases.* 2012:258–260
30. Waters V. *Curr Pharm Des.* 2012;18(5):696–725 PMID: 22229574
31. King P, et al. *Antimicrob Agents Chemother.* 2010;54(1):143–148 PMID: 19805554
32. Horsley A, et al. *Cochrane Database Syst Rev.* 2012;10:CD009529 PMID: 23076960
33. Wiersinga WJ, et al. *N Engl J Med.* 2012;367(11):1035–1044 PMID: 22970946
34. Cheng AC, et al. *Am J Trop Med Hyg.* 2008;78(2):208–209 PMID: 18256414
35. Chetchotisakd P, et al. *Lancet.* 2014;383(9919):807–814 PMID: 24284287
36. Fujihara N, et al. *J Infect.* 2006;53(5):e199–e202 PMID: 16542730
37. American Academy of Pediatrics. *Campylobacter* infections. In: Pickering LK, et al, eds. *Red Book: 2012 Report of the Committee on Infectious Diseases.* 2012:262–264
38. Ternhag A, et al. *Clin Infect Dis.* 2007;44(5):696–700 PMID: 17278062
39. Kirkpatrick BD, et al. *Curr Opin Gastroenterol.* 2011;27(1):1–7 PMID: 21124212
40. Oehler RL, et al. *Lancet Infect Dis.* 2009;9(7):439–447 PMID: 19555903
41. Jolivet-Gougeon A, et al. *Int J Antimicrob Agents.* 2007;29(4):367–373 PMID: 17250994
42. Wang HK, et al. *J Clin Microbiol.* 2007;45(2):645–647 PMID: 17135428
43. Darville T. *Adv Exp Med Biol.* 2013;764:109–122 PMID: 23654060
44. American Academy of Pediatrics. Chlamydial infections. In: Pickering LK, et al, eds. *Red Book: 2012 Report of the Committee on Infectious Diseases.* 2012:272–281
45. Workowski KA, et al. *MMWR Recomm Rep.* 2010;59(RR-12):1–110 PMID: 21160459
46. Blasi F, et al. *Clin Microbiol Infect.* 2009;15(1):29–35 PMID: 19220337
47. Burillo A, et al. *Infect Dis Clin North Am.* 2010;24(1):61–71 PMID: 20171546
48. Beeckman DS, et al. *Clin Microbiol Infect.* 2009;15(1):11–17 PMID: 19220335
49. Campbell JI, et al. *BMC Infect Dis.* 2013;13:4 PMID: 23286235
50. Sirinavin S, et al. *Pediatr Infect Dis J.* 2005;24(6):559–561 PMID: 15933571
51. Nuñez Cuadros E, et al. *J Med Microbiol.* 2014;63(Pt1):144–147 PMID: 24243285
52. Doran TI. *Clin Infect Dis.* 1999;28(2):384–394 PMID: 10064257
53. Jacoby GA. *Clin Microbiol Rev.* 2009;22(1):161–182 PMID: 19136439
54. Sobel J. *Clin Infect Dis.* 2005;41(8):1167–1173 PMID: 16163636
55. American Academy of Pediatrics. Botulism and infant botulism. In: Pickering LK, et al, eds. *Red Book: 2012 Report of the Committee on Infectious Diseases.* 2012:281–284
56. Hill SE, et al. *Ann Pharmacother.* 2013;47(2):e12 PMID: 23362041
57. Pant C, et al. *Curr Med Res Opin.* 2013;29(8):967–984 PMID: 23659563
58. American Academy of Pediatrics. *Clostridium difficile.* In: Pickering LK, et al, eds. *Red Book: 2012 Report of the Committee on Infectious Diseases.* 2012:285–287
59. American Academy of Pediatrics. Clostridial myonecrosis. In: Pickering LK, et al, eds. *Red Book: 2012 Report of the Committee on Infectious Diseases.* 2012:284–285
60. American Academy of Pediatrics. *Clostridium perfringens* food poisoning. In: Pickering LK, et al, eds. *Red Book: 2012 Report of the Committee on Infectious Diseases.* 2012:288–289
61. American Academy of Pediatrics. Tetanus. In: Pickering LK, et al, eds. *Red Book: 2012 Report of the Committee on Infectious Diseases.* 2012:707–712

62. Brook I. *Expert Rev Anti Infect Ther.* 2008;6(3):327–336 PMID: 18588497
63. American Academy of Pediatrics. Diphtheria. In: Pickering LK, et al, eds. *Red Book: 2012 Report of the Committee on Infectious Diseases.* 2012:307–311
64. Fernandez-Roblas R, et al. *Int J Antimicrob Agents.* 2009;33(5):453–455 PMID: 19153032
65. Holdiness MR. *Drugs.* 2002;62(8):1131–1141 PMID: 12010076
66. Dalal A, et al. *J Infect.* 2008;56(1):77–79 PMID: 18036665
67. Anderson A, et al. *MMWR Recomm Rep.* 2013;62(RR-03):1–30 PMID: 23535757
68. Kersh GJ. *Expert Rev Anti Infect Ther.* 2013;11(11):1207–1214 PMID: 24073941
69. Pritt BS, et al. *N Engl J Med.* 2011;365(5):422–429 PMID: 21812671
70. Paul K, et al. *Clin Infect Dis.* 2001;33(1):54–61 PMID: 11389495
71. Ceyhan M, et al. *Int J Pediatr.* 2011;2011:215–237 PMID: 22046191
72. Hsu MS, et al. *Eur J Clin Microbiol Infect Dis.* 2011;30(10):1271–1278 PMID: 21461847
73. Tamma PD, et al. *Clin Infect Dis.* 2013;57(6):781–788 PMID: 23759352
74. Harris PN, et al. *Int J Antimicrob Agents.* 2012;40(4):297–305 PMID: 22824371
75. Livermore DM, et al. *Int J Antimicrob Agents.* 2011;37(5):415–419 PMID: 21429716
76. Arias CA, et al. *Nat Rev Microbiol.* 2012;10(4):266–278 PMID: 22421879
77. American Academy of Pediatrics. Non-group A or B streptococcal and enterococcal infections. In: Pickering LK, et al, eds. *Red Book: 2012 Report of the Committee on Infectious Diseases.* 2012:686–688
78. Hollenbeck BL, et al. *Virulence.* 2012;3(5):421–433 PMID: 23076243
79. Veraldi S, et al. *Clin Exp Dermatol.* 2009;34(8):859–862 PMID: 19663854
80. American Academy of Pediatrics. Tularemia. In: Pickering LK, et al, eds. *Red Book: 2012 Report of the Committee on Infectious Diseases.* 2012:768–769
81. Hepburn MJ, et al. *Expert Rev Anti Infect Ther.* 2008;6(2):231–240 PMID: 18380605
82. Huggan PJ, et al. *J Infect.* 2008;57(4):283–239 PMID: 18805588
83. Riordan T. *Clin Microbiol Rev.* 2007;20(4):622–659 PMID: 17934077
84. Donders G. *Obstet Gynecol Surv.* 2010;65(7):462–473 PMID: 20723268
85. Ahamed SP, et al. *Neurosciences (Riyadh).* 2010;15(1):40–42 PMID: 20677591
86. Agrawal A, et al. *J Clin Microbiol.* 2011;49(11):3728–3732 PMID: 21900515
87. Greenberg ER, et al. *Lancet.* 2011;378(9790):507–514 PMID: 21777974
88. McColl KE. *N Engl J Med.* 2010;362(17):1597–1604 PMID: 20427808
89. Georgopoulos SD, et al. *Expert Opin Pharmacother.* 2013;14(2):211–223 PMID: 23331077
90. Yagupsky P, et al. *Pediatrics.* 2011;127(3):557–565 PMID: 21321033
91. Weiss-Salz I, et al. *Adv Exp Med Biol.* 2011;719:67–80 PMID: 22125036
92. Petrosillo N, et al. *Expert Rev Anti Infect Ther.* 2013;11(2):159–177 PMID: 23409822
93. Nordmann P, et al. *Lancet Infect Dis.* 2009;9(4):228–236 PMID: 19324295
94. Bergen PJ, et al. *Curr Opin Infect Dis.* 2012;25(6):626–633 PMID: 23041772
95. Viasus D, et al. *Medicine (Baltimore).* 2013;92(1):51–60 PMID: 23266795
96. Griffith ME, et al. *Curr Opin Infect Dis.* 2006;19(6):533–537 PMID: 17075327
97. Florescu D, et al. *Pediatr Infect Dis J.* 2008;27(11):1013–1019 PMID: 18833028
98. Bortolussi R. *CMAJ.* 2008;179(8):795–797 PMID: 18787096
99. Murphy TF, et al. *Clin Infect Dis.* 2009;49(1):124–131 PMID: 19480579
100. Falagas ME, et al. *Infection.* 2006;34(6):315–321 PMID: 17180585
101. Milligan KL, et al. *Clin Pediatr (Phila).* 2013;52(5):462–464 PMID: 22267858
102. American Academy of Pediatrics. Diseases caused by nontuberculous mycobacteria. In: Pickering LK, et al, eds. *Red Book: 2012 Report of the Committee on Infectious Diseases.* 2012:759–767
103. Nessar R, et al. *J Antimicrob Chemother.* 2012;67(4):810–818 PMID: 22290346
104. Griffith DE, et al. *Am J Respir Crit Care Med.* 2007;175(4):367–416 PMID: 17277290
105. American Academy of Pediatrics. Tuberculosis. In: Pickering LK, et al, eds. *Red Book: 2012 Report of the Committee on Infectious Diseases.* 2012:736–759
106. Hlavsa MC, et al. *Clin Infect Dis.* 2008;47(2):168–175 PMID: 18532886
107. Hay RJ. *Curr Opin Infect Dis.* 2009;22(2):99–101 PMID: 19276876
108. Uslan DZ, et al. *Arch Dermatol.* 2006;142(10):1287–1292 PMID: 17043183
109. American Academy of Pediatrics. Leprosy. In: Pickering LK, eds. *Red Book: 2012 Report of the Committee on Infectious Diseases.* 2012:466–469

110. Doedens RA, et al. *Pediatr Infect Dis J.* 2008;27(1):81–83 PMID: 18162949
111. American Thoracic Society, et al. *MMWR Recomm Rep.* 2003;52(RR-11):1–77 PMID: 12836625
112. Waites KB, et al. *Antimicrob Agents Chemother.* 2008;52(10):3776–3778 PMID: 18663020
113. Watt KM, et al. *Pediatr Infect Dis J.* 2012;31(2):197–199 PMID: 22016080
114. Bradley JS, et al. *Clin Infect Dis.* 2011;53(7):e25–e76 PMID: 21880587
115. Akaike H, et al. *Jpn J Infect Dis.* 2012;65(6):535–538 PMID: 23183207
116. Centers for Disease Control and Prevention. *MMWR Morb Mortal Wkly Rep.* 2012;61(31):590–594 PMID: 22874837
117. Wu HM, et al. *N Engl J Med.* 2009;360(9):886–892 PMID: 19246360
118. Glikman D, et al. *Pediatrics.* 2006;117(5):e1061–e1066 PMID: 16606681
119. Wilson JW. *Mayo Clin Proc.* 2012;87(4):403–407 PMID: 22469352
120. American Academy of Pediatrics. Nocardiosis. In: Pickering LK, et al, eds. *Red Book: 2012 Report of the Committee on Infectious Diseases.* 2012:521–522
121. Casanova-Román M, et al. *Infection.* 2010;38(4):321–323 PMID: 20376528
122. Goldstein EJ, et al. *Antimicrob Agents Chemother.* 2012;56(12):6319–6323 PMID: 23027193
123. Murphy EC, et al. *FEMS Microbiol Rev.* 2013;37(4):520–553 PMID: 23030831
124. Ozdemir O, et al. *J Microbiol Immunol Infect.* 2010;43(4):344–346 PMID: 20688296
125. Stock I, Wiedemann B. *J Antimicrob Chemother.* 2001;48(6):803–811 PMID: 11733464
126. Brook I, et al. *Clin Microbiol Rev.* 2013;26(3):526–546 PMID: 23824372
127. Nisbet M, et al. *J Antimicrob Chemother.* 2007;60(5):1097–1103 PMID: 17875606
128. Perry A, et al. *Expert Rev Anti Infect Ther.* 2011;9(12):1149–1156 PMID: 22114965
129. Saperston KN, et al. *J Urol.* 2014;191(5Suppl):1608–1613 PMID: 24679887
130. Tumbarello M, et al. *J Antimicrob Chemother.* 2004;53(2):277–282 PMID: 14688041
131. Sun HY, et al. *Chest.* 2011;139(5):1172–1185 PMID: 21540216
132. Grgurich PE, et al. *Expert Rev Respir Med.* 2012:6(5):533–555 PMID: 23134248
133. Tam VH, et al. *Antimicrob Agents Chemother.* 2010;54(3):1160–1164 PMID: 20086165
134. Freifeld AG, et al. *Clin Infect Dis.* 2011;52(4):e56–e93 PMID: 21258094
135. Velkov T, et al. *Future Microbiol.* 2013;8(6):711–724 PMID: 23701329
136. Döring G, et al. *J Cyst Fibros.* 2012;11(6):461–479 PMID: 23137712
137. Mogayzel PJ Jr, et al. *Am J Respir Crit Care Med.* 2013;187(7):680–689 PMID: 23540878
138. Saiman L. *Paediatr Respir Rev.* 2007;8(3):249–255 PMID: 17868923
139. Yamshchikov AV, et al. *Lancet Infect Dis.* 2010;10(5):350–359 PMID: 20417417
140. American Academy of Pediatrics. Rickettsial diseases. In: Pickering LK, et al, eds. *Red Book: 2012 Report of the Committee on Infectious Diseases.* 2012:620–625
141. Woods CR. *Pediatr Clin North Am.* 2013;60(2):455–470 PMID: 23481111
142. American Academy of Pediatrics. *Salmonella* infections. In: Pickering LK, et al, eds. *Red Book: 2012 Report of the Committee on Infectious Diseases.* 2012:635–640
143. Haeusler GM, et al. *Adv Exp Med Biol.* 2013;764:13–26 PMID: 23654054
144. Onwuezobe IA, et al. *Cochrane Database Syst Rev.* 2012;11:CD001167 PMID: 23152205
145. Effa EE, et al. *Cochrane Database Syst Rev.* 2008;(4):CD006083 PMID: 18843701
146. To KK, et al. *Scand J Infect Dis.* 2010;42(10):757–762 PMID: 20524786
147. Shiferaw B, et al. *Clin Infect Dis.* 2012;54(Suppl5):S458–S463 PMID: 22572670
148. American Academy of Pediatrics. *Shigella* infections. In: Pickering LK, et al, eds. *Red Book: 2012 Report of the Committee on Infectious Diseases.* 2012:645–647
149. Sjölund Karlsson M, et al. *Antimicrob Agents Chemother.* 2013;57(3):1559–1560 PMID: 23274665
150. Vinh H, et al. *PLoS Negl Trop Dis.* 2011;5(8):e1264 PMID: 21829747
151. Gaastra W, et al. *Vet Microbiol.* 2009;133(3):211–228 PMID: 19008054
152. American Academy of Pediatrics. Rat bite fever. In: Pickering LK, et al, eds. *Red Book: 2012 Report of the Committee on Infectious Diseases.* 2012:608–609
153. Liu C, et al. *Clin Infect Dis.* 2011;52(3):e18–e55 PMID: 21208910
154. Long CB, et al. *Expert Rev Anti Infect Ther.* 2010;8(2):183–195 PMID: 20109048
155. Cheung GY, et al. *Curr Opin Infect Dis.* 2010;23(3):208–216 PMID: 20179594
156. Marchant EA, et al. *Clin Dev Immunol.* 2013;2013:586076 PMID: 23762094
157. Falagas ME, et al. *J Antimicrob Chemother.* 2008;62(5):889–894 PMID: 1866294

158. Church D, et al. *Scand J Infect Dis.* 2013;45(4):265–270 PMID: 23113657
159. American Academy of Pediatrics. Group A streptococcal infections. In: Pickering LK, et al, eds. *Red Book: 2012 Report of the Committee on Infectious Diseases.* 2012:668–680
160. American Academy of Pediatrics. Group B streptococcal infections. In: Pickering LK, et al, eds. *Red Book: 2012 Report of the Committee on Infectious Diseases.* 2012:680–688
161. Belko J, et al. *Pediatr Infect Dis J.* 2002;21(8):715–723 PMID: 12192158
162. Broyles LN, et al. *Clin Infect Dis.* 2009;48(6):706–712 PMID: 19187026
163. Stelzmueller I, et al. *Eur J Pediatr Surg.* 2009;19(1):21–24 PMID: 19221948
164. Deutschmann MW, et al. *JAMA Otolaryngol Head Neck Surg.* 2013;139(2):157–160 PMID: 23429946
165. Pichichero ME. *Pediatr Clin North Am.* 2013;60(2):391–407 PMID: 23481107
166. American Academy of Pediatrics. Pneumococcal infections. In: Pickering LK, et al, eds. *Red Book: 2012 Report of the Committee on Infectious Diseases.* 2012:571–582
167. Jones RN, et al. *Int J Antimicrob Agents.* 2010;36(3):197–204 PMID: 20558045
168. Kaplan SL, et al. *Pediatr Infect Dis J.* 2013;32(3):203–207 PMID: 23558320
169. Baddour LM, et al. *Circulation.* 2005;111(23):e394–e434 PMID: 15956145
170. American Academy of Pediatrics. Syphilis. In: Pickering LK, et al, eds. *Red Book: 2012 Report of the Committee on Infectious Diseases.* 2012:690–703
171. Turner MA, et al. *Arch Dis Child.* 2012;97(6):573–577 PMID: 21697219
172. American Academy of Pediatrics. Cholera. In: Pickering LK, et al, eds. *Red Book: 2012 Report of the Committee on Infectious Diseases.* 2012:789–791
173. Charles RC, et al. *Curr Opin Infect Dis.* 2011;24(5):472–477 PMID: 21799407
174. Dechet AM, et al. *Clin Infect Dis.* 2008;46(7):970–976 PMID: 18444811
175. Daniels NA. *Clin Infect Dis.* 2011;52(6):788–792 PMID: 21367733
176. Fàbrega A, et al. *Enferm Infecc Microbiol Clin.* 2012;30(1):24–32 PMID: 22019131
177. American Academy of Pediatrics. *Yersinia enterocolitica* and *Yersina pseudotuberculosis.* In: Pickering LK, et al, eds. *Red Book: 2012 Report of the Committee on Infectious Diseases.* 2012:795–797
178. American Academy of Pediatrics. Plague. In: Pickering LK, et al, eds. *Red Book: 2012 Report of the Committee on Infectious Diseases.* 2012:569–571
179. Butler T. *Clin Infect Dis.* 2009;49(5):736–742 PMID: 19606935
180. Kaasch AJ, et al. *Infection.* 2012;40(2):185–190 PMID: 21789525

Chapter 8

1. Cornely OA, et al. *Haematologica.* 2009;94(1):113–122 PMID: 19066334
2. Almyroudis NG, et al. *Curr Opin Infect Dis.* 2009;22(4):385–393 PMID: 19506476
3. Maschmeyer G. *J Antimicrob Chemother.* 2009;63(Suppl1):i27–i30 PMID: 19372178
4. Freifeld AG, et al. *Clin Infect Dis.* 2011;52(4):e56–e93 PMID: 21258094
5. De Pauw BE, et al. *N Engl J Med.* 2007;356(4):409–411 PMID: 17251538
6. Salavert M. *Int J Antimicrob Agents.* 2008;32(Suppl2):S149–S153 PMID: 19013340
7. Eschenauer GA, et al. *Liver Transpl.* 2009;15(8):842–858 PMID: 19642130
8. Stockmann C, et al. *Clin Pharmacokinet.* 2014;53(5):429–454 PMID: 24595533
9. Walsh TJ, et al. *Clin Infect Dis.* 2008;46(3):327–360 PMID: 18177225
10. Thomas L, et al. *Expert Rev Anti Infect Ther.* 2009;7(4):461–472 PMID: 19400765
11. Friberg LE, et al. *Antimicrob Agents Chemother.* 2012;56(6):3032–3042 PMID: 22430956
12. Cornely OA, et al. *Clin Infect Dis.* 2007;44(10):1289–1297 PMID: 17443465
13. Bartelink IH, et al. *Antimicrob Agents Chemother.* 2013;57(1):235–240 PMID: 23114771
14. Ashouri N, et al. *Expert Opin Drug Metab Toxicol.* 2008;4(4):463–469 PMID: 18433348
15. Marr KA, et al. Abstract LB2812. 22nd European Congress of Clinical Microbiology and Infectious Diseases, March 31–April 3, 2012; London
16. Chapman SW, et al. *Clin Infect Dis.* 2008;46(12):1801–1812 PMID: 18462107
17. McKinnell JA, et al. *Clin Chest Med.* 2009;30(2):227–239 PMID: 19375630
18. Walsh CM, et al. *Pediatr Infect Dis J.* 2006;25(7):656–658 PMID: 16804444
19. Pappas PG, et al. *Clin Infect Dis.* 2009;48(5):503–535 PMID: 19191635
20. Goins RA, et al. *Pediatr Infect Dis J.* 2002;21(12):1165–1167 PMID: 12506950
21. Piper L, et al. *Pediatr Infect Dis J.* 2011;30(5):375–378 PMID: 21085048

22. Prasad N, et al. *Perit Dial Int.* 2005;25(3):207–222 PMID: 15981767
23. Sobel JD. *Lancet.* 2007;369(9577):1961–1971 PMID: 17560449
24. Lopez Martinez R, et al. *Clin Dermatol.* 2007;25(2):188–194 PMID: 17350498
25. Ameen M. *Clin Exp Dermatol.* 2009;34(8):849–854 PMID: 19575735
26. Galgiani JN, et al. *Clin Infect Dis.* 2005;41(9):1217–1223 PMID: 16206093
27. Anstead GM, et al. *Infect Dis Clin North Am.* 2006;20(3):621–643 PMID: 16984872
28. Williams PL. *Ann N Y Acad Sci.* 2007;1111:377–384 PMID: 17363442
29. American Academy of Pediatrics. Coccidiodomycosis. In: Pickering LK, et al, eds. *Red Book: 2012 Report of the Committee on Infectious Diseases.* 2012:289–291
30. Homans JD, et al. *Pediatr Infect Dis J.* 2010;29(1):65–67 PMID: 19884875
31. Chayakulkeeree M, et al. *Infect Dis Clin North Am.* 2006;20(3):507–544 PMID: 16984867
32. Jarvis JN, et al. *Semin Respir Crit Care Med.* 2008;29(2):141–150 PMID: 18365996
33. American Academy of Pediatrics. *Cryptococcus neoformans* infections (cryptococcosis). In: Pickering LK, et al, eds. *Red Book: 2012 Report of the Committee on Infectious Diseases.* 2012:294–296
34. Perfect JR, et al. *Clin Infect Dis.* 2010;50(3):291–322 PMID: 20047480
35. Naggie S, et al. *Clin Chest Med.* 2009;30(2):337–353 PMID: 19375639
36. Cortez KJ, et al. *Clin Microbiol Rev.* 2008;21(1):157–197 PMID: 18202441
37. Wheat LJ, et al. *Clin Infect Dis.* 2007;45(7):807–825 PMID: 17806045
38. American Academy of Pediatrics. *Borrelia* infections (relapsing fever). In: Pickering LK, et al, eds. *Red Book: 2012 Report of the Committee on Infectious Diseases.* 2012:254–256
39. Queiroz-Telles F, et al. *Clin Infect Dis.* 2007;45(11):1462–1469 PMID: 17990229
40. Menezes VM, et al. *Cochrane Database Syst Rev.* 2006;(2):CD004967 PMID: 16625617
41. American Academy of Pediatrics. Paracoccidioidomycosis (South American blastomycosis). In: Pickering LK, et al, eds. *Red Book: 2012 Report of the Committee on Infectious Diseases.* 2012:530–531
42. Li DM, et al. *Lancet Infect Dis.* 2009;9(6):376–383 PMID: 19467477
43. Panel on Opportunistic Infections in HIV-Exposed and HIV-Infected Children. Guidelines for the prevention and treatment of opportunistic infections in HIV-exposed and HIV-infected children. http://aidsinfo.nih.gov/contentfiles/lvguidelines/oi_guidelines_pediatrics.pdf. Updated November 6, 2013. Accessed October 14, 2014
44. Kauffman CA, et al. *Clin Infect Dis.* 2007;45(10):1255–1265 PMID: 17968818
45. Walsh TJ, et al. *Clin Infect Dis.* 2008;47(3):372–374 PMID: 18558877
46. Chayakulkeeree M, et al. *Eur J Clin Microbiol Infect Dis.* 2006;25(4):215–229 PMID: 16568297
47. Spellberg B, et al. *Clin Infect Dis.* 2009;48(12):1743–1751 PMID: 19435437
48. Reed C, et al. *Clin Infect Dis.* 2008;47(3):364–371 PMID: 18558882
49. Ali S, et al. *Pediatr Emerg Care.* 2007;23(9):662–668 PMID: 17876261
50. Shy R. *Pediatr Rev.* 2007;28(5):164–174 PMID: 17473121
51. Andrews MD, et al. *Am Fam Physician.* 2008;77(10):1415–1420 PMID: 18533375
52. de Berker D. *N Engl J Med.* 2009;360(20):2108–2116 PMID: 19439745
53. Pantazidou A, et al. *Arch Dis Child.* 2007;92(11):1040–1042 PMID: 17954488

Chapter 9

1. Lenaerts L, et al. *Rev Med Virol.* 2008;18(6):357–374 PMID: 18655013
2. Michaels MG. *Expert Rev Anti Infect Ther.* 2007;5(3):441–448 PMID: 17547508
3. Biron KK. *Antiviral Res.* 2006;71(2–3):154–163 PMID: 16765457
4. Boeckh M, et al. *Blood.* 2009;113(23):5711–5719 PMID: 19299333
5. Vaudry W, et al. *Am J Transplant.* 2009;9(3):636–643 PMID: 19260840
6. Emanuel D, et al. *Ann Intern Med.* 1988;109(10):777–782 PMID: 2847609
7. Reed EC, et al. *Ann Intern Med.* 1988;109(10):783–788 PMID: 2847610
8. *Ophthalmology.* 1994;101(7):1250–1261 PMID: 8035989
9. Musch DC, et al. *N Engl J Med.* 1997;337(2):83–90 PMID: 9211677
10. Martin DF, et al. *N Engl J Med.* 2002;346(15):1119–1126 PMID: 11948271
11. Kempen JH, et al. *Arch Ophthalmol.* 2003;121(4):466–476 PMID: 12695243

12. Studies of Ocular Complications of AIDS Research Group. The AIDS Clinical Trials Group. *Am J Ophthalmol.* 2001;131(4):457–467 PMID: 11292409
13. Dieterich DT, et al. *J Infect Dis.* 1993;167(2):278–282 PMID: 8380610
14. Gerna G, et al. *Antiviral Res.* 1997;34(1):39–50 PMID: 9107384
15. Markham A, et al. *Drugs.* 1994;48(3):455–484 PMID: 7527763
16. Kimberlin DW, et al. *J Infect Dis.* 2008;197(6):836–845 PMID: 18279073
17. Kimberlin DW, et al. Six months versus six weeks of oral valganciclovir for infants with symptomatic congenital cytomegalovirus (CMV) disease with and without central nervous system (CNS) involvement: results of a Phase III, randomized, double-blind, placebo-controlled, multinational study. IDWeek 2013, San Francisco, CA, October 5, 2013; Late-Breaker Abstract #43178
18. Griffiths P, et al. *Herpes.* 2008;15(1):4–12 PMID: 18983762
19. Panel on Opportunistic Infections in HIV-Exposed and HIV-Infected Children. Guidelines for the prevention and treatment of opportunistic infections in HIV-exposed and HIV-infected children. http://aidsinfo.nih.gov/contentfiles/lvguidelines/oi_guidelines_pediatrics.pdf. Updated November 6, 2013. Accessed October 14, 2014
20. Biebl A, et al. *Nat Clin Pract Neurol.* 2009;5(3):171–174 PMID: 19262593
21. Chadaide Z, et al. *J Med Virol.* 2008;80(11):1930–1932 PMID: 18814244
22. American Academy of Pediatrics. Epstein-Barr virus infections (infectious mononucleosis). In: Pickering LK, et al, eds. *Red Book: 2012 Report of the Committee on Infectious Diseases.* 2012:318–321
23. Gross TG. *Herpes.* 2009;15(3):64–67 PMID: 19306606
24. Styczynski J, et al. *Bone Marrow Transplant.* 2009;43(10):757–770 PMID: 19043458
25. Kurbegov AC, et al. *Expert Rev Gastroenterol Hepatol.* 2009;3(1):39–49 PMID: 19210112
26. Jonas MM, et al. *Hepatology.* 2008;47(6):1863–1871 PMID: 18433023
27. Lai CL, et al. *Gastroenterology.* 2002;123(6):1831–1838 PMID: 12454840
28. Honkoop P, et al. *Expert Opin Investig Drugs.* 2003;12(4):683–688 PMID: 12665423
29. Shaw T, et al. *Expert Rev Anti Infect Ther.* 2004;2(6):853–871 PMID: 15566330
30. Elisofon SA, et al. *Clin Liver Dis.* 2006;10(1):133–148 PMID: 16376798
31. Jonas MM, et al. *Hepatology.* 2010;52(6):2192–2205 PMID: 20890947
32. Haber BA, et al. *Pediatrics.* 2009;124(5):e1007–1013 PMID: 19805457
33. Shneider BL, et al. *Hepatology.* 2006;44(5):1344–1354 PMID: 17058223
34. Jain MK, et al. *J Viral Hepat.* 2007;14(3):176–182 PMID: 17305883
35. Sokal EM, et al. *Gastroenterology.* 1998;114(5):988–995 PMID: 9558288
36. Jonas MM, et al. *N Engl J Med.* 2002;346(22):1706–1713 PMID: 12037150
37. Chang TT, et al. *N Engl J Med.* 2006;354(10):1001–1010 PMID: 16525137
38. Liaw YF, et al. *Gastroenterology.* 2009;136(2):486–495 PMID: 19027013
39. Keam SJ, et al. *Drugs.* 2008;68(9):1273–1317 PMID: 18547135
40. Marcellin P, et al. *Gastroenterology.* 2011;140(2):459–468 PMID: 21034744
41. Poordad F, et al. *N Engl J Med.* 2011;364(13):1195–1206 PMID: 21449783
42. Schwarz KB, et al. *Gastroenterology.* 2011;140(2):450–458 PMID: 21036173
43. Nelson DR. *Liver Int.* 2011;31(S1):53–57 PMID: 21205138
44. Strader DB, et al. *Hepatology.* 2004;39(4):1147–1171 PMID: 15057920
45. Soriano V, et al. *AIDS.* 2007;21(9):1073–1089 PMID: 17502718
46. Hollier LM, et al. *Cochrane Database Syst Rev.* 2008;(1):CD004946 PMID: 18254066
47. Pinninti SG, et al. Neonatal herpes disease despite maternal antenatal antiviral suppressive therapy: a multicenter case series of the first such infants reported. 48th Annual Meeting of The Infectious Diseases Society of America; October 22, 2010; Vancouver, British Columbia
48. Pinninti SG, et al. *J Pediatr.* 2012;161(1):134–138 PMID: 22336576
49. Kimberlin DW, et al. *Clin Infect Dis.* 2010;50(2):221–228 PMID: 20014952
50. Abdel Massih RC, et al. *World J Gastroenterol.* 2009;15(21):2561–2569 PMID: 19496184
51. Mofenson LM, et al. *MMWR Recomm Rep.* 2009;58(RR-11):1–166 PMID: 19730409
52. Kuhar DT, et al. *Infect Control Hosp Epidemiol.* 2013;34(9):875–892 PMID: 23917901
53. Acosta EP, et al. *J Infect Dis.* 2010;202(4):563–566 PMID: 20594104
54. Kimberlin DW, et al. *J Infect Dis.* 2013;207(5):709–720 PMID: 23230059
55. McPherson C, et al. *J Infect Dis.* 2012;206(6):847–850 PMID: 22807525

56. American Academy of Pediatrics. Measles. In: Pickering LK, et al, eds. *Red Book: 2012 Report of the Committee on Infectious Diseases.* 2012:489–499
57. American Academy of Pediatrics Committee on Infectious Diseases and Bronchiolitis Guidelines Committee. *Pediatrics.* 2014;134:415–420 PMID: 25070315
58. Whitley RJ. *Adv Exp Med Biol.* 2008;609:216–232 PMID: 18193668

Chapter 10

1. Drugs for parasitic infections. *Medical Letter.* 2013;11(Suppl):e1–31
2. Blessmann J, et al. *J Clin Microbiol.* 2003;41(10):4745–4750 PMID: 14532214
3. Haque R, et al. *N Engl J Med.* 2003;348(16):1565–1573 PMID: 1270037
4. Parasitic infections. In: Abramowicz M, ed. *Handbook of Antimicrobial Therapy.* 2011:221–277
5. Stanley SL Jr. *Lancet.* 2003;361(9362):1025–1034 PMID: 12660071
6. Barnett ND, et al. *Pediatr Neurol.* 1996;15(3):230–234 PMID: 8916161
7. Vargas-Zepeda J, et al. *Arch Med Res.* 2005;36(1):83–86 PMID: 15900627
8. Goswick SM, et al. *Antimicrob Agents Chemother.* 2003;47(2):524–528 PMID: 12543653
9. Slater CA, et al. *N Engl J Med.* 1994;331(2):85–87 PMID: 8208270
10. Deetz TR, et al. *Clin Infect Dis.* 2003;37(10):1304–1012 PMID: 14583863
11. Centers for Disease Control and Prevention. *MMWR Morb Mortal Wkly Rep.* 2013;62(33):666 PMID: 23965830
12. Visvesvara GS, et al. *FEMS Immunol Med Microbiol.* 2007;50(1):1–26 PMID: 17428307
13. Tunkel AR, et al. *Clin Infect Dis.* 2008;47(3):303–327 PMID: 18582201
14. Chotmongkol V, et al. *Am J Trop Med Hyg.* 2006;74(6):1122–1124 PMID: 16760531
15. Lo Re V III, et al. *Am J Med.* 2003;114(3):217–223 PMID: 12637136
16. Jitpimolmard S, et al. *Parasitology Res.* 2007;100(6):1293–1296 PMID: 17177056
17. Checkley AM, et al. *J Infect.* 2010;60(1):1–20 PMID: 19931558
18. Centers for Disease Control and Prevention. Immigrant and refugee health: domestic intestinal parasites guidelines. http://www.cdc.gov/immigrantrefugeehealth/guidelines/domestic/intestinal-parasites-domestic.html. Accessed October 14, 2014
19. American Academy of Pediatrics. *Ascaris lumbricoides* infections. In: Pickering LK, et al, eds. *Red Book: 2012 Report of the Committee on Infectious Diseases.* 2012: 239–240
20. Vannier E, et al. *Infect Dis Clin North Am.* 2008;22(3):469–488 PMID: 18755385
21. Wormser GP, et al. *Clin Infect Dis.* 2006;43(9):1089–1134 PMID: 17029130
22. Boustani MR, et al. *Clin Infect Dis.* 1996;22(4):611–615 PMID: 8729197
23. Fisk T, et al. *Cyclospora cayetanensis, Isospora belli, Sarcocystis* species, *Balantidium coli,* and *Blastocystis hominis.* In: Mandell GL, at al, eds. *Principles and Practice of Infectious Diseases.* 2005:3228–3237
24. American Academy of Pediatrics. *Baylisascaris* infections. In: Pickering LK, et al, eds. *Red Book: 2012 Report of the Committee on Infectious Diseases.* 2012:251–252
25. Park SY, et al. *Pediatrics.* 2000;106(4):e56 PMID: 11015551
26. Shlim DR, et al. *Clin Infect Dis.* 1995;21(1):97–101 PMID: 7578767
27. Udkow MP, et al. *J Infect Dis.* 1993;168(1):242–244 PMID: 8515120
28. Bern C, et al. *JAMA.* 2007;298(18):2171–2181 PMID: 18000201
29. Maguire JH. Trypanosoma. In: Gorbach SL, et al, eds. *Infectious Diseases.* 2004:2327–2334
30. Amadi B, et al. *Lancet.* 2002;360(9343):1375–1380 PMID: 12423984
31. Kosek M, et al. *Lancet Infect Dis.* 2001;1(4):262–269 PMID: 11871513
32. Davies AP, et al. *BMJ.* 2009;339:b4168 PMID: 19841008
33. Bushen OY, et al. Cryptosporidiosis. In: Guerrant RL, et al, eds. *Tropical Infectious Diseases.* 2006:1003–1014
34. Derouin F, et al. *Expert Rev Anti Infect Ther.* 2008;6(3):337–349 PMID: 18588498
35. Jelinek T, et al. *Clin Infect Dis.* 1994;19(6):1062–1066 PMID: 7534125
36. Prociv P, et al. *Acta Trop.* 1996;62(1):23–44 PMID: 8971276
37. Eberhard ML, et al. *Curr Opin Infect Dis.* 2002;15(5):519–522 PMID: 12686886
38. Ortega Yr, et al. *Clin Microbiol Rev.* 2010;23(1):218–234 PMID: 20065331
39. Garcia HH, et al. *N Engl J Med.* 2004;350(3):249–258 PMID: 14724304

40. Garcia HH, et al. *Clin Microbiol Rev.* 2002;15(4):747–756 PMID: 12364377
41. Lillie P, et al. *J Infect.* 2010;60(5):403–404 PMID: 20153773
42. Stark DJ, et al. *Trends Parasitol.* 2006;22(2):92–96 PMID: 16380293
43. Johnson EH, et al. *Clin Microbiol Rev.* 2004;17(3):553–570 PMID: 15258093
44. Smego RA Jr, et al. *Clin Infect Dis.* 2003;37(8):1073–1083 PMID: 14523772
45. Franchi C, et al. *Clin Infect Dis.* 1999;29(2):304–309 PMID: 10476732
46. Grencis RK, et al. *Gastroenterol Clin North Am.* 1996;25(3):579–597 PMID: 8863041
47. Tisch DJ, et al. *Lancet Infect Dis.* 2005;5(8):514–523 PMID: 16048720
48. Ottesen EA, et al. *Annu Rev Med.* 1992;43:417–424 PMID: 1580599
49. Jong EC, et al. *J Infect Dis.* 1985;152(3):637–640 PMID: 3897401
50. Calvopina M, et al. *Trans R Soc Trop Med Hyg.* 1998;92(5):566–569 PMID: 9861383
51. Johnson RJ, et al. *Rev Infect Dis.* 1985;7(2):200–206 PMID: 4001715
52. Graham CS, et al. *Clin Infect Dis.* 2001;33(1):1–5 PMID: 11389487
53. Gardner TB, et al. *Clin Microbiol Rev.* 2001;14(1):114–128 PMID: 11148005
54. Ross AG, et al. *New Engl J Med.* 2013;368(19):1817–1825 PMID: 23656647
55. Abboud P, et al. *Clin Infect Dis.* 2001;32(12):1792–1794 PMID: 11360222
56. Hotez PJ, et al. *N Engl J Med.* 2004;351(8):799–807 PMID: 15317893
57. World Health Organization, Technical Report Series 949. Report of a meeting of the WHO Expert Committee on the Control of Leishmaniases, Geneva, 22–26 March 2010
58. Alrajhi AA, et al. *N Engl J Med.* 2002;346(12):891–895 PMID: 11907288
59. Bern C, et al. *Clin Infect Dis.* 2006;43(7):917–924 PMID: 16941377
60. Ritmeijer K, et al. *Clin Infect Dis.* 2006;43(3):357–364 PMID: 16804852
61. Sundar S, et al. *N Engl J Med.* 2002;347(22):1739–1746 PMID: 12456849
62. Sundar S, et al. *N Engl J Med.* 2007;356(25):2571–2581 PMID: 17582067
63. American Academy of Pediatrics. Pediculosis. In: Pickering LK, et al, eds. *Red Book: 2012 Report of the Committee on Infectious Diseases.* 2012:543–547
64. Foucault C, et al. *J Infect Dis.* 2006;193(3):474–476 PMID: 16388498
65. Fischer PR, et al. *Clin Infect Dis.* 2002;34(4):493–498 PMID: 11797176
66. Freedman DO. *N Engl J Med.* 2008;359(6):603–612 PMID: 18687641
67. Kain KC, et al. *Clin Infect Dis.* 2001;33(2):226–234 PMID: 11418883
68. Kain KC, et al. *Infect Dis Clin North Am.* 1998;12(2):267–284 PMID: 9658245
69. Overbosch D, et al. *Clin Infect Dis.* 2001;33(7):1015–1021 PMID: 11528574
70. Centers for Disease Control and Prevention. Malaria. In: *The Yellow Book: CDC Health Information for International Travel 2014.* http://wwwnc.cdc.gov/travel/yellowbook/2014/chapter-3-infectious-diseases-related-to-travel/malaria. Accessed October 14, 2014
71. American Academy of Pediatrics. Pinworm infection. In: Pickering LK, et al, eds. *Red Book: 2012 Report of the Committee on Infectious Diseases.* 2012:566–567
72. American Academy of Pediatrics. Scabies. In: Pickering LK, et al, eds. *Red Book: 2012 Report of the Committee on Infectious Diseases.* 2012:641–643
73. Usha V, et al. *J Am Acad Dermatol.* 2000;42(2pt1):236–240 PMID: 10642678
74. Brodine SK, et al. *Am J Trop Med Hyg.* 2009;80(3):425–430 PMID: 19270293
75. Doenhoff MJ, et al. *Expert Rev Anti Infect Ther.* 2006;4(2):199–210 PMID: 16597202
76. Fenwick A, et al. *Curr Opin Infect Dis.* 2006;19(6):577–582 PMID: 17075334
77. Centers for Disease Control and Prevention. Parasites—schistosomiasis. Resources for health professionals. http://www.cdc.gov/parasites/schistosomiasis/health_professionals/index.html. Accessed October 14, 2014
78. Marti H, et al. *Am J Trop Med Hyg.* 1996;55(5):477–481 PMID: 8940976
79. Segarra-Newnham M. *Ann Pharmacother.* 2007;41(12):1992–2001 PMID: 17940124
80. Chiodini P, et al. *Lancet.* 2000;355(9197):43–44 PMID: 10615895
81. Marty FM, et al. *Clin Infect Dis.* 2005;41(1):e5–e8 PMID: 15937753
82. Donadello K, et al. *Int J Antimicrob Agents.* 2013;42(6):580–583 PMID: 24269075
83. McAuley JB. *Pediatr Infect Dis J.* 2008;27(2):161–162 PMID: 18227714
84. McLeod R, et al. *Clin Infect Dis.* 2006;42(10):1383–1394 PMID: 16619149
85. Petersen E. *Expert Rev Anti Infect Ther.* 2007;5(2):285–293 PMID: 17402843

86. Adachi JA, et al. *Clin Infect Dis.* 2003;37(9):1165–1171 PMID: 14557959
87. Diemert DJ. *Clin Microbiol Rev.* 2006;19(3):583–594 PMID: 16847088
88. DuPont HL. *Clin Infect Dis.* 2007;45(S1):S78–S84 PMID: 17582576
89. Gottstein B, et al. *Clin Microbiol Rev.* 2009;22(1):127–145 PMID: 19136437
90. American Academy of Pediatrics. *Trichomonas vaginalis* (trichomoniasis). In: Pickering LK, et al, eds. *Red Book: 2012 Report of the Committee on Infectious Diseases.* 2012:729–731
91. Fairlamb AH. *Trends Parasitol.* 2003;19(11):488–494 PMID: 14580959
92. Pepin J, et al. *Adv Parasitol.* 1994;33:1–47 PMID: 8122565
93. Bisser S, et al. *J Infect Dis.* 2007;195(3):322–329 PMID: 17205469
94. Sahlas DJ, et al. *N Engl J Med.* 2002;347(10):749–753 PMID: 12213947
95. American Academy of Pediatrics. Trichuriasis (whipworm infection). In: Pickering LK, et al, eds. *Red Book: 2012 Report of the Committee on Infectious Diseases.* 2012:731–732

Chapter 13

1. Tetzlaff TR, et al. *J Pediatr.* 1978;92(3):485–490 PMID: 632997
2. Weichert S, et al. *Curr Opin Infect Dis.* 2008;21(3):258–262 PMID: 18448970
3. Paakkonen M, et al. *Int J Antimicrob Agents.* 2011;38(4):273–280 PMID: 21640559
4. Rice HE, et al. *Arch Surg.* 2001;136(12):1391–1395 PMID: 11735866
5. Fraser JD, et al. *J Pediatr Surg.* 2010;45(6):1198–1202 PMID: 20620320
6. Hoberman A, et al. *Pediatrics.* 1999;104(1pt1):79–86 PMID: 10390264
7. Bradley JS, et al. *Pediatrics.* 2011;128(4):e1034–e1045 PMID: 21949152
8. Arnold JC, et al. *Pediatrics.* 2012;130(4):e821–e828 PMID: 22966033
9. Zaoutis T, et al. *Pediatrics.* 2009;123(2):636–642 PMID: 19171632

Chapter 14

1. Oehler RL, et al. *Lancet Infect Dis.* 2009;9(7):439–447 PMID: 19555903
2. Wu PS, et al. *Pediatr Emerg Care.* 2011;27(9):801–803 PMID: 21878832
3. Stevens DL, et al. *Clin Infect Dis.* 2014;59(2):147–159 PMID: 24947530
4. Talan DA, et al. *Clin Infect Dis.* 2003;37(11):1481–1489 PMID: 14614671
5. Wilson W, et al. *Circulation.* 2007;116(15):1736–1754 PMID: 17446442
6. Pasquali SK, et al. *Am Heart J.* 2012;163(5):894–899 PMID: 22607869
7. Cohn AC, et al. *MMWR Recomm Rep.* 2013;62(RR-2):1–28 PMID: 23515099
8. American Academy of Pediatrics. Pertussis. In: Pickering LK, et al, eds. *Red Book: 2012 Report of the Committee on Infectious Diseases.* 2012:553–566
9. Centers for Disease Control and Prevention. Pertussis (whooping cough). Postexposure antimicrobial prophylasix. http://www.cdc.gov/pertussis/outbreaks/PEP.html. Accessed October 14, 2014
10. Brook I. *Expert Rev Anti Infect Ther.* 2008;6(3):327–336 PMID: 18588497
11. American Academy of Pediatrics. Tetanus (lockjaw). In: Pickering LK, et al, eds. *Red Book: 2012 Report of the Committee on Infectious Diseases.* 2012:707–712
12. Centers for Disease Control and Prevention. Tuberculosis (TB). Treatment for latent TB infection. http://www.cdc.gov/tb/topic/treatment/ltbi.htm. Accessed October 14, 2014
13. American Academy of Pediatrics. Tuberculosis. In: Pickering LK, et al, eds. *Red Book: 2012 Report of the Committee on Infectious Diseases.* 2012:736–759
14. Centers for Disease Control and Prevention. *MMWR Morb Mortal Wkly Rep.* 2011;60(48):1650–1653 PMID: 22157884
15. ACOG Committee on Practice Bulletins. *Obstet Gynecol.* 2007;109(6):1489–1498 PMID: 17569194
16. Kimberlin DW, et al. *Pediatrics.* 2013;131(2):e635–e646 PMID: 23359576
17. American Academy of Academy Committee on Infectious Diseases. *Pediatrics.* 2013;132(4):e1089–e1104 PMID: 23999962
18. Kimberlin DW, et al. *J Infect Dis.* 2013;207(5):709–720 PMID: 23230059
19. American Academy of Pediatrics. Rabies. In: Pickering LK, et al, eds. *Red Book: 2012 Report of the Committee on Infectious Diseases.* 2012:600–607

20. American Academy of Pediatrics. *Pneumocystis jirovecii* infections. In: Pickering LK, et al, eds. *Red Book: 2012 Report of the Committee on Infectious Diseases.* 2012:582–587
21. Siberry GK, et al. *Pediatr Infect Dis J.* 2013;32(Suppl2):i–KK4 PMID: 24569199
22. Leach AJ, et al. *Cochrane Database Syst Rev.* 2006;(4):CD004401 PMID: 17054203
23. McDonald S, et al. *Cochrane Database Syst Rev.* 2008;(4):CD004741 PMID: 18843668
24. Williams GJ, et al. *Adv Exp Med Biol.* 2013;764:211–218 PMID: 23654070
25. Craig JC, et al. *N Engl J Med.* 2009;361(18):1748–1759 PMID: 19864673
26. RIVUR Trial Investigators, et al. *N Engl J Med.* 2014;370(25):2367–2376 PMID: 24795142
27. American Academy of Pediatrics Subcommittee on Urinary Tract Infection and Steering Committee on Quality Improvement and Management. *Pediatrics.* 2011;128(3):595–610 PMID: 21873693
28. *Treat Guidel Med Lett.* 2012;10(122):73–80 PMID: 22996382
29. Mangram AJ, et al. *Infect Control Hosp Epidemiol.* 1999;20(4):250–280 PMID: 10219875
30. Edwards FH, et al. *Ann Thorac Surg.* 2006;81(1):397–404 PMID: 16368422
31. Hansen E, et al. *J Orthop Res.* 2014;32(Suppl1):S31–S59 PMID: 24464896
32. Bratzler DW, et al. *Surg Infect (Larchmt).* 2013;14(1):73–156 PMID: 23461695
33. Haley RW, et al. *Am J Epidemiol.* 1985;121(2):206–215 PMID: 4014116
34. Dellinger EP. *Ann Surg.* 2008;247(6):927–928 PMID: 18520218
35. Shaffer WO, et al. *Spine J.* 2013;13(10):1387–1392 PMID: 23988461

Chapter 15

1. Best EJ, et al. *Pediatr Infect Dis J.* 2011;30(10):827–832 PMID: 21577177
2. Smyth AR, et al. *Cochrane Database Syst Rev.* 2012;2:CD002009 PMID: 22336782
3. Gruchalla RS, et al. *N Engl J Med.* 2006;354(6):601–609 PMID: 16467547
4. Solensky R. *J Allergy Clin Immunol.* 2012;130(6):1442–1442 PMID: 23195529
5. *Med Lett Drugs Ther.* 2012;54(1406):101 PMID: 23282790
6. Bradley JS, et al. *Pediatrics.* 2009;123(4):e609–e613 PMID: 19289450
7. Wong VK, et al. *Pediatr Infect Dis J.* 1991;10(2):122–125 PMID: 2062603
8. Bradley JS, et al. *Pediatrics.* 2011;128(4):e1034–e1045 PMID: 21949152
9. Jacobs RF, et al. *Pediatr Infect Dis J.* 2005;24(1):34–39 PMID: 15665708
10. American Academy of Pediatrics. Pertussis. In: Pickering LK, et al, eds. *Red Book: 2012 Report of the Committee on Infectious Diseases.* 2012:553–566
11. Nambiar S, et al. *Pediatrics.* 2011;127(6):e1528–e1532 PMID: 21555496

Index

B

C

M

Q

R